PSYCHODYNAMIC PSYCHOTHERAPY

for Personality Disorders

A CLINICAL HANDBOOK

PSYCHODYNAMIC PSYCHOTHERAPY

for Personality Disorders

A CLINICAL HANDBOOK

Edited by

John F. Clarkin, Ph.D.
Peter Fonagy, Ph.D., F.B.A.
Glen O. Gabbard, M.D.

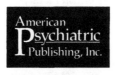

Washington, DC
London, England

Note: The authors have worked to ensure that all information in this book is accurate at the time of publication and consistent with general psychiatric and medical standards, and that information concerning drug dosages, schedules, and routes of administration is accurate at the time of publication and consistent with standards set by the U.S. Food and Drug Administration and the general medical community. As medical research and practice continue to advance, however, therapeutic standards may change. Moreover, specific situations may require a specific therapeutic response not included in this book. For these reasons and because human and mechanical errors sometimes occur, we recommend that readers follow the advice of physicians directly involved in their care or the care of a member of their family.

14   13   12   11   10   5   4   3   2   1
First Edition

Typeset in Adobe's Palatino and ITC's Legacy Sans.

American Psychiatric Publishing, Inc.
1000 Wilson Boulevard
Arlington, VA 22209-3901
www.appi.org

Library of Congress Cataloging-in-Publication Data
Psychodynamic psychotherapy for personality disorders : a clinical handbook / edited by John F. Clarkin, Peter Fonagy, Glen O. Gabbard. — 1st ed.
    p. ; cm.
  Includes bibliographical references and index.
  ISBN 978-1-58562-355-6 (alk. paper)
  1. Personality disorders—Treatment. 2. Psychodynamic psychotherapy. I. Clarkin, John F. II. Fonagy, Peter, 1952- III. Gabbard, Glen O.
  [DNLM: 1. Personality Disorders—therapy. 2. Psychoanalytic Therapy—methods. WM 190 P9733 2010]
  RC554.P757 2010
  616.85'81—dc22

                                2010010066

British Library Cataloguing in Publication Data
A CIP record is available from the British Library.

Contents

  John F. Clarkin, Ph.D.
  Peter Fonagy, Ph.D.
  Glen O. Gabbard, M.D.

Part I
Personality Pathology:
Defining the Focus of Intervention

  Eve Caligor, M.D.
  John F. Clarkin, Ph.D.

  Peter Fonagy, Ph.D., F.B.A.
  Patrick Luyten, Ph.D.
  Anthony Bateman, M.A., F.R.C.Psych.
  György Gergely, Ph.D.
  Lane Strathearn, M.B.B.S., F.R.A.C.P., Ph.D.
  Mary Target, Ph.D.
  Elizabeth Allison, D.Phil.

  Gerhard Roth, Ph.D. (philosophy), Ph.D. (zoology)
  Anna Buchheim, Ph.D.

Part II
Psychodynamic Treatment Approaches

Part III
Research and Future Directions

Contributors

Elizabeth Allison, D.Phil.
Publications Editor, Psychoanalysis Unit, Research Department of Clinical, Educational and Health Psychology, University College London, United Kingdom

Anthony Bateman, M.A., F.R.C.Psych.
Consultant Psychiatrist in Psychotherapy, Halliwick Unit, St. Ann's Hospital, Barnet, Enfield and Haringey Mental Health Trust, London, and Visiting Professor, University College London, United Kingdom; Visiting Consultant, The Menninger Clinic and Menninger Department of Psychiatry and Behavioral Sciences, Baylor College of Medicine, Houston, Texas

Anna Buchheim, Ph.D.
Professor of Clinical Psychology, Institute for Psychology, University of Innsbruck, Innsbruck, Austria

Eve Caligor, M.D.
Clinical Professor of Psychiatry and Associate Director, Residency Training in Psychiatry, New York University School of Medicine, New York, New York

John F. Clarkin, Ph.D.
Clinical Professor of Psychology in Psychiatry, Weill Cornell Medical College, New York, New York

Diana Diamond, Ph.D.
Professor, Department of Psychology, City University of New York and the Weill Medical College of Cornell University, New York, New York

Peter Fonagy, Ph.D., F.B.A.
Freud Memorial Professor of Psychoanalysis and Director of the Sub-Department of Clinical Health Psychology, University College London, and Chief Executive, Anna Freud Centre, London, United Kingdom; Consultant to the Child and Family Program, Menninger Department of Psychiatry and Behavioral Sciences, Baylor College of Medicine, Houston, Texas

Glen O. Gabbard, M.D.
Brown Foundation Chair of Psychoanalysis and Professor of Psychiatry, Baylor College of Medicine, Houston, Texas

György Gergely, Ph.D.
Professor of Psychology, Cognitive Development Center at the Central European University, Budapest, Hungary

Mardi J. Horowitz, M.D.
Professor, Department of Psychiatry, University of California, San Francisco, California

Otto F. Kernberg, M.D.
Professor, Department of Psychiatry, Weill Cornell Medical College, New York, New York

Falk Leichsenring, D.Sc.
Professor of Psychotherapy Research, Department of Psychosomatics and Psychotherapy, University of Giessen, Giessen, Germany

Uma Lerner, M.D.
Clinical Instructor, Department of Psychiatry, University of California, San Francisco, California

Patrick Luyten, Ph.D.
Assistant Professor, Center for Psychoanalysis and Psychodynamic Psychology, Department of Psychology, Catholic University of Leuven, Leuven, Belgium

Leigh McCullough, Ph.D.
Director of Research, Modum Bad Research Institute, Vikersund, Norway; Associate Clinical Professor, Harvard Medical School, Boston, Massachusetts

J. Reid Meloy, Ph.D., A.B.P.P.
Clinical Professor, Department of Psychiatry, University of California, San Diego; Faculty, San Diego Psychoanalytic Institute; Adjunct Professor, University of San Diego School of Law, San Diego, California

John M. Oldham, M.D., M.S.
Senior Vice President and Chief of Staff, The Menninger Clinic; Executive Vice Chairman for Clinical Affairs and Development, Menninger Department of Psychiatry and Behavioral Sciences, Baylor College of Medicine, Houston, Texas

William E. Piper, Ph.D.
Professor, Department of Psychiatry, University of British Columbia, Vancouver, British Columbia, Canada

Gerhard Roth, Ph.D. (philosophy), Ph.D. (zoology)
Professor of Behavioral Physiology and Developmental Biology, Brain Research Institute, University of Bremen, Bremen, Germany

Jonathan Shedler, Ph.D.
Associate Professor, Department of Psychiatry, University of Colorado Denver School of Medicine, Denver, Colorado

Paul I. Steinberg, M.D., F.R.C.P.C.
Psychiatrist, Clinical Professor, Department of Psychiatry, University of British Columbia, Vancouver, British Columbia, Canada

Michael H. Stone, M.D.
Professor of Clinical Psychiatry, Columbia College of Physicians and Surgeons, New York, New York

Lane Strathearn, M.B.B.S., F.R.A.C.P., Ph.D.
Assistant Professor, Department of Pediatrics, Baylor College of Medicine/Texas Children's Hospital, Houston, Texas

Martin Svartberg, M.D., Ph.D.
Private practice, Oslo, Norway

Mary Target, Ph.D.
Professor of Psychoanalysis, Psychoanalysis Unit, Research Department of Clinical, Educational and Health Psychology, University College London, United Kingdom

Drew Westen, Ph.D.
Professor, Department of Psychology and Department of Psychiatry
and Behavioral Sciences, Emory University, Atlanta, Georgia

Paul Williams, Ph.D.
Training and Supervising Analyst, British Psychoanalytical Society,
United Kingdom

Jessica Yakeley, M.B. B.Chir., M.R.C.Psych.
Associate Medical Director and Director of Medical Education, Tavis-
tock and Portman NHS Foundation Trust, London; Honorary Senior
Lecturer, Department of Mental Health and Behavioral Sciences, Uni-
versity College London; Fellow, British Psychoanalytical Society,
United Kingdom

Frank E. Yeomans, M.D., Ph.D.
Clinical Associate Professor, Department of Psychiatry, Weill Medical
College of Cornell University; Lecturer, Columbia Center for Psychoan-
alytic Training and Research, New York, New York

Disclosure of Interests

*The contributors to this volume affirm that they have no competing financial interest in
or other affiliation with a commercial supporter, a manufacturer of a commercial product, a provider of a commercial service, a nongovernmental organization, and/or a government agency, except as stated below:*

Jonathan Shedler, Ph.D., and Drew Westen, Ph.D.: The research described in
Chapter 4 of this volume was supported, in part, by National Institute of Mental
Health Grants MH62377 and MH62378. The authors hold copyrights to the
Shedler-Westen Assessment Procedure (SWAP).

Frank E. Yeomans, M.D., Ph.D., and Diana Diamond, Ph.D.: Chapter 7 of this
volume represents work from the Cornell Psychotherapy Research Project, supported by grants from the National Institute of Mental Health, the International
Psychoanalytic Association, and the Kohler Fund of Munich, and a grant from
the Borderline Personality Disorder Research Foundation.

Preface

Clinicians recognize that symptoms reside within a person whose personality patterns are unique (Westen et al. 2006). All therapeutic interventions, including medication management, involve a complex relationship between a patient, of unique personality, and a clinician. This book is about the individual patient whose personality can be conceptualized as dysfunctional along a continuum from mildly to severely disturbed; its focus is on advances in assessment and treatment of the personality disorders from a psychodynamic orientation.

The prevalence of the personality disorders is high; in the general U.S. population, it ranges from 1.5% for the Cluster B disorders to 5.7% for the Cluster A disorders and 6.0% for the Cluster C disorders, with 9.1% for any personality disorder (Lenzenweger et al. 2007). A reexamination of psychodynamic treatments is timely. Recent empirical evidence indicates that patients with mixed personality disorder and those with severe personality disorders, such as borderline personality disorder, respond to psychodynamic treatments, as documented by Leichsenring in Chapter 15.

This handbook is intended for clinicians with a range of expertise who utilize a psychodynamic orientation in their assessment and/or treatment of patients with personality pathology. The chapters are organized to inform students of psychotherapy (psychology graduate students, psychiatric residents, psychoanalytic candidates) and experienced clinicians. Of special interest to students are the clear statement of intervention principles (Key Clinical Concepts) and the suggested readings section offered in each chapter. Experienced clinicians may find the update of object relations and attachment theory and research, neurocognitive science information, and differentiated chapters on the various personality disorders and constellations helpful in refining their work. The treatment chapters include both principles of intervention and clinical illustrations. Although the chapters cover a particular disorder (e.g., borderline personality disorder) or one of the three clusters of disorders in Axis II, we do not overlook the extensive comorbidity on Axis II and the superiority of a dimensional view of personality pathology over a categorical one (see Chapter 1).

Part I is focused on the nature of personality pathology. The model of personality and personality pathology informs the clinician at every step in the assessment and treatment of patients, whether they be patients with major Axis I disorders with comorbid personality pathology or patients with major difficulties of personality. Caligor and Clarkin (Chapter 1) describe an object relations model of normal and disturbed personality functioning with its implications for a typology and an assessment of personality organization. From this orientation, the assessment of personality pathology for differential treatment planning must take into account not only the descriptive characteristics of the personality pattern, but also the severity of personality pathology in reference to key functions of the individual such as self and other representations, defensive functioning, modulation of affect, and moral functioning. In Chapter 2, Fonagy and colleagues present an attachment theory perspective on personality development and functioning. Attachment theory, with its related methods for empirical assessment of working models of self and others and related interpersonal behavior, has provided a powerful framework for understanding personality from a developmental perspective. Roth and Buchheim (Chapter 3) provide the reader with a current understanding of the neurobiology of personality functioning. They point out that personality disorders are the result of a combination of genetic polymorphisms, deficits in brain development, and adverse developmental experiences. They emphasize that many brain areas are sites of intense interaction between emotional and cognitive processes. Neurobiological data have accumulated particularly on borderline and antisocial personality disorders, revealing dysfunctions in brain networks and in neuronal metabolism. To complete this section, Shedler and Westen (Chapter 4) explore the divide between science and clinical practice in understanding personality disorder, a gap that is most evident in the assessment of personality pathology. Rather than use the semistructured interviews so popular in research, clinicians employ the clinical interview to examine the interpersonal world of the patient, including how the patient relates to the clinician. These authors provide both a method of diagnosis based on a clinical interview that is empirically sound and a description of personality disorder prototypes that is richer than that found on Axis II of DSM-IV-TR (American Psychiatric Association 2000).

The background of models of personality and its pathology comprises Part I. Part II contains chapters on the treatment of specific constellations of personality disorder. Each of the treatment chapters provides information on the relevant empirical research, patient phenomenology and psychodynamics, and treatment strategies and techniques, woven together with clinical illustrations and vignettes.

The DSM-IV-TR Axis II Cluster A personality disorders (schizoid, schizotypal, and paranoid personality disorders) and their treatment are described by Williams (Chapter 5). The therapist is faced with many challenges in patients with these treatment-resistant disorders, especially transference difficulties, which may only be hinted at by the patient. The pathology of these personality disorders demands that the therapist give special attention to building a trusting therapeutic relationship with patience, persistence, and careful attention to the interaction.

Probably the most extensive research, both phenomenological and therapeutic, has been done with the Cluster B personality disorders. Bateman and Fonagy (Chapter 6) describe a treatment for borderline patients that is focused on improving the ability of the patient to understand self and others in terms of thoughts, emotions, and motivation: that is, mentalization skills. This treatment has been shown to significantly reduce symptoms in day hospital and outpatient treatment settings. In addition, the follow-up data indicate that patients who have been treated with mentalization-based therapy maintain their treatment gains, and this result is hypothesized to be related to their increased mentalizing capacities in understanding self and others. Yeomans and Diamond (Chapter 7) describe an alternative psychodynamic treatment for borderline patients called transference-focused psychotherapy (TFP). This intense individual treatment for borderline patients targets the patient's representations of self and others as they are demonstrated in the interaction with the therapist. TFP has been shown to significantly reduce symptoms and to compare favorably with a special supportive treatment and with dialectical behavior therapy. In addition, TFP has been shown to significantly increase reflective functioning, a measure of the ability to conceptually describe self and others with depth of understanding. In Chapter 8, Gabbard raises the central question of current psychotherapy research: If treatments work (i.e., reduce symptoms), how do they work? What are the mechanisms of change? He argues that the clinical and research approaches to the mechanisms of change all have limitations, but that it is quite likely that multiple mechanisms of change are operative. This focus on multiple mechanisms of change is demonstrated in all the treatment chapters in this volume.

In Chapter 9, Kernberg views narcissism as a pathological regulation of self-esteem and self-regard. He explores the complex relationship between self-esteem, moods, and the vicissitudes of internalized object relations. Normal narcissism, infantile narcissism, and pathological narcissism are distinguished, and treatments for different levels of pathological narcissism are examined. In particular, Kohut's self psychology, Rosenfeld's Kleinian approach, and Kernberg's object relations approach are described and contrasted. Horowitz and Lerner (Chapter 10) use an understanding of states of mind and configural analysis to formulate treatment for patients with histrionic personality disorder—that is, individuals with undermodulated states of intense negativity that lead to emotionally impulsive relationship behaviors. Three treatment phases are described: reduction of crises and increase in stability, increasing connections to others, and finally increased self-coherence and improvement of intimacy with others. Meloy and Yakeley (Chapter 11) view antisocial personality disorder from an attachment theory perspective with an emphasis on the dimensionality of the pathology. Whereas specific cognitive-behavioral techniques have been emphasized in the literature, the importance of deficits in internal experiences of these patients leads to the consideration of dynamic approaches to increasing self-reflection and mentalization for a subset of these patients. Svartberg and McCullough (Chapter 12) utilize their empirical work with Cluster C patients (avoidant, dependent, obsessive-compulsive) to describe a treatment that integrates cognitive-behavioral and psychodynamic techniques to assist patients in the management of affect.

The setting of treatment for patients with personality disorders is usually an outpatient one. However, when functioning is compromised and symptoms are severe, inpatient and day hospital settings offer a unique opportunity to treat patients with severe personality disorders. With their extensive clinical and research experience with these treatment settings, Piper and Steinberg (Chapter 13) address the need for day hospital and inpatient treatment for selected patients. Despite advances in the treatment of many of the personality disorders, there are patient characteristics with diagnostic and nondiagnostic features that define the limits of treatability. Stone (Chapter 14) describes these specific factors based on the literature and his own clinical experience.

Part III includes a summary of the existing treatment outcome research and a glimpse of the diagnostic procedures in the near future. The introduction of Axis II in DSM-III (American Psychiatric Association 1980) provided a reliable diagnostic framework that led to many empirical studies on the pathology and treatment of individuals with personality disorders. The growing empirical investigation of psychodynamic treatments for personality pathology is summarized in Chapter 15 by Leichsenring. This research puts dynamic treatments for patients with personality disorders on a firm footing in the current environment of empirically supported treatments.

Empirical research generated since 1980 on the phenomenology of the personality disorders has produced new information that will be utilized in an improved description of personality pathology in the forthcoming DSM-5. Oldham, a member of the committee on Axis II for DSM-5, describes (in Chapter 16) the current thinking of the committee concerning the diagnosis of personality pathology.

The interested reader must legitimately ask: What is it about the treatments in this book that makes them psychodynamic? What are the defining features of psychodynamic treatments across disorders, and, more specifically, psychodynamic treatments for the patients with personality disorders? The latter question is especially relevant in this era of manualized treatments with specified treatment strategies and techniques that provide a much more refined description of the treatment in question than some vague and abstract label of psychodynamic, cognitive-behavioral, or emotion-focused therapy.

The question of what is psychodynamic treatment for the patients with personality disorders can be answered at two levels. First of all, one can consider the definition of psychodynamic treatments and their defining characteristics in contrast to other treatments such as those with a cognitive-behavioral orientation. Second, one can examine the treatments described in this book that claim to be psychodynamic and generalize to commonalities across the treatments. Taking the latter approach, we can readily see that, at a general level, psychodynamic treatments have a number of characteristics in common. There is great attention to the current active relationship between patient and therapist. The psychodynamic therapist uses many sources of information to understand her patient's relationship style, including an observation of the patient's behavior, his conscious understanding of his own interactive style, and his descriptions of relationships, as well as the therapist's own cognitive-emotional reaction to how the patient is relating to her. In trying to understand this relationship in the present, the psychodynamic therapist has a model of the mind that goes beyond the overt behavior and the conscious cognitive statements of the patient to a level of motivation and mental life that is out of the awareness of the patient. The therapist is very interested in the meanings that the patient attributes to his own thoughts, affective states, and actions, as well as his understanding of internal and external experiences. The therapist is interested in understanding the way a patient's experience and actions can be understood by hypothesizing about past experience (the influence of the patient's past upon present attitudes and behavior) and is on the alert for signs of transference—that is, patterns of relating to the therapist in the present that may indicate persistence of or reactions against significant relationship patterns in the past.

How are these psychoanalytic models characterized in relation to patients with personality disorders? Patients with personality disorders are those individuals who, by definition, have difficulties in relating to others to such a degree that it interferes with major areas of adjustment in life such as work, profession, social life, and intimate relations. Therapists who consider themselves psychodynamic are most alert to how the patient structures the present relationship in the initial sessions. This attention to the patient's current interactive style is simultaneously both diagnostic and relevant to the therapist reactions that might be crucial to whether the treatment continues or the patient prematurely ends the relationship. While the dynamic therapist is alert to symptoms that may plague the patient with a personality disorder (e.g., depression, anxiety), the major focus is on the anomalies and distortions, conflicts and deficits in relating to others (including, but not exclusive to, the therapist) that may have a central role in the symptomatic state of the patient.

Dynamic therapists working with personality-disordered patients utilize models of personality pathology (Chapters 1 and 2) that emphasize developmental distortions and anomalies in cognitive and affective processes in the understanding of self and others. It is these poorly articulated, underdeveloped, or distorted internalized representations that are the object of assessment and change. The need to arrive at a diagnosis of the personality pathology, both prototypically (Shedler and Westen, Chapter 4) and dimensionally (Chapter 1) is followed by a shaping of the dynamic treatment to the differential characteristics of the patient.

A careful examination of the psychodynamic treatments for the various personality disorder diagnoses in this book suggests that contemporary psychodynamic researchers and clinicians experience the need to vary the treatment to the specifics of the personality pathology. There is no suggestion in this book that one psychodynamic treatment fits all personality pathology (although this has been frequently assumed to be the case in the past). One could argue that any treatment, whether psychodynamic or cognitive-behavioral, must go beyond the general treatment for a patient with a specific personality disorder to the tailoring of the treatment for the specific patient, who has a personality disorder that is not adequately captured by the category of pathology because it is modified by the patient's strengths and particular social context. In this regard, the various chapters in this book provide psychodynamic templates for approaching patients with prominent (but not exclusive) personality features that match a particular category. These templates can be adapted to the specifics of the individual patient with his or her unique combination of pathology and strengths being played out in a particular environment that the patient helped construct. In contrast to the stereotype of dynamic treatment as focused on the patient's past, the treatments for personality disorders described here focus primarily on the present.

There is a marked overlap between modern dynamic treatments and cognitive-behavioral treatments for patients with personality disorder. This is an indication of historical shifts in both orientations and also of the common constraints that personality disorder places on the therapeutic relationship. The so-called common factors of structure, support, empathic relationship, and therapeutic alliance are active in most treatments. In addition to the common strategies and techniques, some psychodynamic treatments (see, e.g., Chapter 12) describe an explicit combination of what are called psychodynamic and cognitive-behavioral techniques. In general, in putting together this book we have noted a marked convergence of therapeutic approaches and many indications that the era of a strict and clear demarcation between psychodynamic and other treatments may be over. One sees the inclusion of cognitive-behavioral techniques in dynamic treatments, and conversely one sees cognitive-behavioral writers putting more emphasis on the therapeutic relationship and the patient's resistance (see Leahy 2001).

We, the editors of this volume, have enjoyed the collegial support of our accomplished authors. It was only with their enthusiastic response that we could bring together current psychodynamic thinking on the models, assessment, and treatment of patients with personality disorders.

John F. Clarkin, Ph.D.
Peter Fonagy, Ph.D., F.B.A.
Glen O. Gabbard, M.D.

References

American Psychiatric Association: Diagnostic and Statistical Manual of Mental Disorders, 3rd Edition. Washington, DC, American Psychiatric Association, 1980

American Psychiatric Association: Diagnostic and Statistical Manual of Mental Disorders, 4th Edition, Text Revision. Washington, DC, American Psychiatric Association, 2000

Leahy R: Overcoming Resistance in Cognitive Therapy. New York, Guilford, 2001

Lenzenweger MF, Lane MC, Loranger AW, et al: DSM-IV personality disorders in the National Comorbidity Survey Replication. Biol Psychiatry 62:553–564, 2007

Westen D, Gabbard GO, Blagov P: Back to the future: personality structure as a context for psychopathology, in Personality and Psychopathology. Edited by Krueger RF, Tackett JL. New York, Guilford, 2006, pp 335–384

PERSONALITY PATHOLOGY: DEFINING THE FOCUS OF INTERVENTION

CHAPTER 1

An Object Relations Model of Personality and Personality Pathology

Eve Caligor, M.D.
John F. Clarkin, Ph.D.

Clinicians treating patients with personality disorders commonly grapple with several key questions:

- What is the relationship between normal personality functioning and personality pathology?
- What are pathological aspects of personality functioning common to many or most of the personality disorders?
- What relationships exist among the higher-level and the more severe personality disorders?
- How can we evaluate and characterize the severity of pathology among the different personality disorders?
- How can we evaluate and characterize the severity of pathology of individuals within a particular diagnostic group?

The object relations theory model of personality disorders provides a clinically based approach to answering them.

To facilitate what will be a clinically based introduction to the object relations theory model of personality disorders, we present four vignettes of patients with personality disorders:

Ms. N is a 28-year-old single, employed woman who was seen in consultation with the complaint of "problems with men" and "difficulty with confrontation." Ms. N was attractive, charming, and quietly seductive, and she acknowledged that she was often surprised to find herself the center of attention in social settings. Yet she noted that she tended to feel inadequate and unattractive relative to her friends and co-workers, and she described herself as shy with men and sexually inhibited. She felt that these traits explained why she had not had a long-term relationship since college. Ms. N also complained of difficulty with "confrontation," with a tendency to shy away from conflict. She felt that as a result she was at times excessively accommodating. Though she did not have a boyfriend, she had a close-knit group of friends. Ms. N described her work as an elementary school teacher as both challenging and fulfilling. She felt that she was, overall, an optimistic and level-headed person, but she was demoralized about her inability to establish a long-term relationship with a man or to feel better about herself. By the end of an hour-long interview, the consultant found himself feeling warmly toward Ms. N, and he felt that he had a vivid impression of Ms. N, of her difficulties, and of the important people in her life.

Ms. B is a 28-year-old single, employed woman who was seen in consultation with the complaint of "problems with men" and "difficulty with confrontation." Ms. B was attractive and engaging; she wore a short skirt and low-cut blouse, and her manner was sexually provocative in a way that made the consultant vaguely uneasy. She described feeling uncomfortable in settings in which she was not the center of attention. Ms. B told the consultant that she found it difficult to control her anger in the setting of conflicts with her boyfriends and that she was prone to temper tantrums. Since graduating from college, Ms. B had held a series of jobs; she was currently working as a receptionist. She found her work dreary and boring, though she could not think of anything else she would rather be doing. She lived alone and did not have a steady partner. She described a series of relationships with men that, according to Ms. B, always ended badly. She had a scattered group of friends, but her sister was the only person she felt entirely trusting of and attached to. She felt her life was "going nowhere," and she was intermittently plagued by feelings of emptiness and self-loathing. The consultant found himself struck by the apparent contradiction between Ms B's composure in the interview and the history she provided of rageful, accusatory, and manipulative behavior with her boyfriends.

Mr. N is a 38-year-old married lawyer with two young children. He was seen in consultation with a complaint of "problems with work" and problems with self-esteem. Mr. N described his work as a junior partner at a successful law firm as challenging and intellectually fulfilling. Nevertheless, he complained of feeling inadequate in the workplace and not as able as those around him, and he was troubled by a tendency to be "too detail-oriented" and to put things off until the last minute. Mr. N was emotionally constricted and extremely reserved but nevertheless conveyed a deeply felt attachment to his wife and young children. He understood that his loved ones experienced him as emotionally unavailable, but he felt unable to change his behavior. He had a few close friends dating back to high school but was, by his own account, not especially social. After hearing Mr. N's story, the consultant found himself impressed by Mr. N's conscientiousness and his motivation for treatment.

Mr. B is a 38-year-old married, unemployed lawyer. He was seen in consultation with a complaint of "problems with work" and problems with self-esteem. He described himself as "a procrastinator" and complained of being detail-oriented to a fault; he often found himself lost for hours chasing irrelevant information. However, as the interview proceeded, it emerged that since graduating from law school 10 years earlier, Mr. B had been fired from a series of jobs because he had had difficulty completing projects and had often missed deadlines; he also had a history of falsifying time sheets, frequently calling in sick, and getting into power struggles with his bosses. He had most recently worked as a paralegal—a job he found demeaning—and had been fired 6 months earlier. Mr. B described himself as alternating between feeling smarter than everyone and like a "dumb loser." He was emotionally distant and constricted, and his wife complained that he provided neither financial nor emotional support. He explained that he had lost sexual interest in her early in the marriage and that he periodically visited prostitutes. Mr. B complained of feeling empty and restless. He wanted the consultant to tell him how to feel less dysphoric and anxious, and how to have a more stable sense of himself as exceptional. At the end of an hour-long interview, the consultant found himself with only a vague and superficial sense of Mr. B and an even more shadowy image of his wife. The consultant felt overwhelmed by the intractability of Mr. B's difficulties and was concerned that Mr. B had little genuine motivation for treatment.

While all of these patients have personality disorders, the differences among them are both striking and of great significance in a clinical setting. By the end of this chapter, the reader will have a framework within which to consider both the similarities and the differences among these patients; the object relations theory model of personality disorders provides a systematic and coherent approach to assessment, classification, and treatment of personality pathology across the spectrum of severity.

What Is Object Relations Theory?

In psychodynamic psychiatry, the term *object* is used, for historical reasons and rather unfortunately, to refer to a person with whom the subject has a relationship. Similarly, the term *object relations* refers to the quality of the subject's relationships with others. Turning from the external, interpersonal world to the internal world of the subject, we use the term *internal object* to refer to the representation or presence of another within the mind of the subject. *Object relations theory* comprises a cluster of somewhat loosely related psychodynamic and psychoanalytic models of psychological motivation and functioning in which the internalization of early patterns of relating is viewed as a central feature of psychological development and psychological functioning.

The particular object relations theory–based model of personality disorders that we present was developed by Otto Kernberg and his colleagues at the Personality Disorders Institute of the Weill Cornell Medical College (Kernberg and Caligor 2005). This approach represents an integration of major contributions emerging from the Kleinian and British schools of psychoanalysis with developments within American ego psychology—in particular, the work of Edith Jacobson, Margaret Mahler, and Erik Erikson. An offshoot of object relations theory, attachment theory (Shaver and Mikulincer 2005), is discussed in Chapter 2 ("Attachment and Personality Pathology"). In this chapter, we focus on those aspects of Kernberg's model that are most relevant to clinical practice. We cover the basic concepts underlying the object relations theory approach to personality disorders, along with the system of classification of personality pathology at the core of Kernberg's model. We omit discussion of Kernberg's more controversial developmental theory, as well as his exploration of the psychoanalytic construct of "drives." Because the model we present is clinically based, emerging from experience with the psychodynamic treatment of patients with personality disorders, it is not wedded to a specific model of etiology of personality disorders.

Psychological Structures

The cornerstone of the object relations theory approach to personality disorders is that descriptive features of personality pathology that characterize a particular personality disorder can be seen to reflect the nature and organization of underlying psychological structures. Psychodynamic treatments that lead to changes in psychological structures will at the same time lead to changes in descriptive features of personality pathology and to improvement in psychological functioning. This "bottom-up" approach to treatment and therapeutic change can be contrasted with (and can also be advantageously combined with) "top-down" cognitive-behavioral approaches, which focus directly on changing maladaptive behaviors and patterns of thinking.

Before proceeding, we want to say a word about the term *structure* as it is used in psychodynamic psychiatry, as this is often cause for confusion. In a psychodynamic frame of reference, structures are stable patterns of psychological functioning that are repeatedly and predictably activated in particular contexts.[1] This is to say that psychological structures are not structures in the concrete sense but rather are psychological processes that can be conceptualized as dispositions to organize subjective experience and behavior in certain predictable ways. At the level of cognitive neuroscience, the neural correlates of what we think of as psychological structures can be conceptualized as associations among neuronal circuits, or "associational networks," that tend to be activated in concert (Westen and Gabbard 2002). Motivational systems, coping mechanisms, patterns of relating, and processes that function to regulate mood and impulses are all examples of psychological structures. The nature and the organization of psychological structures are characteristic of the individual and tend to be stable over time, though they can be modified as a result of maturation, life experience, and successful treatment.

It is important to appreciate that, in contrast to descriptive features of personality, psychological structures as they are conceptualized within a psychodynamic frame of reference can be neither directly observed by the clinician nor reported by the patient. Rather, at the level of clinical observation, the nature of psychological structures can be inferred and also systematically assessed on the basis of their impact on descriptive aspects of personality functioning, in particular an individ-

---

[1] We distinguish between this usage of the term *structure* and the psychometric concept of structure. In trait theory, *personality structure* refers to a factor structure that fits existing data. This statistical method is used to explore latent variables underlying different personality traits by identifying covariation among traits. Trait theory identifies structures across a population. In contrast, psychodynamics uses structures to refer to how psychological functioning is organized within a particular individual.

ual's behavior, interpersonal relations, and subjective experience. For example, *conscience* is a familiar psychological structure comprising the psychological processes involved in moral functioning. Ethical (and unethical) behavior, feelings of guilt, and commitment to moral values and ideals are descriptive features of personality functioning that are organized by the various processes that constitute the structure termed *conscience*. Similarly, the defensive operation *denial* is a psychological process manifested descriptively in the predictable tendency to minimize the emotional impact of painful experiences.

Our emphasis on the relationship between observable behavior and internal, unobservable cognitive-affective structures is shared by many contemporary theories of personality; one can discern the use of similar and overlapping constructs across a wide array of models, all of which point to the role of certain basic cognitive and emotional processes in both normal personality functioning and personality pathology (see Lenzenweger and Clarkin 2005). In particular, Mischel and Shoda (2008) have conceptualized normal personality as a system of mediating units (e.g., encodings, expectancies, motives, and goals) that operate at various levels of consciousness to enable the individual to interact successfully with the environment. According to this model, termed the *Cognitive-Affective Personality System* (CAPS), particular cognitive-affective mental representations are activated in response to environmental contingencies, including those that emerge in the interpersonal environment. Thus, according to this influential theory, the essential element in personality functioning is the organization of cognitive-affective representations, which are patterned, relate to behavior expression, accrue into a perception of self across situations, and motivate the selection of particular environments that the individual prefers and actively seeks.

Internal Object Relations

In the object relations theory approach, cognitive-affective units consisting of an image of the self interacting with an image of another person, with the entire interaction linked to a particular affect state, are considered to be the most basic psychological structures. These internalized relationship patterns are referred to as *internal object relations*. In the object relations theory model, internal object relations are the building blocks of higher-order structures, and they are also seen to organize subjective experience. For example, the structure *identity* is conceptualized as an organization of internal object relations pertaining to the experience of self and of others; *conscience* comprises object relations pertaining to prohibitions and ideals. Different contexts will lead to the activation of different internal object relations. The particular internal object relations that are activated will organize the individual's behavior and experience of that setting and will be played out in his or her interpersonal relations.

As an example of how we conceptualize internal object relations and their role in psychological functioning and subjectivity, consider an object relation comprising the image of a small, childlike self interacting with an image of a powerful, threatening authority figure in which the interaction is linked to feelings of fear—or, alternatively, the image of a small, childlike self and a caring, protective figure associated with feelings of gratification and safety. In these illustrations, the internal object relations described will become manifest in the adult to the degree that they function to organize the individual's expectations and experience of dependent relations—coloring the experience of the self and of the person depended upon, while activating, in the first case, an affective experience of anxiety and fear and, in the second, an experience of gratification and safety.

Kernberg (Kernberg and Caligor 2005) suggests that internal object relations emerge from the interaction of inborn affect dispositions and attachment relationships; from the earliest days of life, constitutionally determined affect states are activated in relation to, regulated by, and cognitively linked to interactions with caretakers. Over time, these interactions are internalized as relationship patterns, which are gradually organized to form the enduring, affectively charged psychological structures that we refer to as internal object relations.

Our emphasis on internalized patterns of relating as central organizing features of psychological functioning is shared by many other approaches, including cognitive and behavioral theory, interpersonal theory, and attachment theory. However, while there is much overlap among these models, object relations theory is distinguished by virtue of invoking a relatively complex, "dynamic" relationship between early attachment relationships and the psychological structures that come to organize adult experience. In the object relations theory model, we invoke not only early experience—colored by cognitive developmental level—as affecting the nature of internal object relations, but also psychodynamic factors, including the individual's psychological conflicts, defenses, and fantasies.

To illustrate the potential role of conflict and defense in determining the nature of internal object relations, let's return to our earlier example of an internal object relation comprising a small, childlike self and a powerful, threatening authority figure linked to feelings of fear. We are suggesting that for a particular individual, the self experience of powerlessness and fear in the setting of dependent relationships may reflect not only actual early experiences with a frightening parent but also defensive needs or fantasy. For example, for someone like Ms. N, this object relation might be a defensive construction in relation to conflictual wishes to hurt a parental figure. Here we would speak of "projection," as if to say: "She is aggressive and sadistic, not me; I am weak and frightened. Therefore I need not feel guilty for having sadistic feelings." Alternatively, for someone like Ms. B, a more extreme and highly affectively charged version of this same object relation might function as part of a defensive effort to protect a fantasy of a wished-for, perfectly gratifying parental figure. This is an example of "splitting": "This feels terrible, but nevertheless it means that I can still hope to find a perfect caretaker." In sum, the internal object relations that organize subjective experience in a particular setting may at the same time serve defensive functions, protecting the subject from awareness of more threatening or painful, conflictual experiences of self and other. In the object relations theory model, the nature and quality of internal object relations are seen to reflect temperamental factors (e.g., inborn affect dispositions), developmental experience, and also conflict and defense.

An Object Relations Theory–Based Approach to Personality Pathology

A PSYCHODYNAMIC DESCRIPTION OF PERSONALITY AND PERSONALITY PATHOLOGY

From a psychodynamic perspective, a comprehensive description of personality pathology will include 1) the descriptive features of the disorder, 2) a formulation about the structural organization underlying descriptive features, and 3) a theory about the patient's psychodynamics.

Assessment of *descriptive* features provides information about presenting complaints and problems, maladaptive personality traits, and relationships with significant others, and such assessment can be used to formulate a descriptive diagnosis. This is the approach taken by DSM-IV-TR (American Psychiatric Association 2000). A *structural* formulation provides information about the severity of personality pathology through the lens of the individual's experience of himself and his significant others, object relations, defensive operations, and reality testing (Kernberg 1984). Together, descriptive and structural assessments offer the clinician a clear appreciation of the patient's objective and subjective difficulties and provide the information needed to make a diagnosis and to guide treatment planning.

A comprehensive psychodynamic description of psychopathology will also include an understanding of the psychological *conflicts* underlying the disorder. It is by exploring conflicts underlying maladaptive behaviors and subjective states that the psychodynamic clinician gives meaning to the seemingly irrational difficulties that bring patients with personality disorders to treatment. And it is through the exploration and working through of underlying meanings and motivations that psychodynamic clinicians help their patients develop greater flexibility and adaptation. Assessment of the descriptive, structural, and dynamic dimensions of personality functioning (see also Chapter 4, "The Shedler-Westen Assessment Procedure," in this volume) will guide differential treatment planning and enable the clinician to anticipate developments in treatment.

When it comes to assessment, classification, and differential treatment planning, the object relations theory model of personality disorders combines a dimensional classification of personality disorders, according to severity of *structural* pathology, with a second-order categorical or prototypical classification based on *descriptive* traits (i.e., the type of diagnosis provided by DSM-IV-TR). Thus, both clinically and conceptually, the object relations theory approach is first to characterize the severity of personality pathology by assessing the nature, organization, and degree of integration of psychological structures, and then to characterize descriptive features of personality pathology to make a diagnosis of personality "type" or "style."

Our two-axial approach reflects the clinical reality that similar personality styles or maladaptive traits may be seen across a broad spectrum of pathology, with markedly different prognostic implications; from a clinical perspective, the nature and degree of severity of structural pathology are typically of greater importance with regard to prognosis and differential treatment planning than is personality "type." For example, we would suggest that in the clinical setting, the similarities between Ms. N and Mr. N on the axis of structural pathology are of greater significance than are the manifest similarities in presenting complaints and personality style that link Ms. N to Ms. B and Mr. N to Mr. B on the descriptive axis. In this chapter, we focus largely on the structural axis of the model, as this aspect is unique to object relations theory and provides an overarching, integrative approach to personality pathology.

DESCRIPTIVE FEATURES OF PERSONALITY DISORDERS

When we refer to someone's *personality*, we are referring to the enduring and habitual patterns of behavior, cognition, emotion, motivation, and ways of relating to others that are characteristic of the individual. These directly observable components of personality functioning constitute the *descriptive* features of an individual's personality and personality pathology. From a descriptive perspective, an individual's personality is expressed as a particular *personality style.* For example, an individual like Mr. N who has an obsessive-compulsive style is attentive to detail, perfectionistic, risk-averse, and constricted in emotional expression, where each of these descriptors is viewed as a "personality trait."

As personality traits become more rigid and more extreme, we move from a normal "personality style" to pathological personality functioning. When we speak of personality traits as "rigid," we mean that the individual is unable to change his or her behavior, even when he or she would like to do so and even when it is highly maladaptive not to do so. Thus, Mr. N is unable to stop procrastinating, even though he is aware that his behavior causes him unnecessary distress and might make it difficult for him to excel. Rather than learning from experience and modifying maladaptive patterns, the individual will activate the same behaviors, emotional responses, and ways of relating time and time again, and in a broad array of circumstances, regardless of whether or not these behaviors are appropriate to the setting. When we describe personality traits as "extreme," we refer to an increasingly wide deviation from commonly encountered and culturally normative behaviors and ways of functioning. Thus, Mr. B's procrastination routinely led him to miss deadlines, whereas Mr. N's did not; Ms. N's seductiveness is understated and socially appropriate, whereas Ms. B's feels exaggerated and somewhat crude. Personality pathology exists on a spectrum, with traits becoming more rigid and more extreme, and interfering with the individual's functioning more profoundly and more globally, as personality pathology becomes more severe. At the most severe end of the spectrum, we see traits that are not only extreme but also mutually contradictory. For example, Mr. B is excessively detail-oriented, yet at the same time he routinely overlooked glaring typographic and spelling errors in his work. When personality rigidity reaches the point that it significantly, consistently, and chronically interferes with daily functioning, and/or causes significant distress to the individual and those around him or her, we speak of a *personality disorder.*

OVERVIEW OF THE STRUCTURAL APPROACH TO PERSONALITY DISORDERS

The structural approach to personality disorders classifies personality pathology on the basis of the nature of key psychological processes or structures. (This classification is sometimes referred to as *structural diagnosis.*) Specifically, the structural approach examines the following:

1. Identity (sense of self and others)
2. Predominant level of defensive operations (customary ways of coping with external stress and internal conflict)
3. Reality testing (appreciation of conventional notions of reality)
4. Quality of object relations (understanding of the nature of interpersonal relations)
5. Moral functioning (ethical behavior, ideals and values)

This view is consistent with the approach adopted by personality disorder researchers (Livesley 2001; Parker et al. 2004; Verheul et al. 2008), who also focus on aspects of adaptive and maladaptive personality functioning in order to characterize the severity of personality pathology. In particular, these researchers identify a stable self-image, self-reflective functioning, aggression regulation, purposefulness, and a capacity for intimacy as core components of personality functioning relevant to assessing severity of personality pathology.

At a conceptual level, the structural approach to personality pathology is compatible with an emerging consensus among personality disorder researchers that difficulties in relation to a sense of self, or identity, and chronic interpersonal dysfunction are essential elements in personality disorders (Livesley 2001; Pincus 2005). Theoreticians and clinicians representing cognitive (Pretzer and Beck 2005), interpersonal (Benjamin 2005), and attachment (Levy 2005; Meyer and Pilkonis 2005; see also Chapter 2, this volume) perspectives, as well as those working within the model of object relations theory, emphasize the centrality of these key areas of functioning in personality pathology.

LEVELS OF PERSONALITY ORGANIZATION AND CLASSIFICATION OF PERSONALITY PATHOLOGY

The structural approach to personality disorders was first developed by Otto Kernberg and emerged from extensive clinical experience with the psychodynamic treatment of patients with personality disorders. Kernberg (1984) divides the universe of personality pathology into two major groups of disorders or levels of personality organization, the *neurotic level of personality organization* (NPO) and the *borderline level of personality organization* (BPO), based on severity of structural pathology.

In the less severe, neurotic level of personality organization, we see maladaptive personality rigidity in the setting of 1) normal identity;

2) the predominance of higher-level, repression-based, defensive operations; and 3) intact reality testing. This group of "higher-level" personality disorders includes the obsessive-compulsive and depressive personality disorders, the higher-level hysterical personality disorder (omitted from DSM-IV-TR), a relatively healthy subset of patients with avoidant personality disorder, and also the large group of patients seen in clinical practice who present with personality pathology but not of sufficient severity to meet criteria for a DSM personality disorder (Westen and Arkowitz-Westen 1998). Individuals organized at a neurotic level generally function well in many domains, with maladaptive personality traits typically interfering predominantly in focal areas of functioning and/or causing subjective distress. Ms. N and Mr. N are both organized at an NPO. Ms. N's personality rigidity has affected her largely in the domain of romantic relations; she functions well at work, does well socially, and maintains close friendships. Mr. N's personality rigidity causes inhibition in the expression of emotion but does not interfere with his forming deep attachments; his tendencies to get lost in detail and to procrastinate in his work cause distress and handicap him to some degree, but he is nevertheless very successful professionally.

In the personality disorders organized at a borderline level,[2] patients present with severely maladaptive personality rigidity in the setting of 1) clinically significant identity pathology; 2) the predominance of lower-level, splitting-based defensive operations; and 3) variable reality testing in which ordinary reality testing is grossly intact, but the more subtle capacities to appreciate social conventions and to accurately perceive the inner states of others are impaired. In this more severe group of personality disorders we find most of the personality disorders described in DSM-IV-TR, including the dependent, histrionic, narcissistic, borderline, paranoid, schizoid, and antisocial personality disorders. Individuals organized at a borderline level have pervasive difficulties that adversely compromise functioning in many, if not all, domains, and maladaptive traits that are more extreme and more rigid than those of

---

[2]We want to make clear the distinction between DSM-IV-TR borderline personality disorder (BPD) and the borderline level of personality organization (BPO). BPD is a specific personality disorder, diagnosed on the basis of a constellation of descriptive features. BPO is a much broader category based on structural features—in particular, pathology of identity formation. The BPO diagnosis subsumes the DSM-IV-TR BPD as well as all of the severe personality disorders. We refer the reader to Figure 1–1 for further clarification of the relationship between the DSM-IV-TR Axis II diagnostic categories and level of personality organization.

individuals in the NPO group. Ms. B and Mr. B are both illustrative of the difficulties encountered in the BPO group; one can see that their personality pathology affects virtually all areas of functioning. In Figure 1–1, we orient the reader unfamiliar with this system by illustrating the relationship between the structural approach to personality disorders, emphasizing the dimension of severity, and the more familiar DSM-IV-TR personality disorders.

Despite the apparently categorical nature of our framework as it is described above and represented in Figure 1–1, in fact, our approach assumes a dimensional perspective on personality pathology. At the healthiest end of the spectrum are individuals with normal identity, pre-

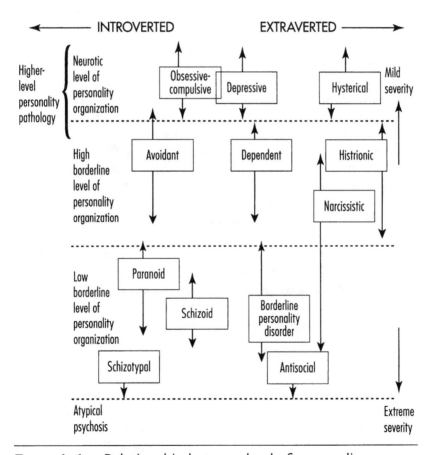

FIGURE 1–1.   Relationship between level of personality organization and DSM-IV-TR Axis II diagnoses.

Severity ranges from mildest, at the top of the figure, to extremely severe, at the bottom. Vertical arrows indicate ranges of severity for each DSM-IV-TR personality disorder.

dominantly higher-level defenses, and stable reality testing, while at the most pathological end are those with severe identity pathology, predominantly lower-level defenses, and shaky reality testing. In between we find a range of psychopathology. This is to say that the classification of personality disorders presented in this chapter is most accurately conceptualized as describing a continuous spectrum of personality pathology. As a result, the demarcation between the neurotic and borderline levels of personality organization is not categorical, and there are patients with very mild identity pathology who present with mixed features.

The structural classification of personality pathology, dividing personality disorders into those associated with a neurotic and those associated with a borderline level of organization, is further refined on the basis of characterization of 1) quality of object relations and 2) moral functioning (Kernberg and Caligor 2005). Within the BPO group, evaluation of these additional dimensions leads to identification of *high-level borderline organization* (i.e., healthier, with less pathology of object relations and more intact moral functioning, and having a better prognosis) and *low-level borderline organization* (i.e., having more severe personality pathology, with grossly impaired object relations and significant pathology of moral functioning, and having a poorer prognosis) (see Figure 1–1; see also Table 1–1). An essential distinction between the high- and low-level borderline groups is the role played by aggression in psychological functioning and pathology. Psychopathology in the low-level borderline group is characterized by the expression of poorly integrated forms of aggression, which may be inwardly and/or outwardly directed; aggression is less central in high-level borderline pathology. The high-level BPO group includes dependent, histrionic, more disturbed avoidant personalities, and the healthier end of the narcissistic spectrum. Ms. B is organized at a high borderline level; she presents with identity pathology, in the setting of some capacity for mutually dependent relations and largely intact moral functioning. Mr. B is organized at a low borderline level; he presents with more severe identity pathology, in the setting of relationships based on exploitation and deficits in moral functioning.

The distinctions between NPO and BPO and between high and low levels of borderline personality organization have important implications for prognosis and differential treatment planning. These three groups of patients (NPO, high-level BPO, low-level BPO) have different clinical needs, and patients in each group benefit from treatments specifically tailored to their psychopathology. At the end of this chapter we address some of these issues, and they are further developed in other chapters in this volume and in our suggested readings.

Table 1–1 outlines the structural approach to the classification of personality pathology. In the rest of this chapter, we elaborate on the material outlined in Table 1–1. We cover the constructs of identity, defenses, reality testing, quality of object relations, and moral functioning, focusing on their differential manifestations among the three levels of personality organization. We then introduce psychodynamic considerations, and we end with comments on implications for treatment.

Identity

The construct of identity anchors the object relations theory model of personality disorders. Normal identity distinguishes the normal personality and neurotic-level personality disorders on the one hand from the personality disorders organized at a borderline level on the other (Table 1–1). *Identity* is the structural correlate of both the subjective sense of self and the experience of significant others, which in this model are viewed as inextricably linked. (The intimate relation between self experience and the experience of others has been empirically examined and supported in a series of studies conducted by Andersen [Andersen and Chen 2002].) As mentioned earlier, in the object relations theory model, internal object relations are conceptualized as the building blocks of higher-order structures. Kernberg (Kernberg and Caligor 2005) suggests that in normal identity formation, internal object relations associated with the experience of self and others are organized in relation to one another in a stable but flexible fashion. This organization corresponds with an integrated sense of self, which is manifested subjectively in experiences of both the self and significant others that are complex, well differentiated, characterized by subtlety and depth, continuous over time and across situations, flexible, and realistic. In addition, normal identity is associated with the ability to accurately appreciate the internal experience of others; to invest, over time, in professional, intellectual, and recreational interests; and to "know one's own mind" with regard to one's values, opinions, tastes, and beliefs.

Kernberg contrasts normal identity with pathological identity formation; following Erikson (1956), he refers to the latter as the syndrome of *identity diffusion*. In identity diffusion, internal object relations making up the sense of self are polarized, by which we mean "all good" or "all bad," associated with strongly positive or strongly negative affect states, and extreme. These highly affectively charged internal object relations are poorly and unstably organized in relation to one another. At a descriptive level, the outcome of this structural organization is the absence of an overarching, coherent sense of self or of significant others.

TABLE 1–1. Structural approach to classification of personality pathology

Structural domain	Normal personality organization	Neurotic personality organization	High-level borderline personality organization	Low-level borderline personality organization
Personality rigidity	None	Mild to moderate	Extreme	Very extreme
Identity	Consolidated	Consolidated	Mild to moderate pathology	Severe pathology
Dominant defensive functioning	Mature	Repression-based	Splitting-based, repression-based	Splitting-based
Reality testing	Intact, stable	Intact, stable	Intact; some social deficits	Intact; social deficits (transient psychotic states)
Object relations	Deep, mutual	Deep, mutual	Some mutual	Need-fulfilling
Moral functioning	Internalized, flexible	Internalized, rigid	Inconsistent	Pathology

Instead, the subjective experience of both self and others is fragmented, lacking in continuity, extreme, and unstable.[3] For example, Ms. B's view of herself and her mood state shifted dramatically depending on whether or not there was a man in her life; a new romantic interest lifted her from dysphoria and self-loathing and left her feeling "like a new person." With his wife, Mr. B was withdrawn and passive, but when he was socializing at his gym he behaved entirely differently—he was outgoing, affable, and funny. In the setting of identity pathology, the individual's subjective experience of others tends to be poorly differentiated (lacking in subtlety and depth), affectively polarized ("black and white"), extreme, and/or superficial. Mr. B described his wife as "boring," "dowdy," "nagging," and "no fun." His image of her was vague and one-dimensional, more of a caricature than a complex and realistic view of another person. When prompted, Mr. B could think of nothing positive to say about her, though he acknowledged that she "makes a lot of money."

Individuals with identity pathology typically lack the capacity to accurately "read" others (Donegan et al. 2003; Wagner and Linehan 1999) and may be unable to respond tactfully to subtle social cues. Poorly consolidated identity is associated with feelings of emptiness and chronic dysphoria, along with a paucity of meaningful investments in professional, intellectual, and recreational pursuits. Tastes, opinions, and values are inconsistent, typically adopted from others in the environment, and may shift easily and dramatically with changes in milieu. For example, Ms. B changed her style of dress, taste in music, and patterns of speech to suit her latest boyfriend. While most clearly evident in DSM-IV-TR borderline personality disorder, some degree of identity pathology characterizes all severe personality disorders (see Table 1–1).

There are different degrees of identity pathology and different ways in which identity pathology may become manifest. Borderline personality disorder is in many ways the prototype of the personality disorders characterized by identity disturbance; both sense of self and sense of others are polarized, vague, unrealistic, and unstable. Temporal discontinuity tends to be an especially prominent subjective manifestation of identity pathology in this group. In contrast, in narcissistic personality disorder, a more stable sense of self, albeit distorted and often fragile,

---

[3]We refer the reader to Westen and Cohen (1993) for empirical support for the transitory, split, poorly integrated, and "black-and-white" quality of the self-representation in severe personality pathology described by Kernberg.

coexists with what is often a dramatically superficial, shadowy, or caricature-like experience of others, even in individuals who are highly intelligent and accomplished. Feelings of inauthenticity tend to be an especially prominent subjective manifestation of identity pathology in the narcissistic group. In the schizoid personality, in contrast, we see a capacity to appraise others in the absence of any integrated or stable sense of self, in conjunction with prominent feelings of emptiness. In personality disorders falling in the high-level BPO range, identity disturbance can be relatively mild, characterized by a sense of self that is less unstable than that characteristic of individuals organized at a low borderline level, along with a better-developed capacity to realistically experience and sustain relationships with significant others.

Clinical Illustration of Identity Pathology

Ms. B had worked at a series of jobs since graduating from college; none had been particularly interesting to her and she couldn't think of anything she wanted to do. She told the consultant when he inquired that, typically, the men she dated seemed wonderful at first but quickly became controlling and abusive. She described herself as having many friends, but her descriptions of the people in her life were vague and general—for example, characterizing someone as "nice," or "pretty," "funny," or "selfish." When the consultant asked Ms. B to describe herself, she could come up with little to say but did comment that she felt empty and aimless.

Comments. Ms. B's poorly developed sense of herself as a person, her lack of investment in her work, and her feelings of emptiness and aimlessness, coupled with the superficial, extreme, poorly differentiated, and at times unstable nature of her experience of the people in her life, are emblematic of identity pathology. These features can be evaluated in the clinical setting by asking the patient to describe himself or herself as a person and to describe a significant other. Patients with identity pathology generally find it difficult to provide a complex and realistic description of themselves, and they typically convey a shadowy or cartoonlike picture of significant others; descriptions of self and other are most often some combination of vague and superficial on the one hand and extreme and contradictory on the other. In contrast, individuals with normal identity, like Ms. N and Mr. N, are able to leave the clinician with a vivid and complex sense of themselves and of their significant others.

Defensive Operations

Defenses are an individual's automatic psychological responses to stressors or emotional conflict. Different levels of personality pathology are associated with different dominant defensive operations, and defenses operate differently in individuals with consolidated identity than in those whose identity is not consolidated. At the healthiest end of the spectrum, defenses are flexible and adaptive and involve little or no distortion of internal or external reality. At the most pathological end of the spectrum, defenses are highly inflexible and maladaptive, involving increasing degrees of distortion of reality (Vaillant 1993). Across the spectrum of personality pathology, defensive operations protect the individual from anxiety and pain associated with the expression of conflictual object relations, but at the same time they introduce maladaptive rigidity and underlying structural pathology into personality functioning.

Kernberg (1976) presents an approach to the classification of defenses that divides them into three groups: 1) mature defenses, 2) repression-based or "neurotic" defenses, and 3) splitting-based or lower-level (also referred to as "primitive") defenses. This classification is in many ways consistent with current consensus within the research community (Perry and Bond 2005), while placing greater emphasis on the psychological mechanisms underlying defensive operations.

Mature defenses[4] are the predominant defensive style in the normal personality and are associated with flexible and adaptive functioning. Mature defenses do not bar any aspect of a conflict from consciousness, nor do they maintain a distance between aspects of emotional life that are in conflict. Rather, mature defenses allow all aspects of an anxiety-provoking situation into subjective awareness, with little or no distortion, but in a fashion that minimizes psychological distress while optimizing coping (Vaillant 1993).

Repression-based, or neurotic, defenses[5] avoid distress by repressing, or banishing from consciousness, aspects of the subject's psychological experience that are conflictual or a potential source of emotional discomfort. Individuals organized at a neurotic level rely predominantly on a combination of repression-based and mature defenses (Kernberg and Caligor 2005). While there are a variety of neurotic

---

[4]Mature defenses include anticipation, suppression, altruism, humor, and sublimation.

[5]Repression-based, or neurotic, defenses include repression, reaction formation, neurotic projection, displacement, isolation of affect, and intellectualization.

defenses that work in different ways, they all involve repression; in the setting of a relatively well-integrated sense of self, repression-based defenses ensure that conflictual aspects of experience are split off from the dominant sense of self and remain more or less permanently out of conscious awareness. This process protects against awareness of conflictual experiences of self and other but at the same time introduces rigidity into personality functioning (e.g., "I never get angry"). Thus, Ms. N is unaware of having competitive or aggressive motivations, which are conflictual, but the rigidity introduced by her repressive defenses leaves her compelled to shy away from confrontation and to have difficulty appropriately asserting herself. Repression-based defenses alter the subject's internal reality, but they typically do so without grossly distorting the subject's sense of external reality. Although repression-based defenses result in personality rigidity, influence cognitive processes, and lead to subtle distortions of experience, and may cause discomfort or distress, they typically do not lead to grossly abnormal or disruptive behaviors.

Whereas neurotic defenses make use of repression, the lower-level, or splitting-based, defenses[6] make use of dissociation,[7] or splitting, to avoid psychological conflict and emotional distress. When we use the terms *dissociation* and *splitting*, we refer to a psychological process in which two aspects of experience that are in conflict are both allowed to emerge fully into consciousness, but either not at the same time as, or not in conjunction with, the same object relation (Kernberg 1976). Thus, splitting-based defenses, in contrast to repression-based defenses, do not banish mental contents from consciousness per se, but instead compartmentalize or maintain at a distance conscious aspects of experience that are in conflict or whose approximation would generate psychological discomfort.

Kernberg (1984) suggests that splitting-based defenses are intimately tied to identity pathology and that splitting is the prototypical defense seen in patients with severe personality disorders. In patients

---

[6]Splitting-based, or lower-level, defenses include splitting, primitive idealization, devaluation, projective identification, omnipotent control, and primitive denial. (These defenses are sometimes referred to as *primitive defenses* in the psychodynamic literature.)

[7]We distinguish between dissociation as a defensive operation and dissociative states. Dissociative states involve the defensive operation of dissociation, but they also involve an altered state of consciousness; dissociation as a defensive operation does not involve an altered state of consciousness.

organized at a borderline level, splitting most commonly involves separating sectors of experience associated with positive affects along with idealized representations of self and others, on the one hand, from sectors associated with negative affects and devalued or paranoid (also referred to as *persecutory*) object relations, on the other. In the setting of identity pathology, splitting-based defenses are responsible for experiences of others that are polarized ("black or white"), experienced as either "all good" (i.e., idealized) or "all bad" (i.e., paranoid or devalued)— loving, gratifying, and secure, on the one hand, or frustrating, frightening, or worthless, on the other. These polarized experiences of self and other are both superficial and unrealistic—for example, a *perfectly* gratifying caretaker or an *unbearably* frustrating caretaker, a *perfect* protector or an object who *threatens to obliterate* the self, an *omnipotent* self or a feeble self devoid of *any* power. Because in the setting of identity pathology these object relations cannot be contextualized in relation to an integrated view of significant others or of the self, these extreme images of self and other are often concretely experienced, as though "how I experience it now is all there is, and there is no room to think about alternative perspectives; it is not that you are frustrating me now, but rather that you are a frustrating person."

Splitting-based defenses in the setting of identity pathology are typically unstable and may lead to abrupt and rather chaotic shifts between idealized and persecutory experiences of self and other (Kernberg 1984). In individuals organized at a BPO, splitting-based defenses cause severe personality rigidity and are responsible for flagrant distortion of interpersonal reality. In this setting, these defenses typically have behavioral manifestations and frequently result in disruptive behaviors.

Individuals falling in the high-borderline range rely on a combination of repression-based and splitting-based defenses. This defensive organization is typically characterized by stable functioning in many domains and relatively well integrated experience much of the time. However, in the setting of stress or in areas of psychological conflict, the individual is subject to the abrupt intrusion into consciousness of more highly affectively charged, "split" internal object relations as they break through repressive defenses.

Individuals organized at an NPO also make use of splitting and dissociation. However, in contrast to the situation in the severe personality disorders, we are now seeing the impact of splitting and dissociation on the psychological experience of an individual who has a consolidated identity and a relatively well integrated sense of self. In this setting, splitting and dissociation are less extreme and more stable than in more severe personality pathology and do not lead to the highly polarized,

rapidly shifting, and affectively charged experiences of internal and external reality characteristic of the severe personality disorders. Thus, in
individuals organized at a neurotic level, splitting and dissociation are
not typically associated with "primitive" mental states, but rather with
the segregation of aspects of psychological experience that are in conflict and with the more or less subtle dissociation of conflictual motivations from dominant self experience (Caligor et al. 2007).

For example, a young woman with conflicts around sexuality was
extremely emotionally and sexually inhibited with men she became
emotionally involved with. She would occasionally pursue brief affairs
with men toward whom she felt no attachment; in this setting she was
both a passionate and a sexually adventurous lover. Here, while conflictual motivations are consciously experienced and enacted, they remain at the same time split off from other motivations and aspects of self
experience with which they are in conflict. As in the severe personality
disorders, splitting and dissociation are supported by denial; the individual organized at a neurotic level denies the significance of dissociated aspects of conscious experience that are incompatible with his or
her dominant sense of self. Thus, the young woman in our example
viewed herself as inhibited and not especially interested in sex, denying
the significance of her sexual adventures: "They don't really mean anything."

Clinical Illustration of Splitting-Based Defenses in Severe Personality Pathology

Mr. B was referred for dynamic therapy. He spent the first month of the
treatment apparently working very happily with his therapist while repeatedly telling the therapist how brilliant she was and how she was the
one who was finally "solving" his problems. In this setting, Mr. B's
mood improved and he felt less anxious. About 4 weeks into the treatment, the therapist had to take care of an emergency and, as a result, began Mr. B's session five minutes late. As soon as Mr. B entered the
therapist's office, he began to viciously attack her: the therapist was
heartless and incompetent, and Mr. B had been a fool to be in treatment
with someone who clearly cared nothing about his welfare and was just
using him to make money. The therapist managed to contain her anger
and her impulse to defend herself. Instead, she listened to Mr. B, put her
understanding of Mr. B's experience into words, and then commented
that she was struck by the contradiction between Mr. B's current experience of her, on the one hand, and, on the other hand, the positive atti-

tude that had characterized their interactions up until this point, and the certainty Mr. B had expressed in previous sessions that she cared about him and was helping him. Mr. B responded that he remembered those sessions, but they were irrelevant now; he now saw the therapist for who she truly was, and that was the only thing that mattered.

Comments.   Mr. B's unstable, widely polarized, superficial, and unrealistic views of his therapist are typical manifestations of splitting, in which "all-good," idealized views of significant others temporarily ward off awareness of "all-bad," paranoid and hateful object relations. Initially, Mr. B enacts an idealized relationship with the therapist. When the therapist keeps Mr. B waiting, we see his view of her, and of himself in relation to her, undergo a dramatic shift, and highly negatively charged, paranoid object relations flood Mr. B's experience. Note that both the idealized and the paranoid images of the therapeutic are consciously experienced, though at different times. This vignette also illustrates how splitting is supported by denial; when the therapist calls Mr. B's attention to the rapid shift in his view of her, Mr. B denies the emotional significance of his earlier, idealized view of their relationship. This enables Mr. B to continue to separate the idealized and paranoid aspects of his experience.

Reality Testing

Sustained loss of perceptual reality testing is not a feature of personality disorders. However, transient loss of reality testing can be seen in some of the more severe personality disorders, especially in highly stressful or affectively charged settings or in the context of alcohol or substance abuse. When a patient presents with frank loss of reality testing, the evaluation and treatment of psychosis becomes the highest priority, and the issue of personality pathology is deferred until psychotic symptoms resolve.

If we turn from reality testing proper to what we refer to as *social reality testing*, we see that individuals organized at a BPO frequently present with deficits in this area. Social reality testing is responsible for the ability to read social cues, understand social conventions, and respond tactfully in interpersonal settings, all of which are characteristic of the normal personality and are also seen in the NPO. Deficits in social reality testing can lead individuals who are organized at a borderline level to behave inappropriately in social settings, typically without being aware of doing so, and misinterpretation of social cues may lead to transient feelings of paranoia or fears of being abandoned.

Clinical Examples of Deficits in Social Reality Testing

In social settings, Mr. B often got into heated political arguments, during which his behavior was inappropriately aggressive for the setting. Ms. B. was routinely late for work, and she often arrived inappropriately dressed, in a fashion that was either excessively casual or excessively revealing.

Comments.   Mr. B was unaware of the inappropriateness of his behavior and of the discomfort he elicited in others, both common manifestations of deficits in social reality testing. Ms. B demonstrated a lack of appreciation of social conventions; she did not understand the importance of arriving on time to work (she felt it "didn't really matter"), and she did not have an appreciation of what is and what is not suitable work attire.

Quality of Object Relations

Quality of object relations refers to the individual's understanding of the nature of relationships and to his or her capacity to establish and sustain mutual and intimate attachments. In the normal personality, we see the capacity to appreciate and care about the needs of the other, independent of the needs of the self, and the ability to maintain mutually dependent relationships based on an understanding of give and take. The NPO is also associated with the capacity for mutual dependency and concern, but often with a failure to fully integrate intimate and mutually dependent relations with sexuality. Thus, Ms. N has deep and mature relationships with her friends, but she is unable to sustain a relationship of this kind in the setting of sexual intimacy.

In contrast, the BPO is characterized by pathology of object relations. In low-level BPO, pathology of object relations is severe, and we see the predominance of a need-fulfilling understanding of interpersonal relations. By this we mean it is assumed that all relations are organized on a quid pro quo basis—that is, "If I do something for you, I expect to receive something in return," and a particular relationship is valued precisely to the degree that it meets the needs of the subject. Pathology of quality of object relations is most extreme in the antisocial personality, for whom all human interactions are based on usage and exploitation of others. Individuals organized at a high level of borderline personality organization are distinguished from the low borderline group by virtue of their demonstration of at least some capacity for mutual dependency and for maintaining relationships that transcend a self-serving orientation. Pathology of object relations that is severe relative to overall level of functioning is characteristic of narcissistic pathology.

Clinical Example of Pathology of Object Relations

Mr. B explained to the consultant that even though he no longer had any positive or sexual feelings for his wife, he stayed with her because she had the means to support him financially; he avoided close friendships because he didn't want anyone to feel he "owed" them anything.

Comments.   Mr. B's relationship with his wife is frankly exploitative. His concerns about the dangers of friendship illustrate a quid pro quo view of relationships; there is no comfortable sense of give and take, but only giving in order to get back. In contrast, though not a social person, Mr. N was deeply attached to his wife and children, and he went to great lengths to ensure that they were well taken care of.

Moral Values

The normal personality is associated with a commitment to values and ideals and a "moral compass" that is consistent, flexible, and fully integrated into the sense of self. In the NPO also, we see commitment to values and ideals and the absence of antisocial behavior, reflecting a fully integrated and internalized sense of values and ideals. However, moral rigidity, a tendency to hold the self to unreasonably high standards—to be excessively self-critical or to anguish over the temptation to stray—is a common feature of personality disorders organized at a neurotic level. In contrast, the BPO is characterized by a variable degree of pathology in moral functioning. At one end of the spectrum, we find a relatively well developed but rigid and excessively severe level of moral functioning characterized by severe anxiety and subjective distress, in the form either of self-criticism or of anticipated criticism from others, in relation to not adhering to internal standards. At the other end of the spectrum, we see the absence of any internal moral compass and a lack of capacity for guilt, characteristic of patients organized at a low borderline level, and in particular those with antisocial personality disorder or severe narcissistic pathology.

Clinical Example of Pathology in Moral Functioning

Mr. B prided himself on having extremely high ethical standards, and he was contemptuous of those who "bend the rules." At the same time, he routinely lied to both his wife and his therapist about using prostitutes. He experienced no discomfort in relation to lying to them, never giving his behavior a second thought. When his therapist brought Mr. B's lying to his attention, Mr. B denied the significance of his behavior and rationalized that he did it to "smooth things out."

Comments.   It is common for individuals organized at a borderline level to demonstrate excessively harsh moral standards that may comfortably coexist with glaring "lacunae" in moral functioning. Splitting and denial underlie the capacity to maintain frankly contradictory attitudes toward moral functioning.

DYNAMIC FEATURES OF PERSONALITY DISORDERS AND THE DEGREE OF INTEGRATION OF MOTIVATIONAL SYSTEMS

In the object relations model, psychological conflicts are seen to be organized around "conflictual motivations"—that is, motivations whose direct expression would be threatening or painful to the individual. Kernberg (Kernberg and Caligor 2005) suggests that an important distinction between the neurotic and borderline levels of personality organization is the degree of integration and accessibility to consciousness of conflictual motivations, and he focuses in particular on the role of aggressive motivations in psychological functioning in the personality disorders. When motivations are well integrated, they are associated with affects that are relatively complex and well modulated, lending subtlety and depth to affective experience. In contrast, poorly integrated motivations are associated with affects that are intense, extreme, shallow, and poorly modulated.

In the normal personality and the NPO, the motivational systems that color conscious experience are relatively well integrated; conflictual motivations that are more poorly integrated are for the most part repressed. In the low-level BPO, in contrast, psychological functioning is dominated by the impact of poorly integrated, aggressive, and destructive motivational systems. Further, the predominance of splitting-based defenses means that highly charged object relations associated with poorly integrated aggression are not repressed, but are fully accessible to consciousness; when splitting and idealization fail, aggressively colored internal object relations flood subjective experience with overwhelming negative affect states. For example, consider the quality of the hatred and paranoia Mr. B experienced in relation to his therapist when he was no longer able to idealize her. Contrast this with the quality of hostility we would expect of Mr. N were he to become angry. In the high-level BPO the quality of aggression is intermediate between that seen in the NPO and in the low-level BPO. The combination of repressive and splitting-based defenses characteristic of the high-level BPO means that much of the time, more highly charged, less well integrated aggressive motivations and associated object relations are repressed. However, in areas of conflict or in times of stress, more poorly integrated, paranoid internal object relations can abruptly emerge into consciousness.

In the NPO, psychological conflicts commonly involve the expression of sexual, dependent, competitively aggressive, and sadistic motivations. For example, if we were to put Ms. N's conflicts around the expression of aggression into words, they might sound like this: "If I were to express hostile or competitive feelings toward people I care about, it would make me a bad or unlovable person. In the face of this conflict, I automatically defend against recognizing hostile feelings by repressing or projecting them. As a result, I do not consciously experience myself as hostile or competitive." Subjectively, we see a dominant sense of self that is relatively complex and realistic but that has been stripped of aggression.

In the BPO, conflicts are typically organized somewhat differently. As has been already described, Kernberg (1984) suggests that the central dynamic feature of the low-level BPO is the predominance of poorly integrated aggression in the setting of splitting-based defenses. The dominant anxiety associated with the low-level BPO is that poorly integrated forms of aggression, associated with powerful negative affect states and paranoid object relations, will overwhelm positive sectors of experience. In this setting, to protect positive object relations, positive and negative feelings toward the same person must be kept apart. This is accomplished by splitting-based defenses, which segregate idealized object relations from negative, aggressively infiltrated object relations. As a result of this process, positively colored object relations are protected, but at the expense of interfering with processes of psychological integration that would lead in the long term to a tempering of aggression by the simultaneous experience of positive object relations and affect states, and to identity consolidation. In this setting, the tendency to project "all-bad" object relations often leads to intense paranoia, overwhelming anxiety and fear, and an inability to assume responsibility for one's affect states or one's actions, which typically feel justified on the basis of perceived (often misperceived) provocation.[8] For example,

---

[8]There is empirical support for the predominance of malevolent representations of relationships in individuals with borderline personality disorder (see Bell et al. 1998; Nigg et al. 1992; Westen et al. 1990).

when Mr. B's therapist frustrated him by starting late, Mr. B felt fully justified in attacking and devaluing her.

Where paranoid concerns are preeminent in the low-level BPO, in individuals organized at a high-level BPO anxieties typically have more to do with fears of closeness and dependency, and paranoid concerns are secondary. Here, in the setting of a combination of repression-based and splitting-based defenses, we typically see condensation of conflicts in relation to dependency, sexuality, and self-esteem maintenance, along with conflicts around aggression. In less conflictual areas of functioning, repressive defenses are generally able to manage anxiety and to protect the individual from the emergence into consciousness of poorly integrated motivational states. However, in settings that activate core conflicts or stimulate significant anxiety (often, depending on the individual, these settings involve dependent relations, sexual intimacy, competitive struggles in relation to authority and power, and/or extreme threats to self-esteem), repressive defenses may fail, at times leading to episodes of intensely felt rage, hatred, and paranoia that seem discontinuous with the individual's overall level of psychological functioning. For example, Ms. B was often able to maintain stable and mutual relations with her friends; with her boyfriends, she would also do well for a time. But as she became more dependent she also became more brittle and volatile; if she felt that her boyfriend was not taking care of her as she would like, she could hatefully turn on him in an instant. In this setting, activation of core conflicts around dependency overwhelmed otherwise stable repressive defenses.

Implications for Treatment

Evaluation of level of personality organization will guide differential treatment planning and enable the clinician to anticipate problems that may arise in treatment, along with the nature of transference and countertransference reactions likely to emerge. Personality pathology falling in the NPO range has an excellent prognosis, and the neurotic-level personality disorders typically do well in conventional psychodynamic psychotherapies. In the clinical setting, patients with consolidated identity typically demonstrate the ability to commit to and invest in a long-term treatment; a fairly well-developed capacity for self-observation and self-reflection; a capacity to establish and maintain a therapeutic relationship with relative ease; an appreciation of the symbolic nature of thought; and adequate impulse control (Caligor et al. 2007). In psychotherapy, transferences generally develop slowly and evolve gradually over the course of treatment, and they are realistic, relatively subtle, and associated with well-modulated affect states; the individual organized at a neurotic level is typically able to maintain a view of his or her therapist that remains anchored in the realistic aspects of the doctor-patient relationship despite transference distortions that may arise. Clinicians generally find individuals falling in the NPO group to be gratifying to work with and relatively easy to understand and to empathize with. Countertransference reactions tend to be mild, chronic, and specific to the therapist's and patient's conflicts. (See McWilliams 1994, in our recommended readings, for a description of transference-countertransference paradigms characteristic of the different personality disorders.)

In contrast, personality pathology in the BPO range has a more variable prognosis. Patients organized at a borderline level generally do poorly in unmodified dynamic therapies; they fare better in modified psychodynamic treatments that provide structure, limit setting, attention to the role of splitting in the patient's difficulties, and careful management of the patient's relationship with the therapist. In the clinical setting, low-level borderline pathology is associated with a high rate of treatment dropout; an impaired capacity for self-reflection; difficulty maintaining a therapeutic alliance; a tendency for concrete thinking with the possibility of transient compromise of reality testing; and a tendency for destructive and self-destructive acting out (Clarkin et al. 2006). The transference and countertransference reactions that characterize treatment of patients organized at a low BPO level reflect the impact of splitting-based defenses, and in particular of projective identification, on the clinical situation. Transferences develop quickly and often chaotically, and they are highly affectively charged, extreme, polarized, unrealistic, unstable, and often paranoid; the concrete quality of these transferences easily compromises the patient's capacity to maintain a realistic sense of the doctor-patient relationship (Caligor et al. 2009). Countertransference reactions tend also to be highly affectively charged, as well as confusing, uncomfortable, and difficult to contain, associated with powerful pressures on the therapist to turn to action. Clinicians generally find individuals organized at a low BPO level to be challenging and emotionally taxing patients, and maintaining empathy with patients in this group can be difficult.

In contrast to the low-level BPO group, patients organized at a high borderline level have a relatively favorable prognosis in modified psychodynamic therapies. These patients may present with complaints that superficially resemble those of patients organized at an NPO. However, as treatment progresses, we often see the emergence of milder versions of the kinds of problems that characterize the treatments of patients with more severe identity pathology; in particular, at times of high affect activation, we often see a tendency toward concrete thinking and compromise of the patient's capacity to self-reflect, especially in relation to emotionally charged interactions with the therapist. Anticipation of these difficulties, in conjunction with attention to splitting-based defenses, can prevent an unexpected crisis in treatment. Countertransference reactions tend to be less overwhelming and confusing than those experienced with patients in the low-level BPO group but are nevertheless more affectively charged and more likely to lead to action than are the countertransferences typically encountered in treatments of patients falling in the neurotic range.

The object relations theory model of personality disorders not only guides treatment planning but also leads naturally to specific approaches to treatment. Our group has developed long-term, twice-weekly psychodynamic psychotherapies for personality disorders on this basis. Transference-focused psychotherapy (TFP), described in this book (see Chapter 7, "Transference-Focused Psychotherapy and Borderline Personality Disorder"), is organized around the clinical needs of patients with a BPO. Also described in this volume is a modified version of TFP for treatment of patients with narcissistic pathology (Chapter 9, "Narcissistic Personality Disorder"). Dynamic psychotherapy for higher-level personality pathology (Caligor et al. 2007) targets the difficulties characteristic of individuals organized at a neurotic level, along with those at the interface between neurotic and high BPO levels of organization, while making use of the psychological assets associated with higher-level personality pathology.

For patients organized at a borderline level, who present with clinically significant identity pathology, treatment is organized around promoting the integration of dissociated, idealized and paranoid, internal object relations, with the goal of establishing a more coherent, stable, better-differentiated, and complex experience of self and others (Kernberg and Caligor 2005). For patients organized at a neurotic level, who present with personality rigidity in the setting of normal identity formation, treatment is organized around promoting the integration of repressed or dissociated internal object relations into an already consolidated, stable, and relatively complex sense of self, with the goal of reducing personality rigidity (Caligor et al. 2007). Across all levels of severity of personality pathology, psychotherapy is organized around exploration of the patient's internal object relations as they are played out in current interpersonal relationships, including the relationship with the therapist. Therapeutic inquiry focuses on the here and now, attending closely to the patient's current life situation and to his or her immediate and affectively dominant experience in the treatment hour.

Key Clinical Concepts

◆ Object relations theory grew out of clinical observation and practice and has led to the development of psychodynamic treatments for personality disorders.

◆ The object relations theory model of personality disorders attends to descriptive, structural, and dynamic aspects of personality disorders.

◆ Structural assessment focuses on identity, defenses, reality testing, object relations, and moral functioning.

◆ Assessment of descriptive and structural features of personality disorders enables the clinician to characterize severity of personality pathology and will guide treatment planning.

◆ The object relations theory model of personality disorders is compatible with many recent developments in personality disorder research.

Suggested Readings

Akhtar S: Broken Structures: Severe Personality Disorders and Their Treatment. Northvale, NJ, Jason Aronson, 1992

Caligor E, Kernberg OF, Clarkin JF: Handbook of Dynamic Psychotherapy for Higher Level Personality Pathology. Washington, DC, American Psychiatric Publishing, 2007

Clarkin JF, Yeomans FE, Kernberg OF: Psychotherapy for Borderline Personality: Focusing on Object Relations. Washington, DC, American Psychiatric Publishing, 2006

McWilliams N: Psychoanalytic Diagnosis. New York, Guilford, 1994

PDM Task Force: Psychodynamic Diagnostic Manual: Personality Patterns and Disorders. Silver Spring, MD, Alliance of Psychoanalytic Organizations, 2006

The Structured Interview for Personality Organization (STIPO). The STIPO is a semistructured interview based on the clinical structural interview described in this chapter. The STIPO is available on the Web site http://www.borderlinedisorders.com.

Symphoratapes: Master Clinicians at Work. A video presentation of Dr. Otto Kernberg conducting a diagnostic interview focusing on structural features of personality can be seen on a DVD that is part of this series produced by Drs. Henk-Jan Dalewijk and Bert van Luyn. This DVD set also includes interviews of the same patient by Marsha Linehan, Michael Stone, Larry Rockland, Solomon Aktar, and Lorna Benjamin. The set of DVDs creates a teaching tool for demonstrating clinical interviewing skills and illustrating different theoretical orientations for understanding severe personality disorders. Information about ordering this set of DVDs can be obtained at http://www.bpdresourcecenter.org.

References

American Psychiatric Association: Diagnostic and Statistical Manual of Mental Disorders, 4th Edition, Text Revision. Washington, DC, American Psychiatric Association, 2000

Andersen SM, Chen S: The relational self: an interpersonal social-cognitive theory. Psychol Rev 109:619–645, 2002

Bell M, Billington R, Cicchetti D, et al: Do object relations deficits distinguish BPD from other diagnostic groups? J Clin Psychol 44:511–516, 1988

Benjamin LS: Interpersonal theory of personality disorders: the structural analysis of social behavior and interpersonal reconstructive therapy, in Major Theories of Personality Disorder, 2nd Edition. Edited by Lenzenweger MF, Clarkin JF. New York, Guilford, 2005, pp 157–230

Caligor E, Kernberg OF, Clarkin JF: Handbook of Dynamic Psychotherapy for Higher Level Personality Pathology. Washington, DC, American Psychiatric Publishing, 2007

Caligor E, Yeomans F, Diamond F, et al: The interpretive process in the psychodynamic psychotherapy of borderline personality. J Am Psychoanal Assoc 57:271–301, 2009

Clarkin JF, Yeomans FE, Kernberg OF: Psychotherapy for Borderline Personality: Focusing on Object Relations. Washington, DC, American Psychiatric Publishing, 2006

Donegan NH, Sanislow CA, Blumberg HP, et al: Amygdala hyperactivity in borderline personality disorder: implications for emotional dysregulation. Biol Psychiatry 54:1284–1293, 2003

Erikson EH: The problem of ego identity, in Identity and the Life Cycle. New York, International Universities Press, 1956, pp 101–164

Kernberg OF: Object Relations Theory and Clinical Psychoanalysis. New York, Jason Aronson, 1976

Kernberg OF: Severe Personality Disorders: Psychotherapeutic Strategies. New Haven, CT, Yale University Press, 1984

Kernberg OF, Caligor E: A psychoanalytic theory of personality disorders, in Major Theories of Personality Disorder, 2nd Edition. Edited by Lenzenweger M, Clarkin JF. New York, Guilford, 2005, pp 114–156

Lenzenweger MF, Clarkin JF (eds): Major Theories of Personality Disorder, 2nd Edition. New York, Guilford, 2005

Levy KN: The implications of attachment theory and research for understanding borderline personality disorder. Dev Psychopathol 17:959–986, 2005

Livesley WJ: Conceptual and taxonomic issues, in Handbook of Personality Disorders: Theory, Research, and Treatment. Edited by Livesley WJ. New York, Guilford, 2001, pp 3–38

Meyer B, Pilkonis PA: An attachment model of personality disorders, in Major Theories of Personality Disorder, 2nd Edition. Edited by Lenzenweger MF, Clarkin JF. New York, Guilford, 2005, pp 231–281

Mischel W, Shoda Y: Toward a unified theory of personality: integrating dispositions and processing dynamics within the cognitive-affective processing system, in Handbook of Personality: Theory and Research, 3rd Edition. Edited by John OP, Robins RW, Pervin LA. New York, Guilford, 2008, pp 208–241

Nigg J, Lohr W, Westen D, et al: Malevolent object representations in borderline personality disorder and major depression. J Abnorm Psychol 101:61–67, 1992

Parker G, Hadzi-Pavlovic D, Both L, et al: Measuring disordered personality functioning: to love and to work reprised. Acta Psychiatr Scand 110:230–239, 2004

Perry JC, Bond M: Defensive functioning, in The American Psychiatric Publishing Textbook of Personality Disorders. Edited by Oldham JM, Skodol AE, Bender DS. Washington, DC, American Psychiatric Publishing, 2005, pp 523–540

Pincus AL: A contemporary interpersonal theory of personality disorders, in Major Theories of Personality Disorder, 2nd Edition. Edited by Lenzenweger MF, Clarkin JF. New York, Guilford, 2005, pp 282–333

Pretzer JL, Beck AT: A cognitive theory of personality disorders, in Major Theories of Personality Disorder, 2nd Edition. Edited by Lenzenweger MF, Clarkin JF. New York, Guilford, 2005, pp 43–113

Shaver PR, Mikulincer M: Attachment theory and research: resurrection of the psychodynamic approach to personality. J Res Pers 39:22–45, 2005

Vaillant G: The Wisdom of the Ego. Cambridge, MA, Harvard University Press, 1993

Verheul R, Andrea H, Berghout CC, et al: Severity Indices of Personality Problems (SIPP-118): development, factor structure, reliability, and validity. Psychol Assess 20:23–34, 2008

Wagner AW, Linehan MM: Facial expression recognition ability among women with borderline personality disorder: implications for emotion regulation? J Pers Disord 12:329–344, 1999

Westen D, Arkowitz-Westen: Limitations of Axis II in diagnosing personality pathology in clinical practice. Am J Psychiatry 155:1767–1771, 1998

Westen D, Cohen RP: The self in borderline personality disorder: a psychodynamic perspective, in The Self inEmotional Distress: Cognitive and Psychodynamic Perspectives. Edited by Segal ZV, Blatt SJ. New York, Guilford, 1993, pp 334–368

Westen D, Gabbard G: Developments in cognitive neuroscience, II: implications for theories of transference. J Am Psychoanal Assoc 50:99–134, 2002

Westen D, Lohr N, Silk K, et al: Object relations and social cognition in borderlines, major depressives, and normals: a TAT analysis. Psychol Assess 2:355–364, 1990

CHAPTER 2

Attachment and Personality Pathology

Peter Fonagy, Ph.D., F.B.A.
Patrick Luyten, Ph.D.
Anthony Bateman, M.A., F.R.C.Psych.
György Gergely, Ph.D.
Lane Strathearn, M.B.B.S., F.R.A.C.P., Ph.D.
Mary Target, Ph.D.
Elizabeth Allison, D.Phil.

In this chapter we will discuss the relevance of attachment theory and research to the understanding and treatment of personality pathology. We will focus on recent developments that have highlighted the vital role played by the parent's understanding of the infant's internal world in enabling the infant to acquire capacities for affect regulation, attentional control, and mentalization and in the infant's development of a sense of self-agency. We will argue that the development of these capacities may be compromised in children who have not benefited from the opportunity to be understood and thought about in this way by a sensitive caregiver. Such individuals are then at greater risk of developing personality pathology, particularly if early neglect is compounded by trauma.

Our model was first outlined in the context of a large empirical study in which security of infant attachment with each parent proved to be strongly predicted not only by that parent's security of attachment during the pregnancy (Fonagy et al. 1991b) but even more by the parents' capacity to understand their own childhood relationship to their own parents in terms of states of mind (Fonagy et al. 1991a). We proposed that there was a vital synergy between attachment processes and the development of the child's ability to understand interpersonal behavior in terms of mental states (Fonagy and Target 1997; Fonagy et al. 2002). We called this ability *mentalization*,[1] and we have tried to describe how our understanding of ourselves and others as mental agents grows out of interpersonal experience, and particularly out of the child-caregiver relationship (Fonagy et al. 2002). We shall see that the ability to mentalize is vital for self-organization and affect regulation.

Our model challenges the Cartesian assumption that the mind is transparent to itself and that our ability to reflect on our own minds is innate. We contend that optimal development of the capacity to mentalize depends on interaction with more mature and sensitive minds and that a consideration of the role played by attachment in this development is indispensable. In this chapter we will review some of the evidence linking mentalization to the quality of attachment relationships and will outline our attachment-theory-inspired psychodynamic model of personality pathology.

We will suggest that the capacity to mentalize is best understood as a multidimensional construct whose core processing dimensions rely on distinct neural systems. Thus, mentalization involves both a self-reflective and an interpersonal component; it is based both on observing others and reflecting on their mental states; it is both implicit and explicit and concerns both feelings and cognitions (Fonagy and Luyten 2009; Lieberman 2007; P. Luyten, P. Fonagy, L. Mayes, and B. Van Houdenhove, "Mentalization as a Multidimensional Concept," 2009, submitted; Saxe 2006). When they are working together in optimal combination, the neural systems underpinning these components enable the child to represent causal mental states, distinguish inner from outer reality, infer others' mental states from subtle behavioral and contextual cues, moderate behavior and emotional experience, and construct representations of his or her own mental states from perceptible cues (arousal, behavior, context). We will discuss how the delicate balance of these systems can

---

[1] For research purposes we have operationalized this construct as *reflective function* (Fonagy et al. 1997).

be disrupted by neglect and trauma and what implications this has for understanding and treating personality pathology.

Introduction to Attachment Theory

Early caregiving relationships are probably key to normal development in all mammals, including humans (Hofer 1995). John Bowlby, the founder of attachment theory, postulated a universal human need to form close bonds. Bowlby originally proposed that the basic evolutionary function of the attachment instinct was to ensure that infants would be protected from predators (Bowlby 1969). The attachment behaviors of the human infant (e.g., proximity seeking, smiling, clinging) are reciprocated by adult attachment behaviors (touching, holding, soothing), and these responses reinforce the attachment behavior of the infant toward that particular adult.

However, the evolutionary role of the attachment relationship goes far beyond giving physical protection to the human infant. The infant's attachment behaviors are activated when something about his environment makes him feel insecure. The goal of the attachment system is an experience of security. Thus, the attachment system is first and foremost a regulator of emotional experience (Sroufe 1996).

None of us are born with the capacity to regulate our own emotional reactions. The caregiver understands and responds to the newborn infant's signals of moment-to-moment changes in his state, and a dyadic regulatory system gradually evolves. The infant learns that while in the caregiver's presence he will not be overwhelmed by his emotional arousal, because the caregiver is there to help him reestablish equilibrium. Thus, when he starts to feel overwhelmed, the infant will seek or signal to the caregiver in the hope of soothing and the recovery of homeostasis. By the end of the first year the infant's behavior seems to be based on specific expectations. His past experiences with the caregiver are aggregated into representational systems that Bowlby (1973) termed *internal working models*.

For the purpose of observing infants' internal working models in action, Mary Ainsworth, the second great pioneer of attachment theory, developed a laboratory-based procedure known as the "Strange Situation" (Ainsworth 1978; Ainsworth et al. 1985). When briefly separated from their caregiver and left with a stranger in an unfamiliar setting, infants show one of four patterns of behavior (Table 2–1). Infants classified as *secure* explore readily in the presence of the primary caregiver, are anxious in the stranger's presence and avoid her, are distressed by their caregiver's brief absence, rapidly seek contact with her afterwards, and

TABLE 2–1.   Patterns of attachment in the Strange Situation

Attachment classification	Characteristics
Secure	Explore readily in primary caregiver's presence
	Anxious in stranger's presence and avoid her
	Distressed by caregiver's brief absence
	Rapidly seek contact with caregiver at reunion
	Reassured by renewed contact and return to exploration
Anxious/Avoidant	Appear to be made less anxious by separation
	May not seek contact with caregiver following separation
	May not prefer caregiver over stranger
Anxious/Resistant	Show limited exploration and play
	Highly distressed by separation
	Difficulty settling at reunion
	Anxiety and anger appear to prevent infant from deriving comfort from contact
Disorganized/Disoriented	Undirected/bizarre behavior (e.g., freezing, hand clapping, head banging)
	Try to escape the situation even in caregiver's presence

are reassured by this contact, returning to their exploration. Some infants, who appear to be made less anxious by separation, may not seek proximity with the caregiver following separation and may not prefer her over the stranger; these infants are designated *anxious/avoidant*. The third category, *anxious/resistant* infants, show limited exploration and play, tend to be highly distressed by the separation, and have great difficulty in settling afterwards. The caregiver's presence or attempts at comforting fail to reassure, and the infant's anxiety and anger appear to prevent him from deriving comfort from being close.

Secure infants' behavior is based on repeated experiences of well-coordinated, sensitive interactions where the caregiver is rarely over-arousing and is able to restabilize the child's disorganizing emotional responses. Therefore, secure infants remain relatively organized in stressful situations. Anxious/avoidantly attached children are presumed to have had experiences where their emotional arousal was not restabilized by the caregiver or where they were overaroused through intrusive parenting; therefore they *over-regulate* their affect and avoid situations that are likely to be distressing. Anxious/resistantly attached children *under-regulate*, heightening their expression of distress, possibly in an effort to elicit a response from the caregiver. The threshold beyond which they start to feel threatened is low and the child becomes preoccupied with having contact with the caregiver, yet he seems frustrated even when this is available (Sroufe 1996).

A fourth group of infants shows seemingly undirected behavior, such as freezing, hand clapping, head banging, and the wish to escape the situation even in the caregiver's presence. These infants are referred to as *disorganized/disoriented* (Main and Solomon 1990). It is generally held that for such infants the caregiver has served as a source of both fear and reassurance, so that the arousal of the attachment system produces strong conflicting motivations. Not surprisingly, histories of prolonged or repeated separation (Chisolm 1998), intense marital conflict (Owen and Cox 1997), and/or severe neglect or physical or sexual abuse are often associated with this pattern (Carlson et al. 1989).

These infants' attachment can be considered "disorganized" in the sense that fear is triggered by an abusive or ill adult figure, which in turn activates the attachment system and the need for closeness; but in these circumstances, closeness will increase exposure to the source of fear (the attachment figure or other adults like the attachment figure). As this in turn increases his fear, the child will experience an ever-increasing need for an attachment figure. His fear is generated, rather than downregulated, by physical and psychological closeness to the caregiver. Thus, under some circumstances maltreatment can lead to overactivation of the attachment system, and disorganization may be an indication that this has occurred (Figure 2–1). In these individuals the attachment system may be quite readily triggered, and they may appear to be constantly preoccupied with attachment relationships.

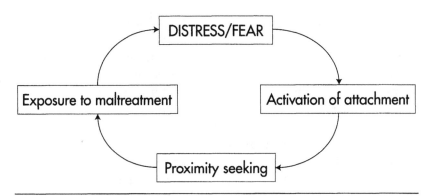

FIGURE 2–1. The vicious cycle of maltreatment.

Bowlby proposed that the internal working models of the self and others established in infancy provide the prototypes for all later relationships. Because internal working models function outside of awareness, they are change resistant (Crittenden 1990). The stability of attachment has been demonstrated by longitudinal studies of infants who were assessed with the Strange Situation and followed up in adolescence or young adulthood with the Adult Attachment Interview (AAI) (C. George, N. Kaplan, and M. Main: "The Adult Attachment Interview," Department of Psychology, University of California at Berkeley, 1985). This structured clinical instrument elicits narrative histories of childhood attachment relationships. The AAI scoring system (M. Main and R. Goldwyn, "Adult Attachment Rating and Classification System, Manual in Draft, Version 6.0," University of California at Berkeley, 1994) classifies individuals into Secure/Autonomous, Insecure/Dismissing, Insecure/Preoccupied, or Unresolved with respect to loss or trauma. Categorization is based on the form rather than the content of subjects' narratives of early experiences (Table 2–2). Whereas *secure/autonomous* individuals value attachment relationships and coherently integrate memories into a meaningful narrative that they regard as formative, *insecure* individuals are poor at integrating memories of experience with the meaning of that experience. Those *dismissing* of attachment show avoidance by denying memories and by idealizing or devaluing early relationships. *Preoccupied* individuals tend to be confused, angry, or fearful in relation to attachment figures and sometimes still complain of childhood slights, echoing the protests of the resistant infant. *Unresolved* individuals have significant disorganization in their attachment relationship representations, as indicated through semantic or syntactic confusions in their narratives concerning bereavements or childhood traumas.

Longitudinal studies have shown a 68%–75% correspondence between attachment classifications in infancy and classifications in adulthood (e.g., Main 1997). This is an unparalleled level of consistency between behavior observed in infancy and outcomes in adulthood, although it is important to remember that such behavior may be sustained by consistent environments as well as by patterns laid down in the first year of life. Moreover, attachment relationships play a key role in the transgenerational transmission of deprivation. Secure adults are three or four times more likely to have children who are securely attached to them (van IJzendoorn 1995). One might wonder if such powerful intergenerational effects are genetically mediated, but evidence from behavior genetic studies offers no support for genetic transmission (e.g., Fearon et al. 2006). Parental attachment patterns predict unique

TABLE 2–2. Characteristics of Adult Attachment Interview (AAI) attachment categories

Attachment category	Characteristics
Secure/Autonomous	Coherently integrate memories into a meaningful narrative
	Demonstrably value attachment relationships
Insecure/Dismissing	Narrative lacks coherence
	Unable to recall specific memories in support of general argument
	Idealize or devalue early relationships
Insecure/Preoccupied	Narrative lacks coherence
	Show confusion, anger, or fear in relation to attachment figures
	Sometimes still complain of childhood slights
Unresolved/Disorganized	Semantic and/or syntactic confusions in narratives concerning bereavements or childhood traumas
	Individuals classified U/D are also assigned to one of the three primary classifications

variance, distinct from that attributable to temperament measures or contextual factors such as life events, social support, and psychopathology (Steele et al. 1996). However, the mechanisms that ensure that securely attached mothers and fathers develop secure attachment relationships with their child have been difficult to pin down (van IJzendoorn 1995).

Insecure, particularly disorganized, infant attachment is a risk factor for suboptimal emotional and social development (Lyons-Ruth and Jacobvitz 2008). But accumulating evidence suggests that the developmental pathway from disorganized infant attachment to later psychological disorder is complex and sometimes circuitous. In building a model of personality disorder using attachment constructs, we cannot hope for a developmentally reductionist model moving directly from infancy to adulthood. Rather, we must anticipate a complex series of steps, each involving factors of risk and resilience interacting with past and future developmental phases. However, infant attachment may be a vulnerability factor that can illuminate the entire developmental process that leads an individual from genetic vulnerability through childhood experience to adult disturbance. Considering the role of attachment in the emergence of personality disorders may highlight mechanisms that define pathways and subgroups within a hetero-geneous population. Although it may be too simplistic to say that per-sonality disorders originate in parent-infant attachment, it is likely that a consideration of attachment at various developmental points will be relevant to understanding their emergence, given that dysfunctional so-cial relationships are central to the definition of personality disorder, at least within the framework of developmental psychopathology (Gun-derson 2007, 2008).

The Neurobiology of Attachment and Its Link to Mentalization

In our view the major evolutionary advantage of attachment in humans is the opportunity that it gives the infant to develop social intelligence. Alan Sroufe (1996) and Myron Hofer (2004) played a seminal role in extending the scope of attachment theory from an account of the devel-opmental emergence of a set of social expectations to a far broader con-ception of attachment as an organizer of physiological and brain regulation. Attachment ensures that the brain processes that serve social cognition are appropriately organized and prepared to enable us to live and work with other people. The brain's development is "experience-expectant" (Siegel 1999), and hence processes as fundamental as gene expression or changes in receptor densities can be influenced by the in-fant's environment (e.g., Meaney and Szyf 2005).

A consideration of drug addiction can provide us with important clues in understanding the neurobiology of attachment. The mesen-cephalic dopaminergic reward system has been implicated in the pro-cess of drug addiction. Substances that lead to dopamine release in this system are also addictive (e.g., psychostimulants). As it is unlikely that a brain system would exist specifically to serve drug and alcohol abuse, addiction is probably parasitic on a biological system that plays some other critical evolutionary role. Jaak Panksepp (1998) was the first to de-lineate a common neurobiology of mother-infant, infant-mother, and ro-mantic attachment relationships linked to the same mesocorticolimbic dopaminergic reward circuit. MacLean (1990) speculated that substance abuse and drug addiction could be understood as attempts to replace opiates or endogenous factors normally provided by social attach-ments. Thomas Insel (2003) has reviewed evidence that suggests addic-tive disorder and social attachment share a common neurobiology.

The dopaminergic reward processing system and the oxytocinergic system have been shown to play key roles in promoting and maintaining maternal behavior (see Fonagy and Luyten 2009, for a detailed review of the evidence). Oxytocin, a neuromodulatory hormone produced in the hypothalamus, has well-described central actions associated with the onset of maternal behavior, as well as peripheral actions in stimulating uterine contraction during labor and milk ejection during lactation. It is released in response to stimuli such as infant suckling, touch, or even the sight or sound of a nursing mother's infant. Oxytocin and vasopressin are released by sociosexual experience. Oxytocin receptors are located in the ventral striatum, a key dopaminergic brain region, and some evidence suggests that oxytocin release may facilitate dopamine release. In this way, social and maternally related cues may be linked with dopamine-associated reinforcement pathways.

Mesocorticolimbic dopamine is an important candidate in the mediation of reward, the capacity for deferred gratification, and addiction, but it is also critical for maternal behavior in rats and for pair bonding in voles. A circuit linking a vasopressin-sensitive mechanism within the anterior hypothalamus (the medial preoptic area) to the ventral tegmental area and the nucleus accumbens shell may be especially important for mediating the rewarding properties of social interaction. There is good evidence that the mesocorticolimbic pathways mediate pair bonding in rodents (Insel and Young 2000). Prairie and pine voles form partner preferences and pair bonds after mating, but montane and meadow voles do not form selective attachments. This seems to be because in prairie but not montane voles, mating is associated with dopamine release in the nucleus accumbens. Dopamine receptor antagonists infused into the nucleus accumbens prevent partner preferences from being formed (Wang et al. 1999). Vole research also suggests the hypothesis that mating releases oxytocin and vasopressin, amplifying the dopamine signal in the nucleus accumbens (Insel 2003).

These suggestions from animal models have been amply confirmed by functional magnetic resonance imaging (fMRI) studies that demonstrate an association between functional brain activity related to attachment and cortical and subcortical sites in the human brain that contain a high density of the neurohormones oxytocin and vasopressin (Swain et al. 2007). Imaging shows that the mesocorticolimbic dopaminergic pathway is activated during processing of attachment-related stimuli (e.g., Nitschke et al. 2004). The most compelling study using this paradigm comes from Bartels and Zeki (2004), who, using the contrast of own versus other child and controlling for age and familiarity, were able to demonstrate activity in almost all of the brain regions critical for the attachment-mediating neuropeptides in the human brain. Because these workers had already reported an fMRI study of romantic love using a similar contrast design (Bartels and Zeki 2000), they were able to confirm that most of the regions activated by maternal love were the same as those that were associated with romantic love.[2]

To what extent can these biological systems explain differences in the quality of human attachment between mothers and infants? Some studies have shown differential brain responses in individuals whose attachment histories and attachment styles differ (e.g., Buchheim et al. 2008; Gillath et al. 2005). There is evidence, for example, that those with insecure/dismissing attachment show reduced ventral striatum activation in responses to smiling adult faces and positive task feedback (Vrticka et al. 2008). Strathearn et al. (2009) aimed to measure differences in maternal brain reward activation and peripheral oxytocin release in response to infant cues, based on the mother's adult attachment classification, and found that first-time mothers with secure patterns of adult attachment, compared with those with an insecure/dismissing pattern, showed increased activation of mesocorticolimbic reward brain regions on viewing their own infant's smiling face. This was true on viewing both happy and sad infant face cues. These findings suggest that for secure mothers, their infants' cues have a more reliable and powerful effect in motivating and reinforcing their caregiving responses.

Secure mothers in the Strathearn et al. (2009) study also showed an increased peripheral oxytocin response while playing with their infants, and this was positively correlated with activation of oxytocinergic and dopamine-associated reward processing regions of the brain (hypothalamus/pituitary and ventral striatum) in the fMRI testing session. As the interactive play session occurred several months earlier than the fMRI testing session, it could be strongly argued that the level of oxytocin released when the mother is close to the infant is a trait (rather than state) effect. In other words, mothers who enter this new relationship with secure (rather than dismissing) attachment histories are more likely to respond consistently to contact with their child with greater oxytocin release. Because oxytocin is a neuropeptide that enhances social sensitivity (e.g., Domes et al. 2007, further discussed below), these mothers are likely to be relatively more responsive to their infants' social cues as a consequence of the oxytocin "surge" and to elicit a positive response from their infant, which may in its turn be felt as rewarding. This means that they are more likely to gain pleasure from their interactions from

---

[2]These regions were in the striatum (the putamen, globus pallidus, caudate nucleus), the middle insula, and the dorsal part of the cingulate cortex.

their babies, potentially yielding a virtuous cycle of increasingly mutually rewarding interactive experiences.

Finally, striking differences in brain activation were seen between secure and insecure mothers in the Strathearn et al. (2009) study in response to the mother's own infant's sad facial affect. This may be important in helping us to understand the intergenerational transmission of attachment security. Securely attached mothers continued to show greater activation in reward processing regions, whereas insecure/dismissing mothers showed increased activation of the anterior insula, a region associated with feelings of unfairness, pain, and disgust (for review, see Montague and Lohrenz 2007). Activation of the anterior insula may signal "norm violations" (Montague and Lohrenz 2007); insecure/dismissing mothers may cognitively appraise their infant's sadness as a violation of an "expected" neutral or positive affect state. This may lead to avoidance or rejection of negative infant cues (Sanfey et al. 2003) rather than the "approach" responses seen in secure mothers. These results are consistent with a number of previously published models of the cortical organization of the attachment system. For example, a number of authors (Crittenden 2008; Leckman et al. 2004; Strathearn 2006) suggest that individuals with insecure/dismissing attachment are biased toward cognitive information processing and tend to inhibit negative affective responses. Similarly, the findings are consistent with the assumption that insecure mothers experience, rather than reflect on, the sadness they see on the faces of their infant and thereby potentially undermine the process of marked mirroring (described in a later section) that we have suggested is critical in enabling the baby to develop both a robust understanding of emotion and the capacity for affect regulation (Fonagy et al. 2002).

Studies published in 2003 and later have highlighted the role played by oxytocin in facilitating social cognition. In randomized, placebo-controlled trials, intranasal oxytocin produces a broad range of social effects, including enhanced social memory, improved eye gaze when viewing faces, increased recognition and memory of facial expressions and identity, and increased manifestations of trust (e.g., Domes et al. 2007; Guastella et al. 2008). Evidence suggests that sensitivity to intentional states as inferred from facial expression increases under the influence of oxytocin compared with placebo (Domes et al. 2007). As we have seen, attachment encounters cause the spontaneous release of oxytocin, and thus there is a plausible neurobiological substrate to link attachment and social cognition. Oxytocin levels have been observed to be reduced in populations where social cognition is also observed to be limited. These characteristics are arguably associated with social adversity (Heim et al. 2008). Negative early caregiving experiences have an impact on the oxytocin system in monkeys and humans, with lower cerebrospinal fluid (CSF) oxytocin levels reported in nursery-reared than mother-reared monkeys (Winslow et al. 2003). Lower CSF oxytocin has been reported in at least one study of women with a history of emotional abuse and/or neglect (Heim et al. 2008). Furthermore, reduced peripheral oxytocin levels have been seen in orphanage-adopted children with histories of early neglect, who also display severe impairments in social reciprocity (Fries et al. 2005).

Thus we can see that the formation of attachment relationships is supported by at least two neurobiological systems: 1) a system linking attachment experiences to reward and pleasure, motivating the caregiver (and in all likelihood the infant as well) to seek experiences of closeness; and 2) a system linking enhanced social understanding to the attachment context, with closer bonds triggering biological systems that are likely to enhance sensitivity to social cues. Given the availability of a neurobiological pathway, what can the psychological developmental literature tell us about the link between attachment and social cognition? Before considering this issue we shall simplify matters by restricting the range of social cognitions under review to a specific set of capacities.

Understanding the Relationship of Attachment and Mentalization

Our focus hereafter will be mentalization, which we define as a form of mostly preconscious imaginative mental activity, namely perceiving and interpreting human behavior in terms of intentional mental states (e.g., needs, desires, feelings, beliefs, goals, purposes, reasons) (Allen et al. 2008). The capacity to infer and represent the mental states of others may be uniquely human. The primary function of mentalizing is to enable humans to predict and interpret others' actions quickly and efficiently in a large variety of competitive and cooperative situations.

Mentalizing must be imaginative because we have to imagine what other people might be thinking or feeling. An important indicator of high quality of mentalization is the awareness that we cannot know absolutely what is in someone else's mind (Fonagy et al. 1997). Furthermore, we suggest that a similar kind of imaginative leap is required to understand our own mental experience, particularly in relation to emotionally charged issues. In order to conceive of ourselves and others as having a mind, we need a symbolic representational system for mental states, and we must also be able to selectively activate states of mind in line with particular intentions, an ability that requires attentional control. We maintain that the ability to mentalize grows out of interpersonal experience, particularly in primary object relationships (Fonagy 2003). If attachment underpins the emergence of mentalization, we would anticipate that secure children would outperform insecure ones in this domain (measured as passing "theory of mind" tasks at an earlier age). Many studies support this hypothesis (see Fonagy and Luyten 2009 for a review). Generally it seems that secure attachment and mentalization may be subject to similar social influences. We briefly consider some of these influences below.

MENTALIZING AND PARENTING

Two decades of research have confirmed that parenting is the key determinant of attachment security. Can aspects of parenting account for the overlap between mentalization and attachment security? In particular, does parental mentalization of the child have an influence? The mother's capacity to think about her child's mind is variously called maternal mind-mindedness, insightfulness, and reflective function. These overlapping attributes appear to be associated with both secure attachment and mentalization in the child (see Sharp et al. 2006).

Elizabeth Meins (Meins et al. 2001), David Oppenheim (Oppenheim and Koren-Karie 2002), and Arietta Slade (Slade et al. 2005) have all been able to link parental mentalization of the infant with the development of affect regulation and secure attachment in the child, mostly by analyzing interactional narratives between parents and children. Although Meins assessed quality of parents' narratives about their children in real time (i.e., while the parents were playing with their children) and Oppenheim's group did this in a more "offline" manner (parent narrating a videoed interaction), both concluded that maternal mentalizing was a more significant predictor of security of attachment than, say, global sensitivity. Slade and colleagues (2005) also observed a strong relationship between attachment in the infant and the quality of the parent's mentalizing about the child. Mothers with low levels of mentalizing were more likely to show atypical maternal behavior as assessed with the AMBIANCE system (Atypical Maternal Behavior Instrument for Assessment and Classification) (E. Bronfman, E. Parsons, K. Lyons-Ruth: "Atypical Maternal Behavior Instrument for Assessment and Classification [AMBIANCE]: Manual for Coding Disrupted Affective Communication, Version 2." Cambridge, MA, Harvard Medical School, 1999), the results of which relate not only to the infant's attachment disorganization but also to unresolved (disorganized) attachment status as determined by the mother's Adult Attachment Interview (AAI) (Grienenberger et al. 2005).

Taken together, these results suggest that mentalizing parents might well facilitate the development of mentalization in their children. Mindful parenting probably enhances both attachment security and mentalization. However, we should bear in mind that these correlations can be just as readily explained as child-to-parent effects as parent-to-child effects. For example, less power-assertive parenting may be associated with mentalization in the child (Pears and Moses 2003) not because this may facilitate independent thinking, but because less-mentalizing children may be more likely to elicit controlling parenting behavior. It may also be that the same aspects of family functioning that facilitate secure attachment also facilitate the emergence of mentalizing.

The process of acquiring mentalization is so ordinary and normal that it may be more appropriate to consider secure attachment as providing an environment that is free of obstacles to its development rather than an active and direct facilitation. The key to understanding the interaction of attachment with the development of mentalization may then be to look at instances where normally available catalysts to the development of mentalization are absent.

Family Discourse

Exposure to normal family conversations appears to be a precondition of mentalization (Siegal and Peterson 2008). Nicaraguan deaf adults who grew up without hearing references to beliefs appear to be incapable of passing false-belief tests (tests of the ability to recognize that another person's belief is false) (Pyers 2001, cited in Siegal and Peterson 2008). Under normal circumstances, conversations in which adults and children talk about the intentions implied by each others' reasonable comments and link these to each others' appropriately interpreted actions may be the "royal road" to understanding minds. The groundbreaking work of Mary Main (Main and Hesse 2000) has linked attachment to this type of verbal communication. Coherent family discourse characteristic of secure attachment (Hill et al. 2003) helps to generate explanatory schemas by means of which other people's behavior can be understood and predicted.

Playfulness

Playfulness is another feature of a secure attachment context. Play may also be important in acquiring mentalizing. The impact of lack of playfulness is most obvious in extreme cases. Blind children's active pretend play is quite limited (Fraiberg 1977), and they also understand pretend play poorly (Lewis et al. 2000). They are delayed in the ability to pass false-belief tests, passing only when they reach a verbal mental age of 11 years as opposed to the more normal 5 years (McAlpine and Moore 1985). Blind infants of course also miss out on access to nonverbal information about inner states. They are deprived of cues to internal states, such as facial expression, and can experience problems of identity that are perhaps associated with mentalization problems (Hobson and Bishop 2003).

MALTREATMENT

Maltreatment disorganizes the attachment system, as we discussed earlier (see Cicchetti and Valentino 2006 for a comprehensive review). Does it disrupt mentalization? The evidence for significant developmental delay in maltreated children's understanding of emotions is consistent, though slightly reduced when IQ and socioeconomic status are controlled for (e.g., Frodi and Smetana 1984; Smith and Walden 1999). As well as problems of emotional understanding, social cognition deficits and delayed theory-of-mind understanding have been reported in maltreated children (e.g., Cicchetti et al. 2003; Pears and Fisher 2005).

As reports of maltreatment are commonly associated with diagnoses of personality disorder, let us pause for a moment to consider the apparent deficit in mentalization in individuals with maltreatment histories. The mentalization deficit associated with childhood maltreatment may be a form of decoupling or inhibition, or even a phobic reaction to mentalizing. Maltreatment can contribute to an acquired partial "mind blindness" by compromising open reflective communication between parent and child. It might undermine the benefit derived from learning about the links between internal states and actions in attachment relationships (for example, the child may be told that she "deserves," "wants," or even "enjoys" the abuse). This will more obviously be destructive if the maltreatment is perpetrated by a family member. Even where this is not the case, the parents' lack of awareness that maltreatment is taking place outside the home may invalidate the child's communications with the parent about how the child is feeling. The child finds that reflective discourse does not correspond to these feelings, a consistent misunderstanding that could reduce the child's ability to understand/mentalize verbal explanations of other people's actions. In such circumstances the child is likely to struggle to detect mental states behind actions accurately and will tend to see actions as inevitable rather than intended.

It would be absurd to suggest (from either a scientific or a common-sense perspective) that positive attachment experience is the only relationship influence on the development of mentalization. Negative experiences (e.g., emotionally charged conflict) may as readily facilitate the rapid development of mentalizing as positive emotions linked with secure attachment (Newton et al. 2000). The reality is that the emergence of mentalizing likely involves numerous aspects of relational influence, some of which probably correlate with secure attachment. But studies of social influence on mentalizing have hitherto mistakenly tended to assume that this social cognitive capacity is unimodal.

Mentalization is probably better considered as a complex, multicomponent capacity with a variety of determinants, some genetic, others more influenced by environmental interference and facilitation. Each correlate of secure attachment may interface with one or more of a range of neuropsychologically defined components of mentalizing. Thus, relationship influences on the development of mentalization should be thought of as limited and specific rather than broad and unqualified (Hughes and Leekham 2004). We will return to this issue later on.

Development of an Agentive Self: Social Acquisition of Social Cognition

So far we have argued that children's caregiving environments are key to their development as social beings. How do these environmental influences have their effect? Our model relies on the child's innate capacity to detect aspects of his (or her) world that react contingently to his own actions. In his first months of life, the baby begins to understand that he is a *physical agent* whose actions can bring about changes in bodies with which he has immediate physical contact (Leslie 1994). At the same time, he begins to understand that he is a *social agent*, as he learns that his behavior affects his caregiver's behavior and emotions (Neisser 1988). Both of these early forms of self-awareness probably evolve through the workings of an innate contingency detection mechanism that enables the infant to analyze the probability of causal links between his actions and stimulus events (Watson 1994). The child's initial preoccupation with perfectly response-contingent stimulation (provided by the proprioceptive sensory feedback generated by his own actions) allows him to differentiate himself from his environment and to construct a primary representation of his bodily self.

At about 3–4 months, infants' preference appears to change. They begin to be drawn to high-but-imperfect contingencies rather than to perfect contingency (Bahrick and Watson 1985)—the level of contingency that characterizes an attuned caregiver's empathic mirroring responses to a baby's emotional displays. Repeated experience of these responses enables the baby to begin to differentiate his internal self-states, a process we have termed *social biofeedback* (Gergely and Watson 1996). A congenial and secure attachment relationship vitally contributes to the emergence of early mentalizing capacities by allowing the infant to "discover" or "find" his psychological self in the social world (Gergely 2001).

At first, infants are not introspectively aware of different emotion states. Rather, their representations of these emotions are primarily based on stimuli received from the external world. Babies learn to differentiate the internal patterns of physiological and visceral stimulation that accompany different emotions by observing their caregivers' facial or vocal mirroring responses to these (e.g., Legerstee and Varghese 2001; Mitchell 1993). The baby comes to associate his control over the parents' mirroring displays with the resulting improvement in his emotional state, and this lays the foundations for his eventual development of the capacity for emotional self-regulation. The establishment of a second-order representation of affect states creates the basis for affect regulation and impulse control: affects can be manipulated and discharged internally as well as through action, and they can also be experienced as something recognizable and hence shared.

Two conditions need to be met if the capacity to understand and regulate emotions is to develop: 1) reasonable *congruency* of mirroring, whereby the caregiver accurately matches the infant's mental state, and 2) *markedness* of mirroring, whereby the caregiver is able to express an affect while indicating that she is not expressing her own feelings (Gergely and Watson 1999). If the caregiver's mirroring is incongruent, the resulting representation of the infant's internal state will not correspond to a constitutional self state, and this might predispose the infant to develop a narcissistic personality structure (perhaps analogous to Winnicott's notion of a "false self" [Winnicott 1965]). If the mirroring is unmarked, the caregiver's expression may seem to externalize the infant's experience and may overwhelm the infant, making his experience seem contagious and escalating rather than regulating his state. A predisposition to experiencing emotion through other people (as in a borderline personality structure) might be established (Fonagy et al. 2002).

TABLE 2–3.   Stages of development of mentalizing capacity

Stage	Characteristics
The teleological agent (6–12 months)	Understanding of self and others as teleological agents:
	– Grasps causal relations between actions, their agents, and the environment
	– Understands agency purely in terms of physical actions and constraints
The intentional agent (12–24 months)	Understanding of self and others as intentional agents:
	– Grasps that actions are caused by prior states of mind (e.g., desires) and that actions can bring about changes in minds as well as bodies
	– Acquires internal-state language and ability to reason non-egocentrically about feelings and desires in others
	– Is not yet able to represent mental states independently of physical reality
	– Sometimes experiences internal reality as far more compelling than the physical world, and at other times as inconsequential to it (psychic equivalence and pretend modes)
The representational agent (3–4 years)	Understanding of self and others as representational agents:
	– Grasps that people's actions are caused by their beliefs
	– Is increasingly likely to be able to pass false-belief task
	– Knows that people do not always feel what they appear to feel and that emotional reactions are influenced by current mood and earlier emotional experiences
Temporally extended self representation (around 6 years)	Ability to relate memories of intentional activities and experiences into a coherent causal-temporal organization
	Establishment of the temporally extended self

Affect Regulation, Attentional Control, and Mentalization

The child is thought to internalize his experience of well-regulated affect in the infant-parent couple to form the basis of a secure attachment bond and internal working model (Sroufe 1996). According to this account, affect regulation is a prelude to mentalization; yet once mentalization occurs, the nature of affect regulation is transformed. Not only does mentalization allow adjustment of affect states, but more fundamentally it is used to regulate the self. The emergence of mentalizing function (Table 2–3) follows a well-researched developmental line that identifies "fixation points":

1. During the second half of the first year of life, the child begins to be able to grasp the causal relations between actions, their agents, and the environment. At around 9 months, infants begin to look at actions in terms of the actor's underlying intentions (Baldwin et al. 2001) and they begin to understand themselves as teleological agents who can choose the most efficient way to bring about a goal from a range of alternatives (Csibra and Gergely 1998). However, at this stage agency is understood purely in terms of physical actions and constraints. Infants expect actors to behave rationally, given physically apparent goal states and the physical constraints of the situation (Gergely and Csibra 2003). The infant does not yet have any idea about the agent's mental state. We have suggested that there is a connection between this focus on understanding actions in terms of their physical as opposed to mental outcomes (a teleological stance) and the mode of experience of agency that we often see in the self-destructive acts of individuals with borderline personality disorder (BPD). For these individuals slight changes in the physical world can trigger elaborate conclusions about states of mind, and only modifications in the realm of the physical can convince them as to the intentions of the other.

2. During the second year, children begin to understand that they and others are intentional agents whose actions are caused by prior states of mind, such as desires (Wellman and Phillips 2000), and that their actions can bring about changes in minds as well as bodies (e.g., by pointing [Corkum and Moore 1995]). At this stage the capacity for emotion regulation comes to reflect the prior and current relationship with the primary caregiver (Calkins and Johnson 1998). Most importantly, children begin to acquire an internal state language and

the ability to reason non-egocentrically about feelings and desires in others (Repacholi and Gopnik 1997). Paradoxically, this ability becomes evident not only through the increase in joint goal-directed activity but also through teasing and provocation of younger siblings (Dunn 1988). However, the child is not yet able to represent mental states independently of physical reality, and therefore the distinction between internal and external, appearance and reality, is not yet fully achieved (Flavell and Miller 1998). This means that internal reality is sometimes experienced as far more compelling and at other times seems inconsequential relative to the child's awareness of the physical world. We have referred to these modes of experiencing internal reality as the *psychic equivalence* and *pretend* modes, respectively.

3. Around 3 to 4 years of age, the child begins to grasp that people's actions are caused by their beliefs. A meta-analytic review of over 500 tests showed that, by and large, children younger than age 3 years fail the false-belief task and as children's age increases they are increasingly likely to pass (Wellman et al. 2001), suggesting that mentalizing abilities take a quantum leap forward around age 4 years. From this point, the child can understand both himself and others as representational agents. He knows that people do not always feel what they appear to feel and that their emotional reactions to an event are influenced by their current mood, or even by earlier emotional experiences that were linked to similar events (Flavell and Miller 1998). Reaching this milestone of understanding transforms his social interactions. His understanding of emotions comes to be associated with empathic behavior (Zahn-Waxler et al. 1992) and more positive peer relations (Dunn and Cutting 1999). His understanding that human behavior can be influenced by transient mental states (such as thoughts and feelings) as well as by stable characteristics (such as personality or capability) creates the basis for a structure to underpin an emerging self-concept (Flavell 1999). His newfound ability to attribute mistaken beliefs to himself and others enriches his repertoire of social interaction with tricks, jokes, and deception (Sodian and Frith 1992; Sodian et al. 1992). Notably, at this time the child also begins to prefer playing with peers to playing with adults (Dunn 1994). This shift brings to a close the time when mentalization was acquired through the agency of an adult mind and opens a lifelong phase of seeking to enhance the capacity to understand self and others in terms of mental state through bonds with individuals who share one's interest and humor.

4. In the sixth year, we see related advances such as the child's ability to relate memories of his intentional activities and experiences to a coherent causal-temporal organization, leading to the establishment of the temporally extended self (Povinelli and Eddy 1995). Full experience of agency in social interaction can emerge only when actions of the self and other can be understood as initiated and guided by assumptions concerning the emotions, desires, and beliefs of both. Further theory-of-mind skills that become part of the child's repertoire at this stage include second-order theory of mind (capacity to understand mistaken beliefs about beliefs), apprehension of mixed emotions (e.g., understanding being in a conflict), capacity to understand that expectations or biases might influence the interpretation of ambiguous events, and capacity for subtle forms of social deception (e.g., white lies). As these skills are acquired, the need for physical violence begins to decline (Tremblay 2000) and relational aggression increases (Cote et al. 2002).

Subjectivity Before Mentalization

In order to make use of this model of the emergence of mentalizing function in understanding the subjective experience of individuals with BPD, we also need a clear conception of what the nonmentalizing mind might be like before the child fully recognizes that his internal states are mere representations of reality. It is important to grasp that at first the small child assumes that what he knows is known by others and vice versa. Our sense of the uniqueness of our own perspective develops only slowly. While infants already possess a distinct sense of their physical integrity by 3 months or so at the latest, we start with the assumption that knowledge is common and that our own thoughts or feelings are shared by others. Young children assume that other children will know facts that they themselves have just learned (Taylor et al. 1994). One reason why toddlers are so prone to outbursts of rage and frustration may be that as the world and individual minds are not yet clearly demarcated; they expect other people to know what they are thinking and feeling, and to see situations in the same way they do. Thus frustration of their wishes seems malign or willfully obtuse rather than the result of a different point of view or alternative priorities.

In describing the normal development of mentalizing in children ages 2 to 5 years (Fonagy and Target 1996; Target and Fonagy 1996), we have suggested that there is a transition from a split mode of experience to mentalization. We hypothesize that the very young child equates the internal world with the external. What exists in the mind must exist out there, and what exists out there must also exist in the mind. At this stage there is no room yet for alternative perspectives: "How I see it is how it is." The toddler's or young preschool child's insistence that "there is a tiger under the bed" is not allayed by parental reassurance. This "psychic equivalence" as a mode of experiencing the internal world can cause intense distress, because the experience of a fantasy as potentially real can be terrifying. The acquisition of a sense of pretend in relation to mental states is therefore essential. While playing, the child knows that internal experience may not reflect external reality, but then the internal state is thought to have no implications for the outside world ("pretend mode").

Normally, at around 4 years old the child integrates these modes to arrive at mentalization, in which mental states can be experienced as representations. Inner and outer reality can then be seen as linked, yet differing in important ways, and no longer have to be either equated to or dissociated from each other (Gopnik 1993). However, under certain circumstances prementalistic forms of subjectivity may still reemerge to dominate social cognition years after the acquisition of full mentalization.

We will discuss these circumstances in the following sections, where we consider the phenomenology of BPD in the light of the developmental theory outlined above.

Borderline Personality Disorder and Attachment

BPD is characterized by a pervasive pattern of difficulties with emotion regulation and impulse control, and by instability both in relationships and in self-image. It is widely agreed that BPD is a dysfunction of self-regulation, particularly in the context of social relationships (e.g., Koenigsberg et al. 2002; Posner et al. 2002). The characteristic difficulties with emotion regulation and intense reactions to the loss of emotional ties both place BPD in the domain of attachment. A number of theorists have drawn on Bowlby's ideas to account for borderline pathology. Most specifically, Gunderson (1984, 1996) suggested that intolerance of aloneness was at the core of borderline pathology and that the inability of those with BPD to invoke a "soothing introject" was due to early attachment failures. He linked typical patterns of borderline dysfunction to the exaggerated reactions of the insecurely attached infant, such as clinging, fearfulness about dependency needs, terror of abandonment, and constant monitoring of the caregiver's proximity. Lyons-Ruth has suggested that disorganization of the attachment system in infancy predisposes to later borderline pathology (Lyons-Ruth 1991; Lyons-Ruth and Jacobvitz 1999). More recently, Gunderson and Lyons-Ruth have advanced the intriguing notion that interpersonal hypersensitivity might be a core feature of BPD (Gunderson and Lyons-Ruth 2008).

Our model of affect regulation, mentalization, and the development of the self also uses the framework of attachment theory, but we emphasize the role of attachment in the development of symbolic function and the way in which insecure disorganized attachment may leave the individual vulnerable to further turmoil and challenges (Fonagy et al. 2000). We also consider the hyperreactivity of the disorganized attachment systems of individuals with severe personality disorder and the way in which intense activation of the attachment system can disrupt mentalization. In this context the impact of maltreatment has had particular importance in our model. Earlier we outlined how *experienced* maltreatment in the context of an attachment relationship might create a vicious cycle of fearful attachment, wherein fear triggers proximity seeking, and proximity, once achieved, in its turn triggers further anxiety (see, e.g., Bartholomew et al. 2001). In our model of intersubjective self development we have also stressed (following Winnicott) that when children are regularly unable to "find" themselves as intentional beings in the reflective stance of the caregiver, because of either neglect or difficulties in infant temperament, they have no choice but to internalize a representation of their caregiver into their self-representation. This inevitably disorganizes the self structure, creating splits, and gives rise to the well-recognized phenomena associated with disorganization of attachment, such as the manipulativeness in middle childhood characteristic of individuals whose attachment was disorganized in infancy (George and Solomon 1999). Manipulativeness (and oppositional behavior as a consequence of attachment disorganization) occurs because the child prefers to externalize the alien part of the self by nudging the caregiver (gently and sometimes not so gently) to experience the angry or anxious states of mind that the child has internalized but experiences as alien (Fonagy et al. 2002). Creating a situation in which unwanted mental states can be felt to belong to somebody else enables the individual with a disorganized attachment history to experience a measure of self-coherence.

Maltreatment creates a further profound complication within this mechanism, when the child uses split-off parts of the self to gain illusory control over the abuser, a process that has been richly described in the psychoanalytic literature as "identification with the aggressor" (Freud 1936/1966). When the child internalizes the mental state of the victimizer into the alien part of the self, he experiences a part of his own mind as torturing, bent on the destruction of the ego. This leads to an unbearably painful emotional state wherein the self is experienced as evil and hateful. In these circumstances it may feel as if the only solution is to turn the attack from within the mind against the body by self-harming. Alternatively, the individual with a history of maltreatment may resort to constantly externalizing the alien, torturing parts of the self structure into a person close by. Through projective identification (as best described by Rosenfeld [1971]) the persecutory parts of the self are located in someone else. In this way the need for the alien experiences to be owned by another mind may lead to the individual's involvement in a sequence of further abusive relationships.

The need for projective identification is a matter of life and death for those with a traumatizing part of the self structure, but the constellation creates a dependence on the object that has many of the features of addiction. This is not surprising given the overlap of the neural structures responsible for mediating intense attachment and addiction (Insel 2003). The urgent need for a container for unacceptable aspects of the self may be part of the reason why the attachment system in BPD appears to be hypersensitive (i.e., too readily triggered). Indications of attachment hyperactivity are among the core symptoms of BPD. They may include frantic efforts to avoid abandonment, with unstable and intense interpersonal relationships that form at a rapidly escalating tempo, moving quickly from acquaintance to great intimacy (Hill and Stein 2002). We shall see below that the triggering of the attachment system might further disorganize the individual by suppressing mentalization. This in turn reduces the chance of either alternative solutions being accepted or a nonteleological (nonphysical) solution being found (see the section "Consequences of the Failure of Mentalization" later in this chapter).

Psychotherapy invariably entails the development of an attachment relationship (Holmes 1996). Given the strong suggestion of abnormal (disorganized) attachment processes in BPD, we suggest that therapeutic change is mediated via the improved regulation of the neuropsychological systems underpinning the organization of interpersonal relationships (Bateman and Fonagy 2004). This is the paradox of therapeutic engagement in psychotherapy with patients with BPD: by engaging, we risk undermining their equilibrium (i.e., causing harm), but if we do not engage, we deprive them of the only mode of intervention that might help them to address the developmental deficits with which they struggle daily.

Deficits in Attachment-Related Mentalization in Borderline Personality Disorder

In 1989 we suggested that we could understand the features of BPD better if we assumed that the capacity of these patients to comprehend their own and others' states of mind and make use of this knowledge was limited (Fonagy 1989). Initially we hypothesized that their apparent difficulty with understanding mental states in an attachment context was a defensive reaction to physical or sexual abuse that had led them to decouple their mentalizing capacity (Fonagy 1991). Later on we concluded that such drastic defensive reactions were more likely in individuals whose capacity for affect regulation had already been weakened by early neglect or perhaps was constitutionally weak, or both (Fonagy and Target 1997).

It is generally agreed that BPD as a category is probably heterogeneous (Krischer et al. 2006; Mervielde et al. 2005; Trull and Durrett 2005), is quite unstable across time (Gunderson 2008), and probably varies across situations and across a number of dimensions of personality functioning (Hill et al. 2008; Tyrer et al. 2007). In recent years, the concept of mentalization when used as a marker for specific forms of psychopathology has been appropriately criticized for being too broad and multifaceted to be operationalized (Choi-Kain and Gunderson 2008; Holmes 2005; Semerari et al. 2005). We have attempted to specify the concept further, identifying a number of components or dimensions of mentalizing, each of which is underpinned by relatively distinct neural systems (Luyten et al. 2009, submitted). Thus, to speak of a loss of mentalization in personality disorder is probably a summary way of describing a more complex and multifaceted picture. Below we distinguish several different components of mentalization. We anticipate that dysfunctions in these different components of mentalization will characterize some of the patients with this diagnosis but not others, and different patterns of dysfunction may identify subgroups of these patients.

Components of Mentalization

Advances in neuroscience and in social and cognitive developmental research, together with accumulating clinical experience, have enabled us to construct a more differentiated picture of mentalization, based on four polarities (Figure 2–2). These four polarities must be balanced appropriately in a given situation if mentalization is to be "fit for purpose" (the interpersonal and self-organizational function for which it was designed). The four polarities are 1) implicit or automatic versus explicit or controlled mentalization; 2) mentalization based on external or sensorially available cues versus mentalization based on internal or largely inferred cues about the internal state of self and others; 3) predominantly cognitive versus predominantly affective mentalization; and 4) a balance between two distinct neural networks, both of which are more or less shared by processes linked to self-knowing and knowing others: namely,

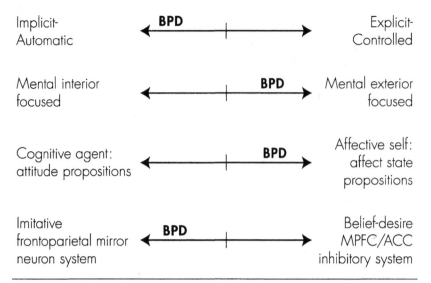

FIGURE 2–2. Mentalizing profile of a prototypical borderline personality disorder patient.

BPD=borderline personality disorder; MPFC/ACC=medial prefrontal cortex/anterior cingulate cortex.

the frontoparietal *mirror neuron system* (Rizzolatti et al. 2006) and the *reflective system* located in the medial prefrontal cortex, the anterior cingulate cortex, and the precuneus (Frith 2007; Frith and Frith 2006).

Explicit mentalization is a conscious, verbal, and reflective process that requires attention, intention, and effort and is relatively slow. *Implicit mentalization* is an automatic process that is nonconscious, nonverbal, and unreflective. It requires little effort or focused attention. An example of implicit mentalization is the automatic parsing of speech, which requires the listener rapidly to compute the speaker's perspective by processing numerous inputs simultaneously in order to understand them. The neural underpinnings of automatic social cognition are phylogenetically older, involving brain circuits that rely heavily on sensory information.[3] By contrast, controlled mentalization involves phylogenetically newer brain circuits involved in processing of linguistic and symbolic material.[4] The distinction between explicit and implicit mentalization can help us to understand personality disorder, in that

---

[3]These include the amygdala, basal ganglia, ventromedial prefrontal cortex, lateral temporal cortex, and dorsal anterior cingulate cortex.

high arousal may facilitate automatic mentalization while inhibiting neural systems associated with controlled mentalization (Mayes 2006, and see later section "The Complex Relationship Between Stress, Attachment, and Mentalization"). Emotional arousal in personality-disordered patients may activate stereotyped, rigid, and automatic assumptions and expectations about relationships, and the ability to reflect on these assumptions may be very limited due to the loss of explicit mentalizing. When not emotionally aroused, these individuals may be able to perform experimental mentalizing tasks as well as control subjects, but they will not be able to understand or respond to mental state explanations under high arousal. This complicates the therapist's attempts to address confusion about mental states, as there will be times of emotional turbulence when patients are unable to bring their explicit mentalizing capacity to bear in order to modify their deeply ingrained implicit preconceptions and expectations of self and others.

Mentalizing can occur on the basis of external cues concerning mental states accessible to the sensory system. Alternatively, it may be based on internal or largely inferred cues. Focusing on mental *interiors* of self and others engages the medial frontoparietal network, whereas focusing on *exteriors* while mentalizing, using physical actions and visible features, recruits a lateral frontotemporal network. Thus, embarrassed self-consciousness, which mostly entails social cognition based on internal self-monitoring, is not apparent in patients with extensive damage to the medial frontoparietal network. However, when *shown* their behavior on a videotape they do become aware that they have behaved inappropriately (Beer et al. 2006) because watching the video recruits externally focused self-reflection, which is underpinned by a different brain system. The separateness of these two systems implies that mind blindness can readily coexist with interpersonal hypersensitivity. Patients with BPD may find it extremely difficult to make inferences about mental interiors, and yet they are often hypersensitive to facial expressions. By contrast, antisocial personality disorder may be characterized by the opposite pattern of mentalization failure. Evidence suggests that those with this diagnosis, particularly more psychopathic individuals, are well able to cope with the task of making inferences about others' mental interiors but fail to respond normally to external visible signals of internal states (Blair 2008).

---

[4] These include the lateral prefrontal cortex, medial prefrontal cortex, lateral parietal cortex, medial parietal cortex, medial temporal lobe, and rostral anterior cingulate cortex.

In distinguishing between *cognitive* and *affective mentalization* we draw on the ideas and findings of Simon Baron-Cohen (e.g., Baron-Cohen et al. 2008). Baron-Cohen distinguishes two relatively high level mentalizing systems, the theory-of-mind mechanism (TOMM) responsible for belief-desire reasoning and the empathizing system (TESS) that works to understand affect within the self. While the TOMM's representations of mental states take the form of *agent-attitude* propositions like "mother believes that John took the cookies," TESS creates *self-affective* state propositions such as "I am sorry you are in pain." In agent-attitude propositions, the statement about the belief may be true even if the belief is inaccurate. Mother may believe that John took the cookies, even if he did not. The importance of the capacity to distinguish internal states from reality is recognized by many psychoanalytic writers in their conceptualizations of the central developmental importance of acquiring a third-person perspective (e.g., Britton 2004; Ogden 1994). According to Baron-Cohen, propositions related to affect never achieve this separateness from a first-person perspective. Emotion is always understood with reference to the self. While it is not grammatically incorrect to say "I am pleased that you are in pain," it is nevertheless socially unacceptable and in most circumstances would indicate significant psychological disturbance. Experiencing and understanding emotion in others always involves the self system and has to achieve consistency with one's own emotional state. It is for this reason that emotions are sensed more than inferred.

In all likelihood TOMM and TESS propositions are processed by different parts of the brain: whereas the TOMM is located in the prefrontal cortex, TESS is part of embodied lateralized systems associated with the inferior prefrontal gyrus. In normal circumstances, mentalizing is likely to involve both systems, as well as other structures. If this is the case, then we might also expect that dysfunction in one system might lead to overcompensation in the other. We hypothesize that in BPD an overly influential empathizing system overcompensates for a dysfunctional theory-of-mind system. This might explain the susceptibility of BPD patients to emotional contagion, their acute sensitivity to certain emotional cues, their predisposition to being overwhelmed by affect, and their inability to integrate affective knowledge with more reflective and cognitive knowledge about both others and themselves (Blatt 2008). The inability to generate agent-attitude propositions might constrain belief-desire reasoning along similar lines to those that appear to operate in emotion understanding. This may help us to understand why mentalization in BPD patients is so strongly dominated by the first-person perspective and lacks the genuine acceptance of a third-person, alternative perspective.

The BPD patient feels strongly that for a belief about another person's state of mind to be true, the patient himself has to feel it to be true.

Two distinct neural networks in the brain appear to be involved in both self-knowing and knowing others. Within each of these networks, it appears that overlapping brain systems are responsible for both envisioning the mind of another and identifying one's own thoughts and feelings, but the two networks achieve these related tasks in rather different ways (Dimaggio et al. 2008; Lombardo et al. 2007).

The first system is the much-publicized frontoparietal mirror neuron "imitative" system (Gallese et al. 2004; Rizzolatti and Craighero 2004), by means of which an understanding of others' experience is generated. When we observe others' actions, the corresponding parts of our own motor cortex are activated, and when we perceive their emotions, this activates our own visceromotor centers. The understanding of others' experience generated by the mirror neuron system has an immediate and intuitive quality, and the representations of others' experience generated in this way are likely to be quite closely fused with our self representations. The mirror neuron system generates involuntary imitative responses that for the most part have to be inhibited in order to avoid the so-called chameleon effect (laughing when other people laugh, yawning when others yawn; see Chartrand and Bargh 1999).

The second system is composed of the medial prefrontal cortex, anterior cingulate, temporoparietal junction, and precuneus. It is activated when we make judgments both about ourselves and about other people's thoughts and feelings. This system is traditionally considered as the key system underpinning the classical belief-desire reasoning aspects of mentalization (Frith and Frith 2006). Emerging evidence suggests that one function of this system may be to inhibit imitative responses, interacting with the mirror neuron system to create an experience of "not-me and therefore me" (Brass and Haggard 2008; Brass et al. 2005, 2007). When we perceive an intention in another, we are "wired" to perform the same behavior in order to achieve an understanding of the other person's intent. But in most instances such automatic imitation must be avoided, and therefore inhibition of imitation plays a key role in generating an experience of selfhood. The inhibition of imitative behavior appears to involve cortical areas that are also related to mentalizing, self-referential processing, and determination of self-agency.[5] Alongside BPD patients' limitations in belief-desire reasoning and perspective taking, we assume that limitations of this inhibitory capacity may explain failures of self/other distinction (identity diffusion), the frequent absence of a sense of "me-ness," the exceptional sensitivity to the "chameleon effect," and the perhaps excessive need to assert the sense of identity by forcing their own state of mind into their interactive partner (what clinicians often note as excessive "projective identification"). When they are unable to mentalize, BPD patients may feel vulnerable to losing their sense of self in interpersonal interchange because they are unable to inhibit the alternative state of mind that social contagion imposes on them. The apparent determination to manipulate and control the minds of others characteristic of BPD patients may be better understood as a defensive reaction, defending the integrity of the self within attachment contexts.

Consequences of the Failure of Mentalization

As we have seen, absence of marked mirroring, lack of a playful, mentalizing environment, and, in the extreme case, maltreatment, might all play a role in weakening mentalizing capacity and making the individual more vulnerable to react to interpersonal stress by losing or strategically reducing the capacity for explicit, internally focused, cognitive mentalizing. We may think of this as an *adaptive* decoupling, because thinking about the state of mind of the perpetrator of maltreatment may well be overwhelming for the helpless child. But there may be more to this than an adaptation. Early trauma may also alter the neural mechanisms of arousal, so that relatively mild emotional stimuli may trigger the arousal system underpinning posterior cortical activation, while taking the frontal mentalizing parts of the brain "offline" (Arnsten 1998; Mayes 2000).

Whatever the immediate cause of this decoupling, its consequence is the reemergence of the psychic equivalence, pretend, and teleological modes of thinking about internal states that antedate fully fledged adult mentalizing capacity. All three are relatively readily observable in typical patterns of thinking of individuals with BPD.

When a patient with BPD is functioning in the *psychic equivalence mode,* the experience of mind can be terrifyingly real (e.g., flashbacks) and can produce intolerance of alternative perspectives ("If I think you had your door shut because [I think] you want to reject me, you just want to reject me").

---

[5]Cortical areas that are also related to mentalizing, self-referential processing, self-agency, and perspective taking (e.g., Aichhorn et al. 2006; Decety and Grèzes 2006; Frith and Frith 2006; Northoff et al. 2006; Ruby and Decety 2003) have been shown to be strongly activated in an imitation-inhibition task (Brass et al. 2007).

Experiences of emptiness, meaninglessness, and dissociation in the wake of trauma show the lack of connection between second-order representations of internal states and their actual experience in relation to something real that is characteristic of the *pretend mode*. In therapy with individuals with BPD, there is always the risk of patient and therapist engaging in endless, inconsequential talk of thoughts and feelings, which is futile because their words lack any true referent: contradictory beliefs can be simultaneously held, and affects do not appropriately accompany thoughts.

The third mechanism brought to the foreground by the decoupling of mentalization is the *teleological stance*. In BPD we also commonly note a focus on understanding actions in terms of their physical as opposed to mental outcomes; patients are not able to accept anything other than a modification in the realm of the physical as a true index of the intentions of the other. The therapist's benign disposition has to be demonstrated by increasingly heroic acts, such as availability on the telephone, extra sessions during weekends, or physical holding, occasionally leading to serious violations of therapeutic boundaries.

Within our theoretical frame of reference, the dysfunctional attachment relationships characteristic of individuals with BPD are not only the consequence of difficulties with holding a stable and consistent representation of others' and one's own mind in mind (Liotti 2002). They are also linked to the disorganization of the self. As we suggested above, when the caregiver's mirroring is not congruent, the infant organizes internal experience by internalizing the caregiver rather than the caregiver's mirroring of the child. Such second-order representations of internal states are by definition "alien." They do not match the constitutional state of the self, and consequently the self-organization evolves in a somewhat flawed manner. In normal development, the capacity to mentalize enables us to create a narrative that "papers over" the discontinuities in self structure that we all have to a greater or lesser degree. If mentalization breaks down, it becomes difficult to generate a coherent narrative (Dimaggio and Semerari 2004), and therefore the alien part of the self can assume greater prominence. Enhancing mentalization and reducing the predominance of nonmentalizing modes of experiencing internal reality represent the path to cure.

The Complex Relationship Between Stress, Attachment, and Mentalization

There seems to be a close link between emotional arousal and activation of the attachment system, and this activation in its turn has an impact on mentalizing capacity. In earlier formulations (e.g., Fonagy and Bateman 2006a) we proposed that at extreme levels, activation of the attachment system deactivates the mentalizing system. Following the model outlined by Mayes (2000, 2006), we suggested that when emotional arousal increases beyond a certain point, there is a switch from cortical to subcortical systems, from controlled to automatic mentalizing and subsequently to nonmentalizing modes (Figure 2–3). We suggested that a tendency to hyperactivation of the attachment system, possibly linked with traumatic experiences, may be one of the pathways to impairments of mentalization in patients with BPD.

Accumulating data suggest that a further elaboration of this already complex relationship may be necessary. It seems that even in nonclinical groups, differences in individuals' responses to the activation of the attachment system may influence the relationship between mentalization, attachment, and stress (Luyten et al., 2009, submitted; P. Luyten, L. Mayes, P. Fonagy, and B. Van Houdenhove, "The Interpersonal Regulation of Stress," University of Leuven, 2009, unpublished).

In the context of *secure* attachment, activation of the attachment system predictably involves a relaxation of normal strategies of interpersonal caution. There is good evidence that intense activation of the attachment system is associated with deactivation of arousal and affect

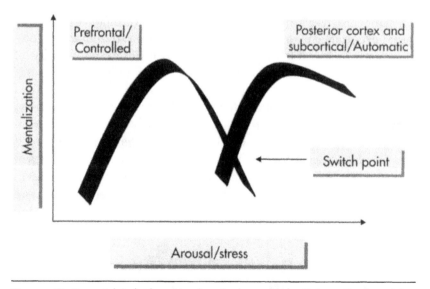

FIGURE 2–3. A biobehavioral switch model of the relationship between stress and controlled versus automatic mentalization.

regulation systems (Luyten et al., 2009, unpublished) as well as deactivation of neurocognitive systems likely to generate interpersonal suspicion—that is, those involved in social cognition or mentalization.

Dismissing individuals tend to deny attachment needs. They assert autonomy, independence, and strength in the face of stress, using attachment deactivation strategies. In contrast, a *preoccupied* attachment classification or an *anxious* attachment style is generally thought to be linked with the use of attachment hyperactivating strategies. Attachment hyperactivating strategies have been consistently associated with the tendency to exaggerate the presence and the seriousness of threats, and with frantic efforts to find support and relief, often expressed in demanding, clinging behavior. AAI and self-report studies have found a predominance of anxious-preoccupied attachment strategies in BPD patients (e.g., Agrawal et al. 2004). The commonly observed trauma history of individuals with BPD supports the hypothesis that attachment history affects the setting of the "switch" that turns the mentalizing system from planned, controlled, and organized cognition to automatic processing with narrowed, poorly sustained attention and increased vigilance for attachment disruptions such as rejection and abandonment.

An individual's switch, in a particular context, from more controlled reflective to automatic mentalization is likely to be determined by a combination of characteristics (Table 2–4 and Figure 2–4; see Luyten et al., 2009, submitted, for a detailed discussion). The anxious-preoccupied attachment strategies that are characteristic of many BPD patients are associated with a lowered threshold for attachment system activation and, simultaneously, a lower threshold for controlled mentalization deactivation. Thus, in BPD patients, more automatic, subcortical systems, including the amygdala, have a low threshold for responding to stress. This hypothesis in and of itself could offer a comprehensive explanation for one of the central dynamic features of BPD patients: their tendency to form attachments easily and quickly, often resulting in disappointments. This pattern would be due to their low threshold for activation of the attachment system and their low threshold for deactivation of neural systems associated with controlled social cognition, including neural systems involved in judging the trustworthiness of others. The vicious interpersonal cycles that are so characteristic of many BPD patients thus can be understood in terms of excitatory feedback loops leading to increased vigilance for stress-related cues in anxious attachment, particularly attachment characterized by high anxiety and high avoidance (Mikulincer and Shaver 2007).

In contrast, individuals who use attachment deactivation strategies are able to keep "online" for longer periods the neural systems involved

TABLE 2–4.   Attachment strategies, arousal, and controlled versus automatic mentalization

Attachment category	Threshold for switch	Strength of automatic response	Recovery of controlled mentalization
Secure	High	Moderate	Fast
Hyperactivating	Low: hyperresponsive to stress	Strong	Slow
Deactivating	Relatively high: hyporesponsive to stress, but with failure under increasing stress	Weak, but moderate to strong under increasing stress	Relatively fast
Disorganized	Incoherent: hyperresponsive to stress, but often with frantic attempts to downregulate	Strong	Slow

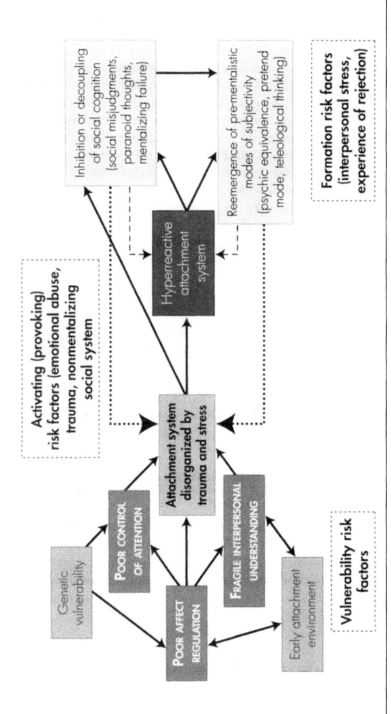

FIGURE 2–4. The hyperactivation of attachment in borderline personality disorder.

in controlled mentalization, including those involved in judging the trustworthiness of other individuals. However, this group can be clearly distinguished from securely attached individuals. Secure individuals are able to keep the controlled mentalizing system "online" even when the attachment system is activated. Although mild stress is not likely to trigger the attachment system for dismissive individuals, when the stress becomes severe their deactivating strategy is likely to fail, leading to a strong reactivation of feelings of insecurity, heightened reactivation of negative self-representations, and increased levels of stress (Mikulincer et al. 2002). If securely attached individuals are those who are able to maintain a relatively high activation of prefrontal areas even when the dopaminergic mesolimbic pathways (attachment and reward system) are activated, then differences in mentalization between securely attached and avoidantly/dismissively attached individuals may only show themselves under increasing stress, and this seems concordant with experimental studies (Mikulincer and Shaver 2007).

These findings imply that treatment should aim to find the optimal balance between attachment activation and mentalization (Fonagy and Bateman 2006a). Moreover, treatments that focus on gaining insight into one's past—and particularly into one's traumatic past, which typically involves high levels of stress—might be contraindicated in patients with serious impairments in mentalization. As trauma is typically associated with attachment insecurity, particularly with anxious and disorganized attachment, insight-oriented treatments might be especially harmful for the subgroup of BPD patients who have experienced trauma (Fonagy and Bateman 2006b).

Relationship-Specific Mentalization: Mentalization in Context

The arguments advanced above imply that deficits in mentalization are not a simple marker of BPD. The association between mentalization, stress, and attachment reviewed in the previous section suggests that we should expect differences in the quality of mentalization depending on the quality of the relationship within which it is observed (Allen et al. 2008; Luyten et al., 2009, submitted).

Thus, some revision of previously held assumptions is called for. Attachment theory and research are largely based on the assumption that cognitive-affective models of relationships (internal working models) are relatively stable over time and are activated in a wide array of interpersonal relationships, including relationships with parents, partners, and friends. Similarly, mentalization has often been assumed to be invariant across different relationships. However, research has called into question the assumption that working models are traitlike.[6] Given the link between the attachment system and mentalization, it is doubtful that individual differences in mentalization are best thought of as essentially traitlike. Mentalization is likely to show considerable fluctuations over time and across relationship contexts, not only as a function of stress but also as a function of the quality of particular relationships. Several sets of empirical observations are relevant to this assumption. First, general and relationship-specific mentalization, although overlapping, appear to be distinct (Humfress et al. 2002; O'Connor and Hirsch 1999). Second, several independent research traditions have suggested that mentalization with regard to one's own infant is a relationship-specific form of mentalization and likely to be specific to this particular child (for a review, see Sharp et al. 2006). Third, and most pertinent in the present context, is the line of evidence suggesting that quality of mentalization of therapists may be specific to particular patients and, even within that limit, may be variable across sessions of psychotherapy (e.g., Diamond and Yeomans 2008; Vermote et al. 2009).

We suggest that any anomalies in mentalizing capacity are unlikely to be manifest in patients with BPD unless the relationship in which mentalization is being observed "pulls" for the activation of these areas. The stronger the attachment in a particular relationship at a particular moment, the more likely it is that anomalies in mentalization will emerge in these patients. Certainly, clinical evidence strongly implies that as the attachment bond between therapist and client intensifies, the quality of BPD patients' mentalization will tend to deteriorate. Thus, initial assessment of clients can leave therapists with the impression that they are working with an individual with relatively high psychological mindedness who is highly suitable for insight-oriented psychotherapy. Typically, as treatment progresses and transference intensifies—activating the patient's internal working models of particular child-parent relationships and the attachment system in general—the quality of psychological mindedness is likely to deteriorate signifi-

---

[6]The substantial within-person variation in internal working models of others (e.g., of father versus mother) (see, e.g., Fraley 2007; Pierce and Lydon 2001) supports a view of internal working models as hierarchically organized networks that contain both global and relationship-specific representations (Fonagy 2001; Overall et al. 2003) or as distributed processes within a connectionistic network (Fraley 2007).

cantly, and the patient's capacity to perceive the therapist's mind as different from his or her own mental state will at times be quite limited.

Treatment Implications

The therapeutic implications of our mentalization-based approach to BPD are extensive and are discussed in greater depth in Chapter 6, "Mentalization-Based Treatment and Borderline Personality Disorder" (see also Allen et al. 2008; Bateman and Fonagy 2004, 2006). Our formulation implies the need to abandon the overvaluation of specific techniques in favor of a generic therapeutic stance that cuts across theoretical modalities. The overarching expectation emerging from this model is that given the generic nature of mentalization as a mental function, most treatments of BPD will be effective to the extent that they include important components facilitating mentalization, even though this capacity may be addressed by using different terms, such as "mindfulness," "validation," or "self states," in the various models of therapy.

From the perspective developed in this chapter, the overall aim of treatment should be to stimulate a patient's attachment and involvement with treatment while helping the patient maintain mentalization. Treatment should avoid situations where patients are expected to talk of mental states that they cannot link to subjectively felt reality. Thus, with regard to dynamic therapies, this implies that there should be 1) a deemphasis on "deep" unconscious interpretations in favor of conscious or near conscious content; 2) a modification of therapeutic aim, especially with severely disturbed patients, from insight to recovery of mentalization (i.e., achieving representational coherence and integration); 3) careful eschewing of descriptions of complex mental states (conflict, ambivalence, unconscious) that are incomprehensible to a person whose mentalizing is vulnerable; and 4) avoidance of extensive discussion of past trauma, except in the context of reflecting on current perceptions of mental states of maltreating figures and changes in mental state from being a victim in the past versus one's experiences now.

The key task of therapy is to promote curiosity about how mental states motivate and explain the actions of self and others. Therapists can achieve this through judicious use of an inquisitive stance, highlighting their own interest in the mental states underpinning behavior, qualifying their own understanding and inferences (showing respect for the opaqueness in mental states), and showing patients how such information can help them to make sense of their experiences. It is not for the therapist to "tell" patients about how they feel, what they think, how they should behave, or what the underlying conscious or unconscious reasons may be for their difficulties. Any therapy approach that moves toward claiming to "know" how patients "are," how they should behave and think, and "why they are the way they are" is likely to be harmful to patients with a vulnerable capacity to mentalize.

The therapist's mentalizing therapeutic stance should include 1) humility derived from a sense of "not knowing"; 2) taking time, whenever possible, to identify differences in perspectives; 3) legitimizing and accepting different perspectives; 4) actively questioning the patient in relation to his or her experience—asking for detailed descriptions of experience ("what" questions) rather than explanations ("why" questions); and 5) eschewing the need to understand what makes no sense (i.e., refraining from saying explicitly that something is unclear). An important component of this stance is monitoring one's own mistakes as a therapist. Acknowledgment of mistakes models honesty and courage and tends to lower arousal because the therapist is taking responsibility. These moments also offer invaluable opportunities to explore how mistakes can arise out of mistaken assumptions about opaque mental states and how misunderstandings can lead to upsetting experiences. In this context, it is important to be aware that the therapist is constantly at risk of losing the capacity to mentalize in the face of a nonmentalizing patient. Consequently, we consider therapists' occasional enactments as an acceptable concomitant of the therapeutic alliance, something that simply has to be owned up to. As with other instances of breaks in mentalizing, such incidents require that the process be "rewound" and the incident explored. Hence, in this collaborative patient-therapist relationship the two partners involved have a joint responsibility to understand enactments.

Key Clinical Concepts

◆ Mentalizing is a form of imaginative mental activity, namely, perceiving and interpreting human behavior in terms of intentional mental states (e.g., needs, desires, feelings, beliefs, goals, purposes, reasons).

◆ Mentalizing is best understood as a multidimensional construct whose core processing dimensions are underpinned by distinct neural systems:

- *Explicit mentalization* is a conscious, verbal, and reflective process that requires attention, intention, and effort and is relatively slow; *implicit mentalization* is an automatic process that is nonconscious, nonverbal, and unreflective.

- Mentalizing can occur on the basis of *external* cues concerning mental states accessible to the sensory system; alternatively, it may be based on *internal* or largely inferred cues.

- *Cognitive mentalizing* takes the form of agent-attitude propositions such as "Mother believes that John took the cookies," whereas in *affective mentalizing,* the empathizing system creates self-affective state propositions such as "I am sorry you are in pain."

- Two distinct neural networks in the brain appear to be involved in both self-knowing and knowing others.

◆ Three developmentally earlier modes of subjectivity antedate mentalization and can characterize its failure:

- In the *teleological stance,* expectations concerning the agency of the other are present, but these are formulated in terms restricted to the physical world. When patients revert to this mode, they become unable to accept anything other than a modification in the realm of the physical as a true index of the intentions of the other.

- In *psychic equivalence,* the very young child equates the internal world with the external; this can cause intense distress, since the experience of a fantasy as potentially real can be terrifying. Both flashbacks and an intolerance for alternative perspectives on what others' intentions might be are characteristic of the reemergence of this mode.

- In the *pretend mode,* the child knows that internal experience may not reflect external reality, but the mental world is decoupled from reality. Indices of the reemergence of this mode in later development are a) feelings of emptiness, meaninglessness, and dissociation in the wake of trauma and b) endless inconsequential talk of thoughts and feelings.

◆ The capacity to mentalize can be undermined by hyperactivation of the attachment system.

- Adverse emotional experience with the caregiver leads to distress and fear, which lead to proximity-seeking in the hope of soothing, but proximity results in further adverse emotional experiences in a vicious cycle.

- The result is that the attachment system becomes hypersensitive (triggered too readily) and the individual is left vulnerable to the failure of mentalizing capacity and reemergence of earlier modes of subjective experience.

Suggested Readings

Bateman AW, Fonagy P: Psychotherapy for Borderline Personality Disorder: Mentalization-Based Treatment. Oxford, UK, Oxford University Press, 2004

Bateman A, Fonagy P: 8-year follow-up of patients treated for borderline personality disorder: mentalization-based treatment versus treatment as usual. Am J Psychiatry 165:631–638, 2008

Fonagy P, Gergely G, Target M: The parent-infant dyad and the construction of the subjective self. J Child Psychol Psychiatry 48:288–328, 2007

Strathearn L, Fonagy P, Amico J, et al: Adult attachment predicts maternal brain and oxytocin response to infant cues. Neuropsychopharmacology 34: 2655–2666, 2009

References

Agrawal HR, Gunderson J, Holmes BM, et al: Attachment studies with borderline patients: a review. Harv Rev Psychiatry 12:94–104, 2004

Aichhorn M, Perner J, Kronbichler M, et al: Do visual perspective tasks need theory of mind? Neuroimage 30:1059–1068, 2006

Ainsworth MD: Attachments across the lifespan. Bull N Y Acad Med 61:792–812, 1985

Ainsworth MD, Blehar MC, Waters E, et al: Patterns of Attachment: A Psychological Study of the Strange Situation. Hillsdale, NJ, Erlbaum, 1978

Allen JG, Fonagy PF, Bateman AW: Mentalizing in Clinical Practice. Washington, DC, American Psychiatric Publishing, 2008

Arnsten AF: The biology of being frazzled. Science 280:1711–1712, 1998

Bahrick LR, Watson JS: Detection of intermodal proprioceptive-visual contingency as a potential basis of self-perception in infancy. Dev Psychol 21:963–973, 1985

Baldwin DA, Baird JA, Saylor MM, et al: Infants parse dynamic action. Child Dev 72:708–717, 2001

Baron-Cohen S, Golan O, Chakrabarti B, et al: Social cognition and autism spectrum conditions, in Social Cognition and Developmental Psychopathology. Edited by Sharp C, Fonagy P, Goodyer I. Oxford, UK, Oxford University Press, 2008, pp 29–56

Bartels A, Zeki S: The neural basis of romantic love. Neuroreport 11:3829–3834, 2000

Bartels A, Zeki S: The neural correlates of maternal and romantic love. Neuroimage 21:1155–1166, 2004

Bartholomew K, Kwong MJ, Hart SD: Attachment, in Handbook of Personality Disorders: Theory, Research, and Treatment. Edited by Livesley WJ. New York, Guilford, 2001, pp 196–230

Bateman A, Fonagy P: Psychotherapy for Borderline Personality Disorder: Mentalization Based Treatment. Oxford, UK, Oxford University Press, 2004

Bateman A, Fonagy P: Mentalization-Based Treatment for Borderline Personality Disorder: A Practical Guide. Oxford, UK, Oxford University Press, 2006

Beer JS, John OP, Scabini D, et al: Orbitofrontal cortex and social behavior: integrating self-monitoring and emotion-cognition interactions. J Cogn Neurosci 18:871–879, 2006

Blair J: Empathic dysfunction in psychopathy, in Social Cognition and Developmental Psychopathology. Edited by Sharp C, Fonagy P, Goodyer I. Oxford, UK, Oxford University Press, 2008, pp 175–198

Blatt SJ: Polarities of Experience: Relatedness and Self-Definition in Personality Development, Psychopathology, and the Therapeutic Process. Washington, DC, American Psychological Association, 2008

Bowlby J: Attachment and Loss, Vol 1: Attachment. London, Hogarth Press and Institute of Psycho-Analysis, 1969

Bowlby J: Attachment and Loss, Vol 2: Separation: Anxiety and Anger. London, Hogarth Press and Institute of Psycho-Analysis, 1973

Brass M, Haggard P: The what, when, whether model of intentional action. Neuroscientist 14:319–325, 2008

Brass M, Derrfuss J, Forstmann B, et al: The role of the inferior frontal junction area in cognitive control. Trends Cogn Sci 9:314–316, 2005

Brass M, Schmitt RM, Spengler S, et al: Investigating action understanding: inferential processes versus action simulation. Curr Biol 17:2117–2121, 2007

Britton R: Subjectivity, objectivity, and triangular space. Psychoanal Q 73:47–61, 2004

Buchheim A, Erk S, George C, et al: Neural correlates of attachment trauma in borderline personality disorder: a functional magnetic resonance imaging study. Psychiatry Res 163:223–235, 2008

Calkins S, Johnson M: Toddler regulation of distress to frustrating events: temperamental and maternal correlates. Infant Behav Dev 21:379–395, 1998

Carlson V, Cicchetti D, Barnett D, et al: Disorganized/disoriented attachment relationships in maltreated infants. Dev Psychol 25:525–531, 1989

Chartrand TL, Bargh JA: The chameleon effect: the perception-behavior link and social interaction. J Pers Soc Psychol 76:893–910, 1999

Chisolm K: A three year follow-up of attachment and indiscriminate friendliness in children adopted from Russian orphanages. Child Dev 69:1092–1106, 1998

Choi-Kain LW, Gunderson JG: Mentalization: ontogeny, assessment, and application in the treatment of borderline personality disorder. Am J Psychiatry 165:1127–1135, 2008

Cicchetti D, Valentino K: An ecological-transactional perspective on child maltreatment: failure of the average expectable environment and its influence on child development, in Developmental Psychopathology, 2nd Edition, Vol 3. Edited by Cicchetti D, Cohen DJ. New York, Wiley, 2006, pp 129–201

Cicchetti D, Rogosch FA, Maughan A, et al: False belief understanding in maltreated children. Dev Psychopathol 15:1067–1091, 2003

Corkum V, Moore C: Development of joint visual attention in infants, in Joint Attention: Its Origins and Role in Development. Edited by Moore C, Dunham P. New York, Erlbaum, 1995, pp 61–83

Cote S, Tremblay RE, Nagin D, et al: The development of impulsivity, fearfulness, and helpfulness during childhood: patterns of consistency and change in the trajectories of boys and girls. J Child Psychol Psychiatry 43:609–618, 2002

Crittenden PM: Internal representational models of attachment relationships. Infant Ment Health J 11:259–277, 1990

Crittenden PM: Raising Parents: Attachment, Parenting and Child Safety. Devon, UK, Willan Publishing, 2008

Csibra G, Gergely G: The teleological origins of mentalistic action explanations: a developmental hypothesis. Dev Sci 1:255–259, 1998

Decety J, Grèzes J: The power of simulation: imagining one's own and other's behavior. Brain Res 1079:4–14, 2006

Diamond D, Yeomans F: The patient-therapist relationship: implications of attachment theory, reflective functioning, and research. Sante Ment Que 33:61–87, 2008

Dimaggio G, Semerari A: Disorganized narratives: the psychological condition and its treatment, in The Handbook of Narrative and Psychotherapy: Practice, Theory, and Research. Edited by Angus L, McLeod J. Thousand Oaks, CA, Sage, 2004, pp 263–282

Dimaggio G, Lysaker PH, Carcione A, et al: Know yourself and you shall know the other...to a certain extent: multiple paths of influence of self-reflection on mindreading. Conscious Cogn 17:778–789, 2008

Domes G, Heinrichs M, Michel A, et al: Oxytocin improves "mind-reading" in humans. Biol Psychiatry 61:731–733, 2007

Dunn J: The Beginnings of Social Understanding. Cambridge, MA, Harvard University Press, 1988

Dunn J: Changing minds and changing relationships, in Children's Early Understanding of Mind: Origins and Development. Edited by Lewis C, Mitchell P. Hove, UK, Lawrence Erlbaum, 1994, pp 297–310

Dunn J, Cutting AL: Understanding others, and individual differences in friendship interactions in young children. Soc Dev 8:202–219, 1999

Fearon P, van IJzendoorn MH, Fonagy P, et al: In search of shared and nonshared environmental factors in security of attachment: a behavior-genetic study of the association between sensitivity and attachment security. Dev Psychol 42:1026–1040, 2006

Flavell JH: Cognitive development: children's knowledge about the mind. Annu Rev Psychol 50:21–45, 1999

Flavell JH, Miller PH: Social cognition, in Handbook of Child Psychology, 5th Edition. Edited by Damon W, Kuhn D, Siegler RS. New York, Wiley, 1998, pp 851–898

Fonagy P: On tolerating mental states: theory of mind in borderline patients. Bulletin of the Anna Freud Centre 12:91–115, 1989

Fonagy P: Thinking about thinking: some clinical and theoretical considerations in the treatment of a borderline patient. Int J Psychoanal 72:1–18, 1991

Fonagy P: The human genome and the representational world: the role of early mother-infant interaction in creating an interpersonal interpretive mechanism. Bull Menninger Clin 65:427–448, 2001

Fonagy P: The development of psychopathology from infancy to adulthood: the mysterious unfolding of disturbance in time. Infant Ment Health J 24:212–239, 2003

Fonagy P, Bateman AW: Mechanisms of change in mentalization-based treatment of BPD. J Clin Psychol 62:411–430, 2006a

Fonagy P, Bateman A: Progress in the treatment of borderline personality disorder. Br J Psychiatry 188:1–3, 2006b

Fonagy P, Luyten P: A developmental, mentalization-based approach to the understanding and treatment of borderline personality disorder. Dev Psychopathol 21:1355–1381, 2009

Fonagy P, Target M: Playing with reality, I: theory of mind and the normal development of psychic reality. Int J Psychoanal 77:217–233, 1996

Fonagy P, Target M: Attachment and reflective function: their role in self-organization. Dev Psychopathol 9:679–700, 1997

Fonagy P, Steele M, Moran GS, et al: Measuring the ghost in the nursery: a summary of the main findings of the Anna Freud Centre/University College London parent-child study. Bulletin of the Anna Freud Centre 14:115–131, 1991a

Fonagy P, Steele H, Steele M: Maternal representations of attachment during pregnancy predict the organization of infant-mother attachment at one year of age. Child Dev 62:891–905, 1991b

Fonagy P, Steele M, Steele H, et al: Reflective-Functioning Manual, Version 4.1, for Application to Adult Attachment Interviews. London, University College London, 1997

Fonagy P, Target M, Gergely G: Attachment and borderline personality disorder: a theory and some evidence. Psychiatr Clin North Am 23:103–122, 2000

Fonagy P, Gergely G, Jurist E, et al: Affect Regulation, Mentalization and the Development of the Self. New York, Other Press, 2002

Fraiberg S: Insights From the Blind. London, Souvenir Press, 1977

Fraley RC: A connectionist approach to the organization and continuity of working models of attachment. J Pers 75:1157–1180, 2007

Freud A: The ego and the mechanisms of defense (1936), Vol 2 in The Writings of Anna Freud, International Universities Press, 1966

Fries AB, Ziegler TE, Kurian JR, et al: Early experience in humans is associated with changes in neuropeptides critical for regulating social behavior. Proc Natl Acad Sci U S A 102:17237–17240, 2005

Frith CD: The social brain? Philos Trans R Soc Lond B Biol Sci 362:671–678, 2007

Frith CD, Frith U: The neural basis of mentalizing. Neuron 50:531–534, 2006

Frodi A, Smetana J: Abused, neglected, and nonmaltreated preschoolers' ability to discriminate emotions in others: the effects of IQ. Child Abuse Negl 8:459–465, 1984

Gallese V, Keysers C, Rizzolatti G: A unifying view of the basis of social cognition. Trends Cogn Sci 8:396–403, 2004

George C, Solomon J: A comparison of attachment theory and psychoanalytic approaches to mothering. Psychoanalytic Inquiry 19:618–646, 1999

Gergely G: The obscure object of desire: "nearly, but clearly not, like me": contingency preference in normal children versus children with autism. Bull Menninger Clin 65:411–426, 2001

Gergely G, Csibra G: Teleological reasoning in infancy: the naive theory of rational action. Trends Cogn Sci 7:287–292, 2003

Gergely G, Watson J: The social biofeedback model of parental affect-mirroring. Int J Psychoanal 77:1181–1212, 1996

Gergely G, Watson J: Early social-emotional development: contingency perception and the social biofeedback model, in Early Social Cognition: Understanding Others in the First Months of Life. Edited by Rochat P. Hillsdale, NJ, Erlbaum, 1999, pp 101–137

Gillath O, Bunge SA, Shaver PR, et al: Attachment-style differences in the ability to suppress negative thoughts: exploring the neural correlates. Neuroimage 28:835–847, 2005

Gopnik A: How we know our minds: the illusion of first-person knowledge of intentionality. Behav Brain Sci 16:1–14, 29–113, 1993

Grienenberger JF, Kelly K, Slade A: Maternal reflective functioning, mother-infant affective communication, and infant attachment: exploring the link between mental states and observed caregiving behavior in the intergenerational transmission of attachment. Attach Hum Dev 7:299–311, 2005

Guastella AJ, Mitchell PB, Mathews F: Oxytocin enhances the encoding of positive social memories in humans. Biol Psychiatry 64:256–258, 2008

Gunderson JG: Borderline Personality Disorder: A Clinical Guide. Washington, DC, American Psychiatric Press, 1984

Gunderson JG: The borderline patient's intolerance of aloneness: insecure attachments and therapist availability. Am J Psychiatry 153:752–758, 1996

Gunderson JG: Disturbed relationships as a phenotype for borderline personality disorder. Am J Psychiatry 164:1637–1640, 2007

Gunderson JG: Borderline personality disorder: an overview. Soc Work Ment Health 6:2008–2012, 2008

Gunderson JG, Lyons-Ruth K: BPD's interpersonal hypersensitivity phenotype: a gene-environment-developmental model. J Pers Disord 22:22–41, 2008

Heim C, Young LJ, Newport DJ, et al: Lower CSF oxytocin concentrations in women with a history of childhood abuse. Mol Psychiatry 14:954–958, 2008

Hill J, Stein H: Revised Adult Personality Functioning Assessment (RAPFA) (Technical Report No 02-0052). Topeka, KS, The Menninger Clinic, Research Department, 2002

Hill J, Fonagy P, Safier E, et al: The ecology of attachment in the family. Fam Process 42:205–221, 2003

Hill J, Pilkonis P, Morse J, et al: Social domain dysfunction and disorganization in borderline personality disorder. Psychol Med 38:135–146, 2008

Hobson RP, Bishop M: The pathogenesis of autism: insights from congenital blindness. Philos Trans R Soc Lond B Biol Sci 358:335–344, 2003

Hofer MA: Hidden regulators: implications for a new understanding of attachment, separation and loss, in Attachment Theory: Social, Developmental, and Clinical Perspectives. Edited by Goldberg S, Muir R, Kerr J. Hillsdale, NJ, Analytic Press, 1995, pp 203–230

Hofer MA: The emerging neurobiology of attachment and separation: how parents shape their infant's brain and behavior, in September 11: Trauma and Human Bonds. Edited by Coates SW, Rosenthal JL, Schechter DS. Hillsdale, NJ, Analytic Press, 2003, pp 191–209

Holmes J: Attachment, Intimacy, Autonomy: Using Attachment Theory in Adult Psychotherapy. Northville, NJ, Jason Aronson, 1996

Holmes J: Notes on mentalization: old hat or new wine? British Journal of Psychotherapy 19:690–710, 2005

Hughes C, Leekham S: What are the links between theory of mind and social relations? Review, reflections and new directions for studies of typical and atypical development. Soc Behav 13:590–619, 2004

Humfress H, O'Connor TG, Slaughter J, et al: General and relationship-specific models of social cognition: explaining the overlap and discrepancies. J Child Psychol Psychiatry 43:873–883, 2002

Insel TR: Is social attachment an addictive disorder? Physiol Behav 79:351–357, 2003

Insel TR, Young LJ: Neuropeptides and the evolution of social behavior. Curr Opin Neurobiol 10:784–789, 2000

Koenigsberg HW, Harvey PD, Mitropoulou V, et al: Characterizing affective instability in borderline personality disorder. Am J Psychiatry 159:784–788, 2002

Krischer M, Sevecke K, Dopfner M, et al: [Personality disorder traits in childhood and adolescence: concepts, methodological approaches and empirical results] (in German). Z Kinder Jugendpsychiatr Psychother 34:87–99, 2006

Leckman JF, Feldman R, Swain JE, et al: Primary parental preoccupation: circuits, genes, and the crucial role of the environment. J Neural Transm 111:753–771, 2004

Legerstee M, Varghese J: The role of maternal affect mirroring on social expectancies in three-month-old infants. Child Dev 72:1301–1313, 2001

Leslie AM: TOMM, ToBy, and agency: core architecture and domain specificity, in Mapping the Mind: Domain Specificity in Cognition and Culture. Edited by Hirschfeld L, Gelman S. New York, Cambridge University Press, 1994, pp 119–148

Lewis V, Norgate S, Collis G, et al: The consequences of visual impairment for children's symbolic and functional play. Br J Dev Psychol 18:449–464, 2000

Lieberman MD: Social cognitive neuroscience: a review of core processes. Annu Rev Psychol 58:259–289, 2007

Liotti G: The inner schema of borderline states and its correction during psychotherapy: a cognitive-evolutionary approach. Journal of Cognitive Psychotherapy 16:349–366, 2002

Lombardo MV, Barnes JL, Wheelwright SJ, et al: Self-referential cognition and empathy in autism. PLoS One 2:E883, 2007

Lyons-Ruth K: Rapprochement or approchement: Mahler's theory reconsidered from the vantage point of recent research in early attachment relationships. Psychoanal Psychol 8:1–23, 1991

Lyons-Ruth K, Jacobvitz D: Attachment disorganization: unresolved loss, relational violence and lapses in behavioral and attentional strategies, in Handbook of Attachment: Theory, Research, and Clinical Applications. Edited by Cassidy J, Shaver PR. New York, Guilford, 1999, pp 520–554

Lyons-Ruth K, Jacobvitz D: Attachment disorganization: genetic factors, parenting contexts, and developmental transformation from infancy to adulthood, in Handbook of Attachment: Theory, Research, and Clinical Applications, 2nd Edition. Edited by Cassidy J, Shaver PR. New York, Guilford, 2008, pp 666–697

MacLean P: The Triune Brain in Evolution: Role in Paleocerebral Functions. New York, Plenum, 1990

Main M: Attachment narratives and attachment across the lifespan. Paper presented at the fall meeting of the American Psychoanalytic Association, New York, 1997

Main M, Hesse E: The organized categories of infant, child, and adult attachment: flexible vs. inflexible attention under attachment-related stress. J Am Psychoanal Assoc 48:1055–1096, 2000

Main M, Solomon J: Procedures for identifying infants as disorganized/disoriented during the Ainsworth Strange Situation, in Attachment During the Preschool Years: Theory, Research and Intervention. Edited by Greenberg M, Cicchetti D, Cummings EM. Chicago, IL, University of Chicago Press, 1990, pp 121–160

Mayes LC: A developmental perspective on the regulation of arousal states. Semin Perinatol 24:267–279, 2000

Mayes LC: Arousal regulation, emotional flexibility, medial amygdala function, and the impact of early experience: comments on the paper of Lewis et al. Ann N Y Acad Sci 1094:178–192, 2006

McAlpine LM, Moore CL: The development of social understanding in children with visual impairments. J Vis Impair Blind 89:349–358, 1985

Meaney MJ, Szyf M: Environmental programming of stress responses through DNA methylation: life at the interface between a dynamic environment and a fixed genome. Dialogues Clin Neurosci 7:103–123, 2005

Meins E, Fernyhough C, Fradley E, et al: Rethinking maternal sensitivity: mothers' comments on infants' mental processes predict security of attachment at 12 months. J Child Psychol Psychiatry 42:637–648, 2001

Mervielde I, De Clercq B, De Fruyt F, et al: Temperament, personality, and developmental psychopathology as childhood antecedents of personality disorders. J Pers Disord 19:171–201, 2005

Mikulincer M, Shaver PR: Attachment in Adulthood: Structure, Dynamics and Change. New York, Guilford, 2007

Mikulincer M, Gillath O, Shaver PR: Activation of the attachment system in adulthood: threat-related primes increase the accessibility of mental representations of attachment figures. J Pers Soc Psychol 83:881–895, 2002

Mitchell RW: Mental models of mirror self-recognition: two theories. New Ideas Psychol 11:295–325, 1993

Montague PR, Lohrenz T: To detect and correct: norm violations and their enforcement. Neuron 56:14–18, 2007

Neisser U: Five kinds of self-knowledge. Philos Psychol 1:35–59, 1988

Newton P, Reddy V, Bull R: Children's everyday deception and performance on false-belief tasks. Br J Dev Psychol 18:297–317, 2000

Nitschke JB, Nelson EE, Rusch BD, et al: Orbitofrontal cortex tracks positive mood in mothers viewing pictures of their newborn infants. Neuroimage 21:583–592, 2004

Northoff G, Heinzel A, de Greck M, et al: Self-referential processing in our brain: a meta-analysis of imaging studies on the self. Neuroimage 31:440–457, 2006

O'Connor TG, Hirsch N: Intra-individual differences and relationship-specificity of social understanding and mentalising in early adolescence. Soc Dev 8:256–274, 1999

Ogden TH: Subjects of Analysis. Northvale, NJ, Jason Aronson, 1994

Oppenheim D, Koren-Karie N: Mothers' insightfulness regarding their children's internal worlds: the capacity underlying secure child-mother relationships. Infant Ment Health J 23:593–605, 2002

Overall NC, Fletcher GJ, Friesen MD: Mapping the intimate relationship mind: comparisons between three models of attachment representations. Pers Soc Psychol Bull 29:1479–1493, 2003

Owen MT, Cox MJ: Marital conflict and the development of infant-parent attachment relationships. J Fam Psychol 11:152–164, 1997

Panksepp J: Affective Neuroscience: The Foundations of Human and Animal Emotions. Oxford, UK, Oxford University Press, 1998

Pears KC, Fisher PA: Emotion understanding and theory of mind among maltreated children in foster care. Dev Psychopathol 17:47–65, 2005

Pears KC, Moses LJ: Demographics, parenting, and theory of mind in preschool children. Soc Dev 12:1–20, 2003

Pierce T, Lydon JE: Global and specific relational models in the experience of social interactions. J Pers Soc Psychol 80:613–631, 2001

Posner MI, Rothbart MK, Vizueta N, et al: Attentional mechanisms of borderline personality disorder. Proc Natl Acad Sci U S A 99:16366–16370, 2002

Povinelli DJ, Eddy TJ: The unduplicated self, in The Self in Infancy: Theory and Research. Edited by Rochat P. Amsterdam, Elsevier, 1995, pp 161–192

Pyers J: Three stages in the understanding of false belief in Nicaraguan signers: the interaction of social experience, language emergence, and conceptual development. Presented at the annual meeting of the Jean Piaget Society, Berkeley, CA, May 31–June 2, 2001

Repacholi BM, Gopnik A: Early reasoning about desires: evidence from 14- and 18-month-olds. Dev Psychol 33:12–21, 1997

Rizzolatti G, Craighero L: The mirror-neuron system. Annu Rev Neurosci 27:169–192, 2004

Rizzolatti G, Ferrari PF, Rozzi S, et al: The inferior parietal lobule: where action becomes perception. Novartis Found Symp 270:129–140 [discussion, 140–145, 164–169], 2006

Rosenfeld H: Contribution to the psychopathology of psychotic states: the importance of projective identification in the ego structure and object relations of the psychotic patient, in Problems of Psychosis. Edited by Doucet P, Laurin C, Amsterdam, Excerpta Medica, 1971, pp 115–128

Ruby P, Decety J: What you believe versus what you think they believe: a neuroimaging study of conceptual perspective-taking. Eur J Neurosci 17:2475–2480, 2003

Sanfey AG, Rilling JK, Aronson JA, et al: The neural basis of economic decision-making in the Ultimatum Game. Science 300:1755–1758, 2003

Saxe R: Uniquely human social cognition. Curr Opin Neurobiol 16:235–239, 2006

Semerari A, Carcione A, Dimaggio G, et al: Metarepresentative functions in borderline personality disorder. J Pers Disord 19:690–710, 2005

Sharp C, Fonagy P, Goodyer I: Imagining your child's mind: psychosocial adjustment and mothers' ability to predict their children's attributional response styles. Br J Dev Psychol 24:197–214, 2006

Siegal M, Peterson CC: Language and theory of mind in atypically developing children: evidence from studies of deafness, blindness, and autism, in Social Cognition and Developmental Psychopathology. Edited by Sharp C, Fonagy P, Goodyer I. Oxford, UK, Oxford University Press, 2008, pp 81–112

Siegel DJ: The Developing Mind: Toward a Neurobiology of Interpersonal Experience. New York, Guilford, 1999

Slade A, Grienenberger J, Bernbach E, et al: Maternal reflective functioning, attachment and the transmission gap: a preliminary study. Attach Hum Dev 7:283–298, 2005

Smith M, Walden T: Understanding feelings and coping with emotional situations: a comparison of maltreated and nonmaltreated preschoolers. Soc Dev 8:93–116, 1999

Sodian B, Frith U: Deception and sabotage in autistic, retarded and normal children. J Child Psychol Psychiatry 33:591–605, 1992

Sodian B, Taylor C, Harris PL, et al: Early deception and the child's theory of mind: false trails and genuine markers. Child Dev 62:468–483, 1992

Sroufe LA: Emotional Development: The Organization of Emotional Life in the Early Years. New York, Cambridge University Press, 1996

Steele H, Steele M, Fonagy P: Associations among attachment classifications of mothers, fathers, and their infants: evidence for a relationship-specific perspective. Child Dev 67:541–555, 1996

Strathearn L: Exploring the neurobiology of attachment, in Developmental Science and Psychoanalysis: Integration and Innovation. Edited by Mayes LC, Fonagy P, Target M. London, Karnac, 2006, pp 117–130

Strathearn L, Fonagy P, Amico J, et al: Adult attachment predicts maternal brain and oxytocin response to infant cues. Neuropsychopharmacology 34:2655–2666, 2009

Swain JE, Lorberbaum JP, Kose S, et al: Brain basis of early parent-infant interactions: psychology, physiology, and in vivo functional neuroimaging studies. J Child Psychol Psychiatry 48:262–287, 2007

Target M, Fonagy P: Playing with reality, II: the development of psychic reality from a theoretical perspective. Int J Psychoanal 77:459–479, 1996

Taylor M, Esbensen BM, Bennett RT: Children's understanding of knowledge acquisition: the tendency for children to report that they have always known what they have just learned. Child Dev 65:1581–1604, 1994

Tremblay RE: The origins of violence. ISUMA Canadian Journal of Policy and Research 1:19–24, 2000

Trull TJ, Durrett CA: Categorical and dimensional models of personality disorder. Annu Rev Clin Psychol 1:355–380, 2005

Tyrer P, Coombs N, Ibrahimi F, et al: Critical developments in the assessment of personality disorder. Br J Psychiatry Suppl 49:S51–S59, 2007

van IJzendoorn MH: Adult attachment representations, parental responsiveness, and infant attachment: a meta-analysis on the predictive validity of the Adult Attachment Interview. Psychol Bull 117:387–403, 1995

Vermote R, Fonagy P, Vertommen H, et al: Outcome and outcome trajectories of personality disordered patients during and after a psychoanalytic hospitalization-based treatment. J Pers Disord 23:293–306, 2009

Vrticka P, Andersson F, Grandjean D, et al: Individual attachment style modulates human amygdala and striatum activation during social appraisal. PLoS One 3:e2868, 2008

Wang Z, Yu G, Cascio C, et al: Dopamine D2 receptor-mediated regulation of partner preferences in female prairie voles (*Microtus ochrogaster*): a mechanism for pair bonding? Behav Neurosci 113:602–611, 1999

Watson JS: Detection of self: the perfect algorithm, in Self-Awareness in Animals and Humans: Developmental Perspectives. Edited by Parker S, Mitchell R, Boccia M. Cambridge, UK, Cambridge University Press, 1994, pp 131–149

Wellman HM, Phillips AT: Developing intentional understandings, in Intentions and Intentionality: Foundations of Social Cognition. Edited by Malle BF, Moses LJ, Baldwin DA. Cambridge, MA, MIT Press, 2001, pp 125–148

Wellman HM, Cross D, Watson J: Meta-analysis of theory-of-mind development: the truth about false belief. Child Dev 72:655–684, 2001

Winnicott DW: Ego distortion in terms of true and false self, in The Maturational Process and the Facilitating Environment. New York, International Universities Press, 1965, pp 140–152

Winslow JT, Noble PL, Lyons CK, et al: Rearing effects on cerebrospinal fluid oxytocin concentration and social buffering in rhesus monkeys. Neuropsychopharmacology 28:910–918, 2003

Zahn-Waxler C, Radke-Yarrow M, Wagner E, et al: Development of concern for others. Dev Psychol 28:126–136, 1992

CHAPTER 3

Neurobiology of Personality Disorders

Gerhard Roth, Ph.D. (philosophy), Ph.D. (zoology)
Anna Buchheim, Ph.D.

From the perspective of psycho-neuroscience, affective and personality disorders correlate with structural and functional deficits of limbic and paralimbic brain centers, and their interactions among themselves, and with cognitive-executive brain centers. It is generally assumed that these disorders result from a combination of 1) genetic polymorphisms affecting predominantly the serotonin system and the hypothalamic-pituitary-adrenal (HPA) (i.e., stress) axis, 2) deficits in brain development, 3) early adverse (traumatizing) childhood experience, and 4) later (adolescent) adverse experience.

On the basis of this general assumption, we present and critically discuss experimental-empirical data concerning the possible neurobiological basis of personality disorders, particularly borderline personality disorder (BPD) and antisocial personality disorder (APD)/psychopathy.

Borderline Personality Disorder

Psychophysiological Studies

Measures of the Autonomic Nervous System

Autonomic responses in the context of diagnosis of psychiatric disorders, including BPD and APD, are usually measured by 1) potentiation of startle response; 2) changes in skin conductance response (SCR; also called *electrodermal response*, or EDR); (3) eye-blink magnitude, as indicated by electromyography of the orbicularis oculi muscle; 4) activity of the corrugator supercilii muscle (frowning); and 5) changes in heart rate. These measurements are taken at the time of or after presentation of pictures from the International Affective Picture Series (IAPS; Lang et al. 1998) that differ in the emotional values "pleasant," "neutral," and "unpleasant." The startle response is usually elicited by a sudden loud tone or noise (around 100 dB), which was preceded by the presentation of IAPS pictures, and the modulation ("potentiation") of the startle response by viewing these pictures is measured.

Rosenthal and colleagues (2008), in their excellent review of the literature on BPD and emotional responding, found that across the studies reviewed, the data on heart rate were inconclusive. It was suggested that the different findings with respect to emotional hyperresponsiveness in BPD patients across studies reflect the use of different procedures. For example, Ebner-Priemer et al. (2005) did not present emotionally evocative stimuli, and there is evidence that cardiovascular indices typically respond differently during imagery conditions that involve viewing of affective slides (Herpertz et al. 1999, 2000).

Similarly, patterns of SCR results varied across studies. Herpertz et al. (1999, 2000) found that individuals with BPD, compared with healthy control subjects, were characterized by lower electrodermal arousal in response to both affective and neutral pictures. Other studies, however (e.g., Ebner-Priemer et al. 2005; Herpertz et al. 2001a), have not provided evidence for SCR hypoarousal among BPD participants in response to laboratory stimuli.

Rosenthal et al. (2008) concluded, from their review of the literature on BPD and emotional responding, that

1. There is no consistent support for elevated physiological responsivity to emotionally evocative stimuli in individuals with BPD, in contrast to theoretical models and studies using self-report methodologies (Koenigsberg et al. 2002), both of which suggest that heightened affect intensity/reactivity is a key characteristic of BPD.

2. Most studies provide some evidence of greater emotional reactivity in BPD across certain indices of emotional responding but not others, suggesting the possibility of mixed or discordant emotional responding among individuals with BPD. For example, in some cases, BPD participants evidenced heightened arousal on some psychophysiological measures but not on others, and in other cases, they reported heightened arousal while exhibiting the same or lower levels of physiological arousal compared with control subjects.

3. Individuals with BPD may be more likely to dissociate during the emotionally evocative laboratory-based paradigms, attenuating the impact of their negative affective experiences. Given the fact that dissociation under stress is a diagnostic criterion for BPD, and that the intercorrelations between a history of traumatic stress, BPD, and dissociation are high (Watson et al. 2006), these results suggest the possibility that individual differences in dissociation among subjects with BPD may help to explain the apparent discrepancies in the patterns of findings across studies.

4. Because BPD is a disorder with considerable symptom heterogeneity, differences in findings across studies may reflect differences in the BPD symptom profiles across samples. For example, not all studies required that BPD participants meet the affective instability or emotional reactivity criteria.

Electroencephalographic Studies

A characteristic feature of BPD is self-injurious behavior in conjunction with a reduction of pain perception. One of the first studies on electroencephalographic (EEG) theta activity and *pain insensitivity* in self-injurious borderline patients was by Russ et al. (1999), who compared results from a 10°C *cold pressor test* among four groups: female inpatients with BPD who did (BPD-P group) or did not (BPD-NP group) report pain during self-injury; female inpatients with major depression; and healthy female subjects. The BPD-NP group reported less pain intensity during the test compared with women in the other groups. Unexpectedly, the total absolute theta power was significantly higher in the BPD-NP group compared with the depressed and healthy groups, with a trend toward being significantly higher compared with the BPD-P group. The authors concluded that the increased theta activity in these borderline patients might be a characteristic of BPD-NP patients and may be indicative of diffuse brain dysfunction.

Schmahl et al. (2004) examined the *differential nociceptive deficits* in patients with BPD and self-injurious behavior, using *laser-evoked potentials* (LEPs), spatial discrimination of noxious stimuli, and pain ratings.

BPD patients had significantly higher heat pain thresholds (23%) and lower pain ratings (67%) than did control subjects. Nevertheless, LEP amplitudes were either normal (N1, P2, P3) or moderately enhanced in BPD patients (N2). LEP latencies and task performance also did not differ between patients and control subjects. P3 amplitudes, the vertex potential (N2–P2), and N1 amplitudes, which are generated near the secondary somatosensory cortex, were significantly reduced during distraction by mental arithmetic in both groups. In addition, P3 amplitudes reflected task difficulty. This study confirmed previous findings of attenuated pain perception in BPD. Normal nociceptive discrimination task performance, normal LEPs, and normal P3 potentials indicate that this attenuation is related neither to a general impairment of the sensory-discriminative component of pain, nor to hyperactive descending inhibition, nor to attention deficits. These findings suggest that hypoalgesia in BPD may primarily be due to altered intracortical processing similar to certain meditative states.

Two other studies, using event-related potentials (ERPs), focused on *executive control* in BPD. Ruchsow et al. (2006) focused on the electrophysiological correlates of *error processing* in BPD patients. Patients with BPD and healthy control subjects were rated with the Barratt Impulsiveness Scale, Version 10 (BIS-10). Participants performed a Go/No go task while a multichannel electroencephalogram was recorded. One main ERP component of interest here was *error-related negativity* (ERN), which reflects brain response of error processing in a forced-choice reaction-time paradigm. At central electrode positions, patients with BPD had significantly smaller ERN amplitudes compared with the control subjects. In addition, increased impulsiveness (nonplanning) was positively correlated with ERN amplitudes in BPD patients. This result can be interpreted as indicative of a dysfunctional system that mirrors deficits in strategic reasoning and intentionality in BPD patients. It remains an open question how ERP signals of BPD patients would differentiate them from healthy controls in successful inhibition.

In the second study, on *response inhibition* in BPD, Ruchsow et al. (2008), using ERPs, investigated patients with BPD and age-, sex-, and education-matched control participants with no history of Axis I or II psychopathology. Participants performed a hybrid flanker–Go/No go task during EEG recording. This study focused on two ERP components: the No go–N2 and the No go–P3, which have been discussed in the context of response inhibition and response conflict. ERPs were computed separately on correct Go trials (button press) and correct No-go trials (no button press). Groups did not differ with regard to the No go–N2. In contrast, BPD patients showed reduced No go–P3 amplitudes. For the entire group, including patients and controls, the authors found a negative correlation of the No go–P3 amplitudes with BIS-10 and the Beck Depression Inventory. The study provides further evidence for impaired response inhibition in BPD patients.

Philipsen et al. (2005) found that BPD patients displayed higher levels of delta power in the sleep electroencephalogram during non–rapid eye movement (REM) sleep compared with healthy control subjects. There was a marked discrepancy between objective and subjective sleep measurements, which indicates an altered perception of sleep in BPD.

Hegerl et al. (2008) examined *EEG-vigilance* (i.e., arousal, wakefulness) differences among patients with BPD, patients with obsessive-compulsive disorder (OCD), and healthy controls. Lowered EEG-vigilance states were associated with emotional instability in older studies, but EEG-vigilance has not been systematically studied in BPD patients. BPD patients were compared with unmedicated OCD patients as well as healthy control subjects in terms of their EEG-vigilance regulation over a period of 5 minutes. The BPD patients showed significantly lower rates of EEG-vigilance awakeness compared with the OCD patients. Hegerl et al. interpreted this as evidence for an instable regulation of EEG-vigilance in BPD patients compared with in OCD patients. This interpretation would be in line with concepts postulating that the behavioral pattern with sensation seeking and impulsivity in BPD has a compensatory and autoregulatory function to stabilize activation of the central nervous system.

NEUROIMAGING STUDIES

Neuroimaging investigations may be helpful to understand the underlying neural basis of the relationship between individual trauma and BPD. They show that a network of regions is involved in emotional regulation, including the amygdala, hippocampus, and prefrontal cortex. The crucial function of these brain regions in the expression, control, and modulation of emotion and impulsivity in animals, including humans, has led to the hypothesis that dysfunctions in these regions may underlie some of the psychopathological symptoms seen in BPD.

Structural Imaging: Volumetric Studies

Studies using magnetic resonance imaging (MRI) scans have found structural brain differences between individuals with and without BPD. Lyoo et al. (1998) found significantly smaller frontal lobe volumes among individuals with BPD who did not have additional co-occurring diagnoses compared with age- and gender-matched control subjects.

Although the authors did not report volumetric data specific to subregions within the frontal lobe, other studies using structural MRI have identified specific regions of dysfunction.

Irle et al. (2007) examined size abnormalities of the superior parietal cortex in young women with BPD compared with healthy control subjects. Structural MRI (3D-MRI) was used to assess volumes of the superior (precuneus, postcentral gyrus) and inferior parietal cortex. BPD subjects had significantly smaller right-sided precuneus (–9%) volumes compared with control subjects. The left postcentral gyrus of BPD subjects with the comorbid diagnosis of dissociative amnesia or dissociative identity disorder was significantly increased relative to that in the controls (+13%) and in the BPD subjects without these disorders (+11%). In BPD subjects, stronger depersonalization was significantly related to larger right precuneus size. Possibly, larger precuneus size in BPD is related to symptoms of depersonalization. Increased postcentral gyrus size in BPD may be related to the development of dissociative amnesia or dissociative identity disorder in the presence of severe childhood abuse.

In addition to the volumetric studies described above, which focused on changes in *neocortical structure* volumes, volumetric studies have focused on the *limbic system*. Driessen et al. (2000) measured hippocampal and amygdala volumes in a sample of BPD patients with a history of childhood physical or sexual abuse and found reduced hippocampal volumes among participants with BPD, as well as a nonsignificant trend for reduced amygdala volumes.

Brambilla et al. (2004) likewise found that BPD subjects had significantly smaller right and left hippocampal volumes, marked in subjects with childhood abuse, and significantly increased volumes of the right and left putamen (as part of the corpus striatum, an important executive center), especially in subjects with substance use disorders. No significant differences between groups were found for the caudate nucleus (another part of the corpus striatum), amygdala, temporal lobes, dorsolateral prefrontal cortex, and total brain volumes. This study replicated prior findings of diminished hippocampal volumes in subjects with BPD. Also, increased putamen volumes were found in BPD, which had not been previously reported. Early traumatic experiences may play a role in hippocampal atrophy, whereas substance use disorders may contribute to putamen enlargement.

Tebartz van Elst et al. (2003) examined orbitofrontal cortex (OFC), anterior cingulate cortex (ACC), dorsolateral prefrontal cortex, amygdala, and hippocampal volumes in medication-free women with BPD with no current substance abuse or major depression and in healthy women. The researchers found, consistent with other studies, a significant reduction of hippocampal and amygdala volumes, as well as significant reductions in the left OFC and right ACC, in the BPD patients compared with control subjects. The authors argued that while volume loss of a single brain structure like the hippocampus seems to be a rather unspecific finding in neuropsychiatry, the volume loss of amygdala, hippocampus, right OFC, and left ACC in the presence of normal overall brain volume might be a pattern that differentiates BPD from other neuropsychiatric conditions.

Finally, Rusch et al. (2003) reported significantly less gray matter volume in the left amygdala among women with BPD compared with control subjects.

Minzenberg et al. (2008) examined structural changes in BPD patients and tested the hypothesis that the patients exhibit gross structural changes that parallel the respective increases in amygdala activation and impairment of rostral/subgenual ACC activation. The BPD group had significantly higher relative gray matter concentration (GMC) in the amygdala compared with the control subjects. In contrast, the BPD group showed significantly lower GMC in left rostral/subgenual ACC. This sample of BPD patients exhibited gross structural changes in gray matter in cortical and subcortical limbic regions that paralleled the regional distribution of altered functional activation to emotional stimuli in these same subjects. The authors concluded that BPD patients have characteristic changes in frontolimbic activity in the processing of fear stimuli, with exaggerated amygdala response and impaired emotion modulation of ACC activity.

In a study comparing teenagers with first presentation of BPD with control subjects, Chanen et al. (2008) identified OFC, but not hippocampal or amygdala, volumetric differences early in the course of BPD. The OFC is involved in conscious perception of emotions, emotional preparation and motivation of actions, assessment of consequences of one's own behavior and of individual and social risks, and identification of emotional expression and of the meaning in the actions of others (empathy), as well as learning and control of socially adequate behavior. Hippocampal and amygdala volume reductions observed in adult BPD samples might develop during the course of the disorder, although longitudinal studies are needed to examine this possibility.

Jovev et al. (2008) examined the relationship between the volume of the pituitary gland (hypophysis) and lifetime number of parasuicidal behaviors in a sample of teenagers with BPD at first presentation and minimal exposure to treatment. Hierarchical regression analysis revealed that age and number of parasuicidal behaviors were significant predictors of the volume of the pituitary. These findings indicate that parasuicidal behavior in individuals with BPD might be associated with greater activation of the HPA axis. Further studies are required, using direct neuroendocrine measures and exploring other parameters of self-injurious behavior, such as recency of self-injurious behavior, intent to die, and medical threat.

The above-mentioned studies suggest that BPD is associated with abnormalities in the limbic structures and that these abnormalities strongly underlie emotional dysfunction in BPD symptoms.

In a study integrating genetic and neuroimaging methodology, Zetzsche et al. (2008) examined 5-HT$_{1A}$ receptor gene C –1019 G polymorphism and amygdala volume in right-handed women with BPD. While no difference in allelic distribution between patients and controls was detected, the described effect of the 5-HTR(1A) genotype on amygdala volume was found for the whole group of patients, as well as for the subgroup of patients with comorbid major depression, but not for the control subjects. In contrast to the significant amygdala volume differences in these subgroups of BPD patients, the mean amygdala volume of the group of BPD patients as a whole was not significantly different from that of the control subjects. In summary, this study provided first evidence that the 5-HTR(1A) gene C –1019 G polymorphism is associated with structural changes in the limbic system of BPD patients—a finding that might be disease-related and that might partly explain the previous discrepant results regarding amygdala volume changes in BPD.

Functional Imaging: Baseline/Resting Studies

Functional brain imaging studies using ^{18}F-labeled fluorodeoxyglucose positron emission tomography (FDG-PET) under resting conditions to assess baseline cerebral glucose metabolism have found differences in metabolism in the prefrontal cortex of patients with BPD compared with healthy control subjects (for review, see Rosenthal et al. 2008).

De la Fuente et al. (1994) found decreased metabolism in the dorsolateral prefrontal cortex, ACC, and several basal ganglia regions among patients with BPD compared with healthy control subjects. Soloff et al. (2000) used FDG-PET imaging procedures to compare serotonergic functioning in the prefrontal cortex of individuals with BPD and healthy control subjects. Compared with the controls, the BPD patients evidenced diminished glucose intake in the orbital and medial regions of the prefrontal cortex. This finding is particularly noteworthy given that the BPD participants were not depressed, providing preliminary evidence that serotonergic uptake in BPD is not solely the result of co-occurring major depression.

In another study, Juengling et al. (2003) used FDG-PET under resting conditions to compare brain metabolism in female inpatients with BPD, who had been medication free for at least 4 weeks and did not have current substance abuse or depression, and healthy female control subjects. Results indicated a hypometabolism in the left hippocampus of the BPD patients compared with controls, whereas increased metabolism was observed in the ACC, superior frontal gyrus, right inferior frontal gyrus, and right precentral gyrus of the BPD patients.

Proton magnetic resonance spectroscopy ([^{1}H]MRS) studies also provide a measure of baseline neuronal function by measuring levels of metabolite concentration. Tebartz van Elst et al. (2001) conducted a pilot [^{1}H]MRS study assessing N-acetylaspartate (NAA) concentration (a marker of neuronal integrity) in left dorsolateral prefrontal cortex and left striatum in patients with BPD and no co-occurring psychiatric illnesses versus healthy controls. NAA concentration was significantly reduced in the dorsolateral prefrontal cortex of BPD patients compared with controls—a finding consistent with deficits in executive function, working memory, or the ability to integrate emotion and cognition.

Functional Imaging: Emotional and Cognitive Stimuli Studies

In general, neuroimaging studies measuring responsivity to emotional stimuli provide support for the presence of a heightened responsivity to emotional stimuli among individuals with BPD. Herpertz et al. (2001a) examined amygdala and prefrontal cortex functioning in response to standardized emotional stimuli among right-handed female inpatients with BPD, all of whom met the affective instability criterion for BPD, had no current Axis I disorder, and were medication free, and age-matched, right-handed female healthy volunteers with no history of psychiatric treatment. Participants were confronted with emotional stimuli consisting of arousing, unpleasant IAPS slides and neutral IAPS slides twice, first while in the functional magnetic resonance imaging (fMRI) scanner and then again immediately after the imaging session, in order to assess self-reported valence and arousal dimensions. Contrary to the findings of Herpertz et al. (1999, 2000), the two groups did not differ in their self-reported emotional response to the slides, suggesting that the BPD group did not consider the slides to be more arousing or more negative. Providing support for increased responsivity to negative emotional stimuli, however, BPD participants displayed a significantly greater activation of the amygdala in response to the negative stimuli compared with the neutral stimuli. In the control group, no such differences in amygdala activation occurred in response to the negative emotional stimuli.

In a related study, Donegan et al. (2003) examined amygdala reactivity to pictures of human facial expressions of emotion in participants with BPD and control subjects. Unlike most other studies in this area, this study included both female and male participants. All BPD patients had co-occurring Axis I disorders (most commonly major depressive disorder, posttraumatic stress disorder [PTSD], or alcohol abuse), and most of them were currently taking psychotropic medications. Compared with the control group, BPD participants evidenced greater levels of left amygdala activation to sad, neutral, and fearful faces. Interestingly, the most striking difference between the groups occurred in response to neutral expressions. In evaluating the ambiguous "neutral" expressions, some of the BPD subjects disambiguated these expressions by projecting emotions or intentions into their descriptions of the neutral faces. Importantly, their attributions were uniformly negative, threatening, and untrustworthy. The strong negative reactions of these subjects to the neutral faces are consistent with the notion of transference in psychotherapy. Findings from this study provide a foundation for elucidating the neural substrates of behavioral and emotional facets of BPD that contribute to disturbed interpersonal relations.

Another study tested a model of frontolimbic dysfunction in facial emotion processing in BPD (Minzenberg et al. 2007), focusing on emotions like fear and anger. BPD patients showed a significantly larger deactivation (relative to control subjects) in the bilateral rostral/subgenual ACC to fear stimuli, and in the left ACC to fear in contrast to neutral stimuli, and significantly greater activation in the right amygdala to fear in contrast to neutral stimuli. There were no significant between-group differences in these areas in response to anger. The authors concluded that BPD patients exhibit changes in frontolimbic activity in the processing of fear stimuli, with exaggerated amygdala response and impaired emotion modulation of ACC activity. The relative hyporesponsivity of the amygdala to anger might be related to an inability of BPD patients to manage socially undesirable behavior, including their own expressions of antagonistic thoughts and behaviors, in interpersonal settings.

Affective dysregulation in BPD in response to both external stimuli and memories has been shown to be associated with functional alterations of limbic and prefrontal brain areas. In an fMRI study, Schnell et al. (2007) used pictures from the Thematic Apperception Test (TAT) to examine neuronal networks involved in autobiographical memory retrieval in BPD patients and control subjects. In both groups, TAT stimuli activated brain areas known to be involved in autobiographical memory retrieval. BPD subjects lacked differential amygdala, OFC, and ACC activations for TAT versus neutral stimuli. In the TAT condition, compared with control subjects, BPD subjects displayed increased BOLD responses in the bilateral orbitofrontal and insular regions and in the left ACC and medial prefrontal cortex, as well as in the parietal and parahippocampal areas, consistent with a more aversive and arousing experience assessed by self-reports. The authors concluded that increased blood oxygen level–dependent (BOLD) responses during TAT processing in BPD subjects were in line with previously reported changes in ACC and OFC, which are known to be involved in memory retrieval. However, BPD subjects displayed hyperactivation in these areas for both TAT and neutral stimuli. The lack of selective activation of areas involved in autobiographical memory retrieval suggests a general tendency toward a self-referential mode of information processing in BPD, or a failure to switch between emotionally salient and neutral stimuli.

The presence or absence of traumatic experiences or PTSD diagnosis has been shown to play an important role. Driessen et al. (2004) recruited women with BPD who had experienced trauma (ages 21–40 years, mean=33 years) and who had various comorbid disorders. The authors interviewed the participants to obtain cues about *traumatic* memories and aversive but nontraumatic memories, and observed them via fMRI during recall of those memories. The authors found OFC activation in both hemispheres and activation of Broca's area in patients with BPD without PTSD, and only a minor OFC activation and no activation of Broca's area in patients with BPD and PTSD. Because all BPD patients tested had experienced trauma, but not all had PTSD, the authors argued that presence or absence of comorbid PTSD may constitute an important subgroup.

In BPD patients listening to personalized scripts of their own trauma (e.g., childhood sexual or physical abuse), Schmahl et al. (2004) found an activation in right dorsolateral prefrontal cortex and deactivation in left dorsolateral prefrontal cortex in women without BPD. There was also activation in right ACC and left OFC in these women. Women with BPD failed to show an activation in the anterior cingulate gyrus and OFC. No activity was seen in dorsolateral prefrontal gyrus in women with the diagnosis and treatment of BPD. This study suggested that a dysfunction of the dorsolateral and medial prefrontal cortex, including ACC, is correlated with the recall of traumatic memories in women with BPD. Here, these brain areas might mediate trauma-related symptoms, such as dissociation or affective instability.

Beblo et al. (2006) aimed at investigating the neural correlates of the recall of unresolved life events in patients with BPD and healthy control subjects. During fMRI, subjects recalled unresolved and resolved negative life events. Individual cue words were used to stimulate autobiographical memory. When unresolved and resolved life events were contrasted, patients showed significant bilateral activation of fronto-temporal areas, including the insula, amygdala, and ACC; left posterior cingulate cortex; right occipital cortex; bilateral cerebellum; and midbrain. In healthy subjects, no differential brain activation was related to these conditions. The authors concluded that the activation of both amygdala and prefrontal areas might reflect an increased effortful but insufficient attempt to control intensive emotions during the recall of unresolved life events in patients with BPD.

The functional neuroimaging studies summarized above measured brain activation patterns in response to visual stimuli (e.g., standardized pictures, faces), passively presented scripts, or recall of unresolved life events. One of us (Buchheim et al. 2008) has developed an fMRI paradigm to examine the functional neuroanatomy of *attachment trauma* while BPD patients are telling individual stories in response to attachment-relevant picture stimuli during a validated narrative-based assessment for attachment, the Adult Attachment Projective (AAP; George and West 2003). Female BPD patients and healthy female control subjects, matched for age and education, told stories in response to the AAP while being scanned. Group differences in narrative and neural responses to "monadic" pictures (characters facing attachment threats alone) and "dyadic" pictures (interaction between characters in an attachment context) were analyzed. Behavioral narrative data showed that monadic pictures were significantly more traumatic for BPD patients than for controls, and BPD patients exhibited significantly more anterior mid-cingulate cortex activation in response to monadic pictures than did controls. In response to dyadic pictures, the BPD patients showed more activation of the right superior temporal sulcus and less activation of the right parahippocampal gyrus compared with controls. These results give evidence for potential neural mechanisms of attachment trauma underlying interpersonal symptoms of BPD—that is, fearful and painful intolerance of aloneness, hypersensitivity to social environment, and reduced positive memories of dyadic interactions.

Functional Imaging: Regulation of Executive Function

It has become increasingly common for BPD to be examined in terms of its core symptoms, rather than as a disorder of its own. This has proven to be true in the study of *impulsivity*, which is a feature of several personality disorders. Völlm et al. (2004) examined patients with BPD or APD or both (with some overlap between disorders), and scanned them during a Go/No go task in which participants had to restrain their behavior. While healthy control participants demonstrated activity in their right dorsolateral and left OFC, patients with impulsive personality disorders exhibited more widespread activity, with more bilateral activation from their medial, superior, and inferior frontal gyri to their anterior cingulate gyri. The implication of this study is that BPD patients may not only demonstrate abnormal metabolism in normal cortical areas but also activate improper cortical areas entirely or, because of inefficient cortical processing, activate a wider cortical area to achieve the same regulation.

Another fMRI study using a Go/No go task to examine failure of frontolimbic inhibitory function in the context of negative emotion in BPD tested the hypothesis that in BPD patients, the ventromedial prefrontal cortex (vmPFC) and associated regions would not be activated during a task requiring motor inhibition (Silbersweig et al. 2007). A specifically designed fMRI activation probe was used, with statistical parametric mapping analyses, to test hypotheses concerning decreased prefrontal inhibitory function in the context of negative emotion in patients with BDP and healthy comparison subjects. The results confirmed that under conditions associated with the interaction of behavioral inhibition and negative emotion, BPD patients show relatively decreased vmPFC (including medial OFC and subgenual ACC) activity compared with healthy subjects. In BPD patients, under conditions of behavioral inhibition in the context of negative emotion, decreasing vmPFC and increasing extended amygdalar–ventral striatal activity correlated highly with measures of decreased constraint and increased negative emotion, respectively. These findings suggest specific frontolimbic neural substrates associated with core clinical features of *emotional and behavioral dyscontrol* in BPD.

SUMMARY

The cause of BPD is complex, with several factors that interact in various ways with each other. Genetic factors and adverse childhood experiences (e.g., attachment trauma, emotional neglect, abuse) might cause emotional dysregulation and impulsivity, leading to dysfunctional behaviors and psychosocial conflicts and deficits, which again might reinforce emotional dysregulation and impulsivity.

Structural and functional neuroimaging revealed a dysfunctional frontolimbic network of brain regions that seems to mediate many of the BPD symptoms. Taken together, these findings suggest that BPD patients exhibit reduced hippocampal, OFC, and amygdala volumes and increased activation in the amygdala in response to emotional stimuli.

However, the extent to which these vulnerabilities underlie the emotional and cognitive dysfunction clinically described in BPD is not well enough understood to make firm conclusions regarding the specificity in BPD compared with other psychiatric disorders.

Moreover, patients with BPD show deficiencies in NAA concentrations in the dorsolateral prefrontal cortex in magnetic resonance spectroscopy, suggesting a lower density of neurons and disturbed neuronal metabolism.

Research has most strongly implicated the serotonin transporter gene (*5HTT*) in the development of BPD; shorter alleles of this gene have been associated with lower levels of serotonin and greater impulsive aggression. Genes for dopamine and monoamine oxidase A (MAO-A) may yet prove to have an etiological role. Genetic findings further consolidate the evidence that there are biological (not only psychological) differences between people with and without BPD.

Neurobiological Basis of Antisocial Personality Disorder and Psychopathy

A review of the neurobiological basis of APD and psychopathy suffers from the fact that there is no universally accepted definition of personality disorders related to "antisocial" behavior. A much-used definition is given in DSM-IV-TR (American Psychiatric Association 2000, p. 706), where APD is classified as a Cluster B personality disorder. The individual with APD exhibits "a pervasive pattern of disregard for and violation of the rights of others occurring since age 15 years, as indicated by three (or more) of the following":

1. Failure to conform to social norms with respect to lawful behaviors as indicated by repeatedly performing acts that are grounds for arrest
2. Deceitfulness, as indicated by repeatedly lying, use of aliases, or conning others for personal profit or pleasure
3. Impulsivity or failure to plan ahead
4. Irritability and aggressiveness, as indicated by repeated physical fights or assaults
5. Reckless disregard for safety of self or others
6. Consistent irresponsibility, as indicated by repeated failure to sustain consistent work behavior or honor financial obligations
7. Lack of remorse, as indicated by being indifferent to or rationalizing having hurt, mistreated, or stolen from another

This definition only partially overlaps with that of "dissocial personality disorder" as defined by the World Health Organization in ICD-10 (World Health Organization 1992):

1. Callous unconcern for the feelings of others and lack of the capacity for empathy
2. Gross and persistent attitude of irresponsibility and disregard for social norms, rules, and obligations
3. Incapacity to maintain enduring relationships
4. Very low tolerance to frustration and a low threshold for discharge of aggression, including violence
5. Incapacity to experience guilt and to profit from experience, particularly punishment
6. Marked proneness to blame others or to offer plausible rationalizations for the behavior bringing the subject into conflict
7. Persistent irritability

Experts state that the DSM-IV definition includes predominantly aspects of aggressive, delinquent, and criminal behavior, whereas the ICD-10 definition emphasizes personal-affective and interpersonal aspects. In this regard, the ICD-10 definition is more closely related to the notion of "psychopathy." *Psychopathy*, as usually defined by the Psychopathy Checklist—Revised (PCL-R; Hare 1991; for a recent discussion see Hare and Neuman 2008), includes the following criteria:

◆ *Factor 1—Aggressive narcissism:* 1) glibness/superficial charm; 2) grandiose sense of self-worth; 3) pathological lying; 4) cunning/manipulative; 5) lack of remorse or guilt; 6) shallow emotions; 7) callous/lack of empathy; 8) failure to accept responsibility for own actions; 9) promiscuous sexual behavior.
◆ *Factor 2—Socially deviant lifestyle:* 1) need for stimulation/proneness to boredom; 2) parasitic lifestyle; 3) poor behavioral control; 4) lack of realistic, long-term goals; 5) impulsivity; 6) irresponsibility; 7) juvenile delinquency; 8) early behavior problems; 9) revocation of conditional release.

Traits *not* correlated with factor 1 or factor 2 are 1) many short-term marital relationships and 2) criminal versatility.

A number of experts offer the view that the notion of "antisocial personality disorder" includes subgroups differing in one or more dimensions, with "psychopaths" as a specific subgroup particularly characterized by "manipulative," "callous," "arrogant," "superficial charm," "pathological lying," "shallow affect," and "lack of guilt, remorse, and empathy." These traits are covered by PCL-R factor 1, "aggressive narcissism," which is not dominant in the DSM-IV definition of APD (see also Kernberg 1984). Nonpsychopathic individuals with APD would be characterized mostly by PCL-R factor 2, "socially deviant lifestyle." Another important difference appears to consist in the type of antisocial-aggressive behavior—namely, whether or not the individuals exhibit mostly *reactive-impulsive aggression* or *proactive-instrumental aggression*. Both types have in common a deficit in self-control, which in the former type is of a reactive-impulsive nature in the sense of motor impulsivity, and in the latter is of a proactive-instrumental nature in the sense of purely egoistic and selfish behavior. The former largely includes intermittent explosive disorder (IED) and conduct disorder as conceptualized by DSM-IV.

REACTIVE-IMPULSIVE AGGRESSION

Reactive-impulsive (also labeled "hostile" or "affective") aggression and violence is the dominant type of antisocial behavior and is positively correlated with increased levels of anger and impulsivity. It occurs as a reaction to perceived threat or provocation, and it is often followed by remorse. Correspondingly, expressions of anger and aggression take an impulsive form (Barratt et al. 1999). Impulsive aggression and uncontrollable temperament are also characteristic of IED (Coccaro 2003).

Autonomic Responses

In healthy individuals, an increase in startle response, eye-blink magnitude, corrugator supercilii muscle activity, and skin conductance and a decrease in initial heart rate are found upon exposure to unpleasant pictures, but not (or not significantly) to neutral or pleasant pictures (Lang et al. 2002). In contrast, in antisocial individuals characterized by a high degree of impulsive-reactive aggression, these autonomic responses are significantly increased (Herpertz et al. 2001b; Lang et al. 2000)—that is, these persons typically "overreact" to unpleasant or threatening pictures.

Functional Neuroanatomy and Imaging Data

There is strong evidence that a structural or functional impairment of the frontal cortex, especially OFC and vmPFC, is associated with impulsive aggression and violent behavior. Indications of a relationship between impulsive aggression and a *reduced* volume of the frontal lobe or other dysfunctions of the prefrontal cortex are found in patients with a variety of psychiatric disorders, such as BPD (New et al. 2002, 2004; Soloff et al. 2000, 2003), IED (Best et al. 2002), and APD in the sense of DSM-IV (Laakso et al. 2002; Raine et al. 2000); in individuals with suicidal behavior (Mann 2003); and in murderers pleading not guilty by reason of insanity (Raine et al. 1994, 1997). This relationship is not surprising given the general function ascribed to OFC and vmPFC—that is, regulation of emotional responses, especially in the context of threatening and risky situations.

OFC and vmPFC are massively interconnected with other limbic brain areas, such as the rostral ACC and the amygdala (Kringelbach and Rolls 2004). Accordingly, when it comes to impulsive aggression and violence, the relative balance of activity between the prefrontal cortex and limbic structures might be disturbed, rather than impairments being present in one or the other structure alone (Bufkin and Luttrell 2005). There are, however, relatively few studies specifically examining the interaction between OFC and amygdala in impulsive aggression and violence. In a PET study, Raine et al. (1997) assessed the ratio of prefrontal-to-subcortical brain functioning in a group of murderers compared with controls. Reduced prefrontal and increased subcortical activity (the latter including the amygdala) were found specifically in those murderers who committed their violent acts in an unplanned and impulsive manner. Similarly, patients with IED showed an exaggerated amygdala reactivity and reduced OFC activation in response to angry faces (Coccaro et al. 2007). These latter fMRI findings by Coccaro et al. provide evidence for an amygdala-OFC dysfunction in response to a social threat signal in individuals with impulsive aggression. Dougherty et al. (2004) demonstrated an aberrant functional relationship between the vmPFC and the amygdala during anger-inducing script imagery in depressed patients with anger attacks.

These data suggest a link between a disturbed frontolimbic circuitry and a state of subcortical hyperarousal (primarily mediated by the amygdala), leading to impulsive aggression and emotional dysregulation. The amygdala and OFC are key structures in the so-called ventral system of emotion perception, which includes the amygdala, insula, ventral striatum, rostral ACC, OFC, and vmPFC (Phillips et al. 2003). According to this concept, the ventral system is important for the rapid appraisal of emotional material, the production of affective states, and the automatic regulation of autonomic responses to emotional stimuli.

A relationship between increased impulsivity and deficits in the ventral system is found in healthy subjects as well. Brown et al. (2006) found that dispositional impulsivity, as measured by a Go/No go paradigm and a face-processing task, was correlated negatively with activations of the lateral OFC and the dorsal amygdala and positively with activations of the bilateral ventral amygdala, parahippocampal gyrus, dorsal ACC, and bilateral caudate nucleus. Patients with conduct disorder and APD, likewise characterized by heightened impulsivity, showed markedly decreased activation in the dorsal ACC when viewing negative pictures (Brown et al. 2006; Sterzer et al. 2005). Thus, we have to assume that activation of the dorsal ACC and OFC/vmPFC in normal impulsive individuals operates as a compensatory mechanism, which is absent in clinical populations (Brown et al. 2006).

This view is in line with the assumption that in *patients* exhibiting excessive aggressive behavior, the OFC is sufficiently activated in response to experienced anger. Coccaro et al. (2007) found a hypofunction of the OFC in response to angry faces in patients with IED. Similarly, depressed patients with increased levels of anger and aggression failed to show vmPFC activation during anger induction (Dougherty et al. 2004).

In conclusion, the combination of prefrontal *hypofunction* with amygdalar *hyperfunction* consistently occurs across anatomical and functional studies with a wide range of healthy subjects characterized by increased impulsivity, as well as clinical and forensic populations characterized by emotional dyscontrol and impulsivity/aggression; this is underlined by a hyperreactivity of autonomic responses.

PROACTIVE-INSTRUMENTAL AGGRESSION AND PSYCHOPATHY

Persons satisfying the criteria of *psychopathy* as defined by the PCL-R are characterized by a dominance of instrumental, proactive, premeditated, or "predatory" aggression in the sense of planned, goal-directed (achieving money, status, drugs, etc.) activity, which is not, or not predominantly, combined with motor impulsivity. On the contrary, psychopaths often exhibit a high degree of self-control at lying, deceiving, and manipulating others, simulating empathy, and so forth, while hiding their true motives. Psychopathy is considered a reliable predictor for violence, high rates of recidivism, and poor treatment responsivity (R.J. Blair 2005; Hare and Neuman 2008).

Autonomic Responses

Some of the earliest and most robust findings in psychopaths are an impairment of autonomic responses to acute or anticipated threat (Hare 1982; Herpertz et al. 2001b; Patrick et al. 1993), startle response (Levenston et al. 2000; Pastor et al. 2003), passive avoidance learning (Lykken

1957; Newman and Kosson 1986), and affective priming (K.S. Blair et al. 2006). In accordance with these findings is the fact that psychopaths exhibit little facial modulation. This indicates a lack of fear, deficits in processing of negative emotional information, and generally emotional hyporesponsivity (cf. R.J. Blair 2005).

Functional Neuroanatomical and Imaging Data

In adult psychopaths, as in individuals with impulsive-reactive aggression, there is a *combined* amygdala-OFC dysfunction; the dysfunction in psychopaths, however, differs in the kind of impairment (i.e., concentrating on deficits in associative learning and emotionality) (K.S. Blair et al. 2006; Budhani et al. 2006; Mitchell et al. 2002, 2006a, 2006b). Regrettably, neuroimaging data on amygdala and OFC activation in psychopaths are somewhat inconsistent. While some studies, using aversive conditioning (Birbaumer et al. 2005; Veit et al. 2002) or affective memory tasks (Kiehl et al. 2001), reported *reduced* activation of limbic centers in psychopaths compared with control subjects, others found *enhanced* activations in the amygdala, OFC, and dorsolateral prefrontal cortex during emotional learning (Schneider et al. 2000) and the processing of negative emotional pictures (Müller et al. 2003). And, using a facial emotion processing task, Deeley et al. (2006) failed to detect any amygdala or OFC activity in criminal psychopaths.

There are several possible reasons for these discrepancies. First, the use of different stimulation paradigms across studies, together with generally small sample sizes ($N < 10$ in most of the studies), raises the possibility that some of the reported effects may be sample-specific. Second, there are large differences in the mean PCL-R total scores (ranging between 0 and 40); the PCL-R was used to assess psychopathy in the studies cited. For example, Birbaumer et al. (2005) reported an overall PCL-R score of about 30 (range 15–31) among the psychopaths studied, whereas Müller et al. (2003) found a mean score of about 37 (range 34–40). Thus, these two samples of psychopaths do not overlap in their PCL-R score. Third, as noted earlier, the PCL-R indexes two distinct, albeit interrelated, facets of psychopathy: factor 1 reflects the emotional-interpersonal features (e.g., shallow affect, lack of remorse or empathy), and factor 2 represents a chronically unstable and antisocial lifestyle. It is therefore conceivable that conflicting results on brain activations in psychopaths might partly be due to sample-specific differences in the relation of these two aspects of psychopathy that do not become apparent when categorization is based solely on the total PCL-R score.

Lack of empathy has often been assumed in the context of both reactive and proactive psychopathic aggression and violence. Empathy can be conceived as a capacity to understand others' actions, emotions, and sensations. The difference between empathic and violent behavior was analyzed in an fMRI study by King et al. 2006, who, using a customized video game, varied the social appropriateness of aggressive and empathic behavior. Participants were supposed to either shoot an aggressive humanoid assailant or bandage a wounded conspecific, both considered *appropriate* behavior. *Inappropriate* behavior demanded the converse combination—namely, shooting the injured conspecific and healing the humanoid attacker. Surprisingly, identical activations were observed in a circuit including the vmPFC and the amygdala for the appropriate situations, irrespective of whether the behavior was violent or compassionate. This finding suggests that context-appropriate behavior is guided by a common neural system including the vmPFC and amygdala. These data also suggest that dysfunction in this system underlies the presentation of inappropriate social behavior.

In another interactive fMRI study, Lotze et al. (2007) examined the role of the prefrontal cortex in the regulation of reactive aggression in high or low callous subjects (in the normal range). In a competitive reaction time task, participants were provoked by a virtual opponent who was allowed to administer aversive pain stimuli to the subjects when he won the challenge. However, when the opponent lost, there was the opportunity for revenge, whereby the participants could determine the intensity of the penalty and watch the opponent suffer on videotape. Increased activity was observed in the vmPFC during retaliation, and in the dorsomedial prefrontal cortex (dmPFC), when subjects had to select the revenge intensity. The dmPFC activation also correlated positively with the intensity of the selected stimulus strength when taking revenge, but not when watching the opponent suffering. The OFC/vmPFC was active during the time the subject watched the opponent suffering; however, this effect was stronger for low callous (i.e., more empathic) participants. The amygdala was also found to be active throughout the different phases of the experiment, and the activity of the right amygdala during watching the opponent correlated positively with the intensity of pain of the opponent.

According to the authors, the results are indicative for a participation of the dmPFC in *cognitive* aspects of social interaction, while the OFC/vmPFC is involved in *affective* processes associated with compassion for the suffering opponent. With regard to activations of OFC/vmPFC and amygdala during viewing an opponent's suffering, the findings resemble those of King et al. (2006) in that punishing an opponent for his or her *unjustified* aggression might be experienced as an *appropriate* social behavior, irrespective of being aggressive. Interestingly, Lotze et al. (2007) reported stronger OFC/vmPFC activations for more empathic participants and a positive correlation between amygdala activity and pain of the opponent. These findings point toward a higher responsiveness of the OFC/vmPFC to distress cues signaled by the amygdala in more empathic individuals and may relate to a neural basis of empathy deficits as seen in psychopaths.

Two other fMRI studies further investigated the link between empathy and psychopathy. Müller et al. (2008) specifically compared individuals diagnosed on the basis of the PCL-R and of ICD-10 ("dissocial personality disorder") with healthy subjects. Pictures taken from the IAPS were taken as positive, neutral, and negative stimuli. A Simon task was run under different emotional conditions induced by the IAPS pictures. In both groups, subjects had significantly longer reaction times during incompatible trials than during compatible tasks, as expected, but there was no influence of emotions on the reaction time. However, in the control group, error rates were significantly higher for incompatible compared with compatible conditions, and the error rate was higher for negative compared with positive conditions—a finding that is consistent with the assumption that negative emotions represent a higher "load" on more demanding cognitive tasks. However, in the psychopathy group, there was *no* such effect of negative conditions on error rate, while both groups did not differ regarding compatible trials. These findings indicate that negative emotions do not disturb cognitive tasks in psychopaths.

As to BOLD response in fMRI, psychopaths exhibited reduced activity in the superior temporal gyrus, as opposed to increased activity in control subjects, at presentation of negative emotional stimuli. This result is in line with those of other studies showing increased temporoparietal activity and decreased prefrontal activity at presentation of incompatible material in healthy subjects that reflects a "load" of more challenging cognitive tasks (Peterson et al. 2002). According to Müller et al., the evidence indicates that the interaction between the superior temporal gyrus and the vmPFC (playing a central role in empathy) is disturbed in psychopaths.

The other study, by Fecteau et al. (2008), addresses the important question of what precisely is the "empathy deficit" in psychopaths. Are these individuals unable to recognize the pain of others, or are they simply indifferent to it? Fecteau et al. here distinguish between "motor empathy," including the mere *recognition* of pain of others, and "affective empathy," which involves *caring* for it. The authors found that painful treatment of a person being observed by subjects during fMRI led to an activation of motor centers. The excitability of motor cortex during passive observation of needle penetration was significantly reduced in both controls and psychopathic patients, but this reduction was greatest in psychopathic patients with the strongest coldheartedness. This could indicate that psychopathic patients can better understand the suffering of others but that they have no concern for the pain of others. This coincides with the finding that mentalizing abilities are spared in psychopaths (R.J. Blair 2005; Dolan and Fullam 2004). The same was found by Munro et al. (2007)—namely, there was no difference in general response inhibition as assessed by a Go/No go experiment and frontal N2/P3 between healthy control subjects and psychopaths (as assessed by the PCL-R). In both groups, the N2 and P3 waves increased above the ACC and left OFC in response inhibition. Thus, general motor impulsivity is not impaired in psychopaths, and the deficit of psychopaths appears to specifically affect emotional empathy (i.e., exhibiting a concern for the pain and suffering of others).

In summary, the neurobiological findings on psychopathy suggest that the condition is due to dysfunctions of ventral and ventromedial prefrontal regions (vmPFC, OFC, ACC), insular cortex, temporoparietal cortical areas, and subcortical limbic centers (predominantly the amygdala), which, however, differ characteristically from those in individuals exhibiting reactive-impulsive aggression. According to Yang and Raine (2008), core psychopathy deficits impair the 1) evaluation of positive or negative reinforcers (OFC/vmPFC), 2) processing of affective stimuli plus their context (amygdala, hippocampus), 3) assessment of emotional salience and regulation of emotional responses (ACC), and 4) pain and empathy system (insula, superior temporal gyrus).

Successful Versus Unsuccessful Psychopaths

The general assumption that psychopathy is characterized by a hyporesponsivity of autonomic stress response has been questioned by studies on distinct subgroups of criminal psychopaths who either have been convicted for their crimes ("unsuccessful" psychopaths) or have remained undiscovered so far ("successful" psychopaths). In one study, these subgroups were compared with respect to their autonomic stress reactivity and executive functioning (Ishikawa et al. 2001). Compared with control subjects, unsuccessful psychopaths showed reduced cardiovascular stress reactivity, which is in line with previous research. However, successful psychopaths demonstrated even greater autonomic reactivity and stronger executive function than both the unsuccessful psychopaths and the control subjects.

Both autonomic and executive functional deficits can result from structural damage to the prefrontal cortex (Bechara et al. 1997). Therefore, in another study with the same sample of psychopaths as in the Ishikawa et al. (2001) study, subjects were tested for prefrontal volumes (Yang et al. 2005). The investigators found a more than 22% reduction in prefrontal gray matter volumes specific to the unsuccessful psychopaths compared with the control subjects and successful psychopaths. Decreased prefrontal volume may render unsuccessful psychopaths particularly susceptible to poor decision making, impulsive aggression, and unregulated antisocial behavior, thus raising the probability of "getting caught." In contrast, successful psychopaths showed a relative sparing of prefrontal gray matter that might provide them with normal executive functioning and intact capacities for the control of affective states. Together with high autonomic functioning, this may allow successful psychopaths to react sensitively to environmental cues signaling danger and, therefore, to avoid conviction (Ishikawa et al. 2001; Yang et al. 2005). Successful psychopaths appear to be good at internalizing anger and response inhibition. They show no impairment in intelligence, insight, understanding of norms, or motor empathy, as opposed to emotional empathy, which is characteristically lacking. Major deficits in these individuals appear to be lack of concern for the pain and negative emotions of others and inability to take into account the long-range negative consequences of their behavior.

NEUROPHARMACOLOGICAL AND GENETIC DEFICITS IN INDIVIDUALS WITH ANTISOCIAL PERSONALITY DISORDER

Increased impulsivity and impulsive aggression have long been associated with a central serotonin deficit both in healthy subjects and in various clinical populations as assessed by a variety of methods (Bjork et al. 2000; Bond et al. 2001; R. Lee and Coccaro 2001; Lesch and Merschdorf 2000; Manuck et al. 2002; Marsh et al. 2002; Placidi et al. 2001; Soloff et al. 2000; Stanley et al. 2000). Furthermore, a number of studies have described a reduced serotonergic modulation of frontal brain areas in the context of impulsivity and aggression (Frankle et al. 2005; New et al. 2002, 2004; Rubia et al. 2005; Soloff et al. 2003). These studies provide neurofunctional evidence for the suggested link between OFC/ACC activity, serotonin function, and inhibitory control. More specifically, they suggest that OFC and adjacent regions exert an inhibitory effect on impulsive aggression through a serotonergic mechanism.

A genetic contribution to the relationship between serotonin function and impulsive aggression is supported by numerous studies that demonstrate an influence exerted by various serotonin-related gene polymorphisms. Most studies refer to the serotonin transporter gene (Beitchman et al. 2003; Davidge et al. 2004; J. H. Lee et al. 2003; Retz et al. 2004; Zalsman et al. 2001) and the tryptophan hydroxylase (TPH) gene (Hennig et al. 2005; New et al. 1998; Rujescu et al. 2003; Staner et al. 2002; Zill et al. 2004). The enzyme TPH is involved in the synthesis of serotonin from the amino acid tryptophan, whereas the serotonin transporter removes serotonin from the synaptic cleft. Another enzyme, MAO-A, selectively degrades serotonin, norepinephrine, and dopamine following reuptake from the synaptic cleft, and therefore plays a major role in the regulation of serotonin levels. As well, the allelic variant of the MAO-A–uVNTR (upstream variable number of tandem repeats) polymorphism coding for high MAO-A activity has been reported to have a positive association with self-reported aggression and impulsivity in men (Manuck et al. 2002).

These findings may be indicative of a higher genotypic risk for impulsivity and aggression in males, conferred by serotonin-related polymorphisms. Caspi et al. (2002) were the first to demonstrate that a polymorphism in the MAO-A gene (*MAOA*) moderates the capacity of experienced abuse in childhood to bring about the "cycle of violence," in which being maltreated as a child increases a person's risk for becoming the perpetrator of violence later in life. Childhood maltreatment led to increased adult violence only in those children whose genotype conferred low levels of *MAOA* expression, while children with high-activity *MAOA* genotype were protected against the negative effects of the same experience. This gene–environment interaction was confirmed by a replication study with a new sample of 975 seven-year-old boys and a meta-analysis across four studies (Kim-Cohen et al. 2006). A study by Passamonti et al. (2006) showed a significantly greater response in the right lateral OFC for the high-activity allele carriers (*MAOA-H*) compared with the low-activity allele carriers (*MAOA-L*).

Passamonti et al. (2006) concluded that genetic variation in the serotonin system drives the brain response related to dispositional impulsivity. These findings raise the possibility that inconsistent results regarding the correlation between prefrontal activations and dispositional impulsivity (Brown et al. 2006; Horn et al. 2003) might be partially related to genetic variations in *MAOA*. In support of this suggestion, the positive correlation between impulsivity and lateral OFC in *MAOA-H* carriers is consistent with the findings of Horn et al. (2003), whereas the negative association between impulsivity and lateral OFC in *MAOA-L* carriers fits the results of Brown et al. (2006) during the face-matching task. Recently, Meyer-Lindenberg et al. (2006) found that carriers of

MAOA-L had volume reductions averaging around 8% relative to the volume in *MAOA-H* subjects in the rostral and dorsal ACC, amygdala, insula, and hypothalamus. With fMRI, it was shown that *MAOA-L* carriers had increased amygdala activation and diminished reactivity of regulatory prefrontal areas (rostral ACC, OFC) compared with *MAOA-H* carriers in a face-matching task.

Meyer-Lindenberg et al. (2006) postulate that their data identify differences in limbic circuitry for emotion regulation and cognitive control that may be involved in the association of *MAOA* with impulsive aggression. However, they also emphasize that their study was performed on psychiatrically healthy volunteers, who were not characterized by increased levels of aggressive or violent behavior, so that they were not studying the relationship of *MAOA* and violence per se. Nonetheless, the work of Meyer-Lindenberg et al. (2006) is the first neuroimaging study that relates impulsive aggression to *MAOA* genotype–dependent reactivity of the neural circuitry of emotion regulation.

Importantly, the findings of Meyer-Lindenberg et al. (2006) demonstrate a possible neural substrate of the gene–environment interaction observed by Caspi et al. (2002). It is plausible to suggest that genetic risk factors act through brain regions implicated in the regulation of emotional behavior and modulated by serotonergic inputs to bring about individual differences in the vulnerability to environmental stress. However, it seems implausible to assume that the described differences in brain function are solely based on genetic variation in *MAOA*. For example, amygdala hyperreactivity to emotionally provocative stimuli in normal volunteers has also been demonstrated as a consequence of genetic variation in the serotonin transporter (Hariri and Holmes 2006), suggesting the need for considering gene–gene effects on emotion.

SUMMARY

The neurobiological data regarding APD and psychopathy confirm the hypothesis that two major types of antisocial behavior exist—namely, reactive-impulsive aggression and proactive-instrumental aggression. While the former best describes the majority of violent criminals, the latter is characteristic of psychopaths. Both groups are characterized by dysfunctional autonomic responses, disturbances of the serotonin system, and deficits in the interaction of limbic cortical-frontal and subcortical centers in the context of impulse control, empathy, and the processing of affects and emotions, particularly fear and anger. However, both groups differ remarkably in the specific kinds of disturbances and deficits.

In antisocial individuals characterized by a high degree of impulsive-reactive aggression, autonomic responses to unpleasant stimuli are significantly increased. From a neurobiological perspective, there is strong evidence that structural or functional impairments (i.e., volume loss and decreased activity) of the frontal cortex, especially of the OFC and vmPFC, are associated with impulsive aggression and violent behavior. This line of evidence goes along with increased activity of subcortical areas, including the amygdala.

In psychopaths characterized by proactive-instrumental aggression and psychopathy, reduced autonomic responses to aversive stimuli are found, indicating lack of fear, deficits in processing of negative emotional information, and generally emotional hyporesponsivity. However, whereas the majority of studies, using aversive conditioning, have reported reduced activation of limbic centers in psychopaths compared with control subjects, others have found enhanced activations in the amygdala, OFC, and dorsolateral prefrontal cortex during emotional learning. Most remarkably, in most studies, psychopaths exhibit no impairment in intellectual-cognitive abilities, empathy, or theory of mind; they simply appear to have no concern for the pain and emotions of others.

While these latter findings hold for "unsuccessful" psychopaths, "successful" psychopaths demonstrate an even greater autonomic reactivity and stronger executive function than both unsuccessful psychopaths and control subjects. They appear to be specifically good at internalizing anger and response inhibition and show no impairment in intelligence, insight, or understanding of norms, which makes them particularly dangerous. Their specific neurobiological deficits remain to be elucidated.

Increased impulsivity and impulsive aggression are generally associated with deficits in serotonin metabolism. Most studies refer to the serotonin transporter gene and the enzyme MAO-A. Genetic variation in the serotonin system appears to drive the brain response related to dispositional impulsivity. Decreased serotonin *and* increased testosterone are found in violent individuals, but not increased testosterone *alone*. Testosterone appears to be linked more specifically to dominance, while a combination of dominance and frustration is likely to lead to increased impulsivity and violence.

Conclusion

Individuals with borderline personality disorder and those with antisocial personality disorder of a psychopathic or nonpsychopathic nature reveal characteristic abnormalities in their autonomic responses, dysfunctions in the interaction of cortical and subcortical centers, and deficits in the serotonin system. BPD patients and nonpsychopathic individuals with reactive-impulsive aggression exhibit many commonalities—namely, hyperresponsivity of the HPA axis in combination with heightened responses to emotional (especially unpleasant) stimuli, decreased level of serotonin, and characteristic polymorphisms in the serotonin transporter gene and the MAO-A enzyme, but also smaller volumes of frontal brain areas and hippocampus, decreased frontal metabolism (including OFC and ACC), and increased amygdala activity, which may explain the deficits in impulse control characteristic of both groups. In psychopaths, we mostly find decreased autonomic responses and deficits in emotionality, including emotional learning and empathy, while intellectual and cognitive functions are unimpaired.

Despite these findings, there are many inconsistencies, especially with respect to the activity of cortical limbic areas. These inconsistencies could be the result of 1) heterogeneity of disorders (BPD, as well as APD, most probably comprises several subgroups); 2) comorbidities; 3) poor or inconsistent diagnoses; 4) small sample sizes; 5) methodological and technical insufficiencies, especially with respect to relating fMRI data to neuroanatomical boundaries; or 6) lack of understanding of the dynamics of the interaction between cognitive and limbic centers as well as between cortical and subcortical limbic centers. Thus, we are far from understanding the neurobiological basis of personality disorders beyond the superficial insight presented in this chapter. However, combined fMRI-EEG techniques are rapidly evolving, in both their spatial and their temporal resolution, and the techniques to better understand brain dynamics, as well as the diagnostic means and experimental-empirical settings, are becoming much more sophisticated.

Key Clinical Concepts

- ◆ From the perspective of psychoneuroscience, personality disorders are associated with structural and functional deficits of limbic and paralimbic brain centers, their interactions among themselves, and cognitive-executive brain centers.
- ◆ Neuroimaging studies are helpful to understand the neural basis of the relationship between individual trauma and borderline personality disorder, demonstrating a network of brain regions involved in emotional regulation that includes the amygdala, hippocampus, and prefrontal cortex.

- ◆ Research has strongly implicated the serotonin transporter gene *5HTT* in the development of BPD, and shorter alleles of this gene have been associated with lower levels of serotonin and greater impulsive aggression; genes for dopamine and MAO-A may yet prove to have an etiological role. Genetic findings further consolidate the evidence that there are biological (not only psychological) differences between between patients with and without BPD.

- ◆ There is strong evidence that a structural or functional impairment of the frontal cortex, especially orbitofrontal cortex and ventromedial prefrontal cortex, is associated with impulsive aggression and violent behavior. The neurobiological data regarding antisocial personality disorder and psychopathy confirm the hypothesis that two major types of antisocial behavior exist: reactive-impulsive aggression on the one hand, and proactive-instrumental aggression on the other.

- ◆ Individuals with BPD and those exhibiting antisocial personality disorders of a psychopathic or nonpsychopathic nature reveal characteristic abnormalities in their autonomic responses; dysfunctions in the interaction of cortical and subcortical centers; and deficits in the serotonergic system.

Suggested Readings

Gabbard GO: Mind, brain, and personality disorders. Am J Psychiatry 162:648–655, 2005. [A highly readable overview bridging neuroscience and personality disorders.]

Herman JL, Perry JC, Van der Kolk BA: Childhood trauma in borderline personality disorder. Am J Psychiatry 146:490–495, 1989. [An important, often-cited work on developmental aspects of borderline personality disorders.]

Rosenthal MZ, Gratz KL, Kosson DS, et al: Borderline personal disorder and emotional responding: a review of the research literature. Clin Psychol Rev 28:75–91, 2008. [An excellent review on that topic summarizing most recent studies in a highly precise way.]

Silbersweig D, Clarkin JF, Goldstein M, et al: Failure of frontolimbic inhibitory function in the context of negative emotion in borderline personality disorder. Am J Psychiatry 164:1834–1841, 2007. [A beautifully designed study with impressive results.]

Yang Y, Raine A: Functional neuroanatomy of psychopathy. Psychiatry 7:133–136, 2008. [An excellent introduction to the neurobiology of psychopathy.]

References

American Psychiatric Association: Diagnostic and Statistical Manual of Mental Disorders, 4th Edition. Washington, DC, American Psychiatric Association, 1994

Barratt ES, Stanford MS, Dowdy L, et al: Impulsive and premeditated aggression: a factor analysis of self-reported acts. Psychiatry Res 86:163–173, 1999

Beblo T, Driessen M, Mertens M, et al: Functional MRI correlates of the recall of unresolved life events in borderline personality disorder. Psychol Med 36:845–856, 2006

Bechara A, Damasio H, Tranel D, et al: Deciding advantageously before knowing the advantageous strategy. Science 275:1293–1295, 1997

Beitchman JH, Davidge KM, Kennedy JL, et al: The serotonin transporter gene in aggressive children with and without ADHD and nonaggressive matched controls. Ann N Y Acad Sci 1008:248–251, 2003

Best M, Williams JM, Coccaro EF: Evidence for a dysfunctional prefrontal circuit in patients with an impulsive aggressive disorder. Proc Natl Acad Sci U S A 99:8448–8453, 2002

Birbaumer N, Veit R, Lotze M, et al: Deficient fear conditioning in psychopathy: a functional magnetic resonance imaging study. Arch Gen Psychiatry 62:799–805, 2005

Bjork JM, Dougherty DM, Moeller FG, et al: Differential behavioral effects of plasma tryptophan depletion and loading in aggressive and nonaggressive men. Neuropsychopharmacology 22:357–369, 2000

Blair KS, Newman C, Mitchell DG, et al: Differentiating among prefrontal substrates in psychopathy: neuropsychological test findings. Neuropsychology 20:153–165, 2006

Blair RJ: Responding to the emotions of others: dissociating forms of empathy through the study of typical and psychiatric populations. Conscious Cogn 14:698–718, 2005

Blair RJ, Peschardt KS, Budhani S, et al: The development of psychopathy. J Child Psychol Psychiatry 47:262–276, 2006

Bond AJ, Wingrove J, Critchlow DG: Tryptophan depletion increases aggression in women during the premenstrual phase. Psychopharmacology (Berl) 156:477–480, 2001

Brambilla P, Soloff PH, Sala M, et al: Anatomical MRI study of borderline personality disorder patients. Psychiatry Res 131:125–133, 2004

Brown SM, Manuck SB, Flory JD, et al: Neural basis of individual differences in impulsivity: contributions of corticolimbic circuits for behavioral arousal and control. Emotion 6:239–245, 2006

Buchheim A, Erk S, George C, et al: Neural correlates of attachment trauma in borderline personality disorder: a functional magnetic resonance imaging study. Psychiatry Res 163:223–235, 2008

Budhani S, Richell RA, Blair RJR: Impaired reversal but intact acquisition: probabilistic response reversal deficits in adult individuals with psychopathy. J Abnorm Psychol 115:552–558, 2006

Bufkin JL, Luttrell VR: Neuroimaging studies of aggressive and violent behavior. Current findings and implications for criminology and criminal justice. Trauma Violence Abuse 6:176–191, 2005

Caspi A, McClay J, Moffitt TE, et al: Role of genotype in the cycle of violence in maltreated children. Science 297:851–854, 2002

Chanen AM, Velakoulis D, Carison K, et al: Orbitofrontal, amygdala and hippocampal volumes in teenagers with first-presentation borderline personality disorder. Psychiatry Res 163:116–125, 2008

Coccaro EF: Intermittent explosive disorder. Curr Psychiatry Rep 2:42–60, 2003

Coccaro EF, McCloskey MS, Fitzgerald DA, et al: Amygdala and orbitofrontal reactivity to social threat in individuals with impulsive aggression. Biol Psychiatry 62:168–178, 2007

Davidge KM, Atkinson L, Douglas L, et al: Association of the serotonin transporter and 5HT1D beta receptor genes with extreme, persistent and pervasive aggressive behaviour in children. Psychiatr Genet 14:143–146, 2004

Deeley Q, Daly E, Surguladze S, et al: Facial emotion processing in criminal psychopathy: preliminary functional magnetic resonance imaging study. Br J Psychiatry 189:533–539, 2006

de la Fuente JM, Lotstra F, Goldman S, et al: Temporal glucose metabolism in borderline personality disorder. Psychiatry Res 55:237–245, 1994

Dolan M, Fullam R: Theory of mind and mentalizing ability in antisocial personality disorders with and without psychopathy. Psychol Med 34:1093–1102, 2004

Donegan NH, Sanislow CA, Blumberg HP, et al: Amygdala hyperreactivity in borderline personality disorder: implications for emotional dysregulation. Biol Psychiatry 54:1284–1293, 2003

Dougherty DD, Rauch SL, Deckersbach T, et al: Ventromedial prefrontal cortex and amygdala dysfunction during an anger induction positron emission tomography study in patients with major depressive disorder with anger attacks. Arch Gen Psychiatry 61:795–804, 2004

Driessen M, Herrmann J, Stahl K, et al: Magnetic resonance imaging volumes of the hippocampus and the amygdala in women with borderline personality disorder and early traumatization. Arch Gen Psychiatry 57:1115–1122, 2000

Driessen M, Beblo T, Mertens M, et al: Posttraumatic stress disorder and fMRI activation patterns of traumatic memory in patients with borderline personality disorder. Biol Psychiatry 55:603–611, 2004

Ebner-Priemer UW, Badeck S, Beckmann C, et al: Affective dysregulation and dissociative experience in female patients with borderline personality disorder: a startle response study. J Psychiatr Res 39:85–92, 2005

Fecteau S, Pascual-Leone A, Théoret H: Psychopathy and the mirror neuron system: preliminary findings from a non-psychiatric sample. Psychiatry Res 160:137–144, 2008

Frankle WG, Lombardo I, New AS, et al: Brain serotonin transporter distribution in subjects with impulsive aggressivity: a positron emission study with [11C]McN 5652. Am J Psychiatry 162:915–923, 2005

George C, West M: The Adult Attachment Projective: measuring individual differences in attachment security using projective methodology, in Comprehensive Handbook of Psychological Assessment, Vol 2: Personality Assessment. Edited by Hilsenroth M. New York, Wiley, 2003, pp 431–448

Hare RD: Psychopathy and physiological activity during anticipation of an aversive stimulus in a distraction paradigm. Psychopathology 19:266–271, 1982

Hare RD: The Hare Psychopathy Checklist–Revised. Toronto, Ontario, Canada, Multi-Health Systems, 1991

Hare RD, Neuman CS: Psychopathy as a clinical and empirical construct. Annu Rev Clin Psychol 4:217–246, 2008

Hariri A, Holmes A: Genetics of emotional regulation: the role of the serotonin transporter in neural function. Trends Cogn Sci 10:182–191, 2006

Hegerl U, Stein M, Mulert C, et al: EEG-vigilance differences between patients with borderline personality disorder, patients with obsessive-compulsive disorder and healthy controls. Eur Arch Psychiatry Clin Neurosci 253:137–143, 2008

Hennig J, Reuter M, Netter P, et al: Two types of aggression are differentially related to serotonergic activity and the A779C TPH polymorphism. Behav Neurosci 119:16–25, 2005

Herpertz SC, Kunert HJ, Schwenger UB, et al: Affective responsiveness in borderline personality disorder: a psychophysiological approach. Am J Psychiatry 156:1550–1556, 1999

Herpertz SC, Schwenger UB, Kunert HJ, et al: Emotional responses in patients with borderline as compared with avoidant personality disorder. J Pers Disord 14:339–351, 2000

Herpertz SC, Dietrich TM, Wenning B, et al: Evidence of abnormal amygdala functioning in borderline personality disorder: a functional MRI study. Biol Psychiatry 50:292–298, 2001a

Herpertz SC, Werth U, Lukas G, et al: Emotion in criminal offenders with psychopathy and borderline personality disorder. Arch Gen Psychiatry 58:737–745, 2001b

Horn NR, Dolan M, Elliott R, et al: Response inhibition and impulsivity: an fMRI study. Neuropsychologia 41:1959–1966, 2003

Irle E, Lange C, Weniger G, et al: Size abnormalities of the superior parietal cortices are related to dissociation in borderline personality disorder. Psychiatry Res 156:139–149, 2007

Ishikawa SS, Raine A, Lencz T, et al: Autonomic stress reactivity and executive functions in successful and unsuccessful criminal psychopaths from the community. J Abnorm Psychol 110:423–432, 2001

Jovev M, Garner B, Phillips L, et al: An MRI study of pituitary volume and para-suicidal behavior in teenagers with first-presentation borderline personality disorder. Psychiatry Res 162:273–277, 2008

Juengling FD, Schmahl C, Hesslinger B, et al: Positron emission tomography in female patients with borderline personality disorder. J Psychiatr Res 37:109–115, 2003

Kernberg OF: Severe Personality Disorders: Psychotherapeutic Strategies. New Haven, CT, Yale University Press, 1984

Kiehl KA, Smith AM, Hare RD, et al: Limbic abnormalities in affective processing by criminal psychopaths as revealed by functional magnetic resonance imaging. Biol Psychiatry 50:677–684, 2001

Kim-Cohen J, Caspi A, Taylor A, et al: MAOA, maltreatment, and gene-environment interaction predicting children's mental health: new evidence and a meta-analysis. Mol Psychiatry 11:903–913, 2006

King JA, Blair RJR, Mitchell DG, et al: Doing the right thing: a common neural circuit for appropriate violent or compassionate behavior. Neuroimage 30:1069–1076, 2006

Koenigsberg HW, Harvey PD, Mitropoulou V, et al: Characterizing affective instability in borderline personality disorder. Am J Psychiatry 159:784–788, 2002

Kringelbach ML, Rolls ET: The functional neuroanatomy of the human orbitofrontal cortex: evidence from neuroimaging and neuropsychology. Prog Neurobiol 72:341–372, 2004

Laakso MP, Gunning-Dixon F, Vaurio O, et al: Prefrontal volumes in habitually violent subjects with antisocial personality disorder and type 2 alcoholism. Psychiatry Res 114:95–102, 2002

Lang PJ, Bradley MM, Cuthbert BN: Emotion and motivation: measuring affective perception. J Clin Neurophysiol 15:397–408, 1998

Lang PJ, Davis M, Ohman A: Fear and anxiety: animal models and human cognitive psychophysiology. J Affect Disord 61:137–159, 2000

Lee JH, Kim HT, Hyun DS: Possible association between serotonin transporter promoter region polymorphism and impulsivity in Koreans. Psychiatry Res 118:19–24, 2003

Lee R, Coccaro E: The neuropsychopharmacology of criminality and aggression. Can J Psychiatry 46:35–44, 2001

Lesch KP, Merschdorf U: Impulsivity, aggression, and serotonin: a molecular psychobiological perspective. Behav Sci Law 18:581–604, 2000

Levenston GK, Patrick CJ, Bradley MM, et al: The psychopath as observer: emotion and attention in picture processing. J Abnorm Psychol 109:373–385, 2000

Lotze M, Veit R, Anders S, et al: Evidence for a different role of the ventral and dorsal medial prefrontal cortex for social reactive aggression: an interactive fMRI study. Neuroimage 34:470–478, 2007

Lykken DT: A study of anxiety in the sociopathic personality. J Abnorm Soc Psychol 55:6–10, 1957

Lyoo IK, Han MH, Cho DY: A brain MRI study in subjects with borderline personality disorder. J Affect Disord 50:235–243, 1998

Mann JJ: Neurobiology of suicidal behaviour. Nat Rev Neurosci 4:819–828, 2003

Manuck SB, Flory JD, Muldoon MF, et al: Central nervous system serotonergic responsivity and aggressive disposition in men. Physiol Behav 77:705–709, 2002

Marsh DM, Dougherty DD, Moeller FG, et al: Laboratory measured aggressive behavior of women: acute tryptophan depletion and augmentation. Neuropsychopharmacology 26:660–671, 2002

Meyer-Lindenberg A, Buckholtz JW, Kolachana BR, et al: Neural mechanisms of genetic risk for impulsivity and violence in humans. Proc Natl Acad Sci USA 103:6269–6274, 2006

Minzenberg MJ, Fan J, New AS, et al: Fronto-limbic dysfunction in response to facial emotion in borderline personality disorder: an event-related fMRI study. Psychiatry Res 155:231–243, 2007

Minzenberg MJ, Fan J, New AS, et al: Frontolimbic structural changes in borderline personality disorder. J Psychiatr Res 42:727–733, 2008

Mitchell DG, Colledge E, Leonard A, et al: Risky decisions and response reversal: is there evidence of orbitofrontal cortex dysfunction in psychopathic individuals? Neuropsychologia 40:2013–2022, 2002

Mitchell DG, Avny SB, Blair RJ: Divergent patterns of aggressive and neurocognitive characteristics in acquired versus developmental psychopathy. Neurocase 12:164–178, 2006a

Mitchell DG, Fine C, Richell RA, et al: Instrumental learning and relearning in individuals with psychopathy and in patients with lesions involving the amygdala or orbitofrontal cortex. Neuropsychology 20:280–289, 2006b

Müller JL, Sommer M, Wagner V, et al: Abnormalities in emotion processing within cortical and subcortical regions in criminal psychopaths: evidence from a functional magnetic resonance imaging study using pictures with emotional content. Biol Psychiatry 54:152–162, 2003

Müller JL, Sommer M, Weber T, et al: Disturbed prefrontal and temporal brain function during emotion and cognition interaction in criminal psychopathy. Behav Sci Law 26:131–150, 2008

Munro GES, Dywan J, Harris GT, et al: Response inhibition in psychopathy: the frontal N2 and P3. Neurosci Lett 418:149–153, 2007

New AS, Gelernter J, Yovell Y, et al: Tryptophan hydroxylase genotype is associated with impulsive-aggression measures: a preliminary study. Am J Med Genet 81:13–17, 1998

New AS, Hazlett EA, Buchsbaum MS, et al: Blunted prefrontal cortical 18fluorodeoxyglucose positron emission tomography response to meta-chlorophenylpiperazine in impulsive aggression. Arch Gen Psychiatry 59:621–629, 2002

New AS, Buchsbaum MS, Hazlett EA, et al: Fluoxetine increases relative metabolic rate in prefrontal cortex in impulsive aggression. Psychopharmacology (Berl) 176:451–458, 2004

Newman JP, Kosson DS: Passive avoidance learning in psychopathic and non-psychopathic offenders. J Abnorm Psychol 95:252–256, 1986

Passamonti L, Fera F, Magariello A, et al: Monoamine oxidase–A genetic variations influence brain activity associated with inhibitory control: new insight into the neural correlates of impulsivity. Biol Psychiatry 59:334–340, 2006

Pastor MC, Moltó J, Vila J, et al: Startle reflex modulation, affective ratings and autonomic reactivity in incarcerated Spanish psychopaths. Psychophysiology 40:934–938, 2003

Patrick CJ, Bradley MM, Lang PJ: Emotion in the criminal psychopath: startle reflex modulation. J Abnorm Psychol 102:82–92, 1993

Peterson BS, Kane MJ, Alexander GM, et al: An event-related functional MRI study comparing interference effects in the Simon and Stroop tasks. Brain Res Cogn Brain Res 13:427–440, 2002

Philipsen A, Feige B, Al-Shajlawi A, et al: Increased delta power and discrepancies in objective and subjective sleep measurements in borderline personality disorder. J Psychiatr Res 39:489–498, 2005

Phillips ML, Drevets WC, Rauch SL, et al: Neurobiology of emotion perception, I: the neural basis of normal emotion perception. Biol Psychiatry 54:504–514, 2003

Placidi GP, Oquendo MA, Malone KM, et al: Aggressivity, suicide attempts, and depression: relationship to cerebrospinal fluid monoamine metabolite levels. Biol Psychiatry 50:783–791, 2001

Raine A, Buchsbaum MS, Stanley J, et al: Selective reductions in prefrontal glucose metabolism in murderers. Biol Psychiatry 36:365–373, 1994

Raine A, Buchsbaum M, Lacasse L: Brain abnormalities in murderers indicated by positron emission tomography. Biol Psychiatry 42:495–508, 1997

Raine A, Lencz T, Bihrle S, et al: Reduced prefrontal gray matter volume and reduced autonomic activity in antisocial personality disorder. Arch Gen Psychiatry 57:119–127, 2000

Retz W, Junginger P, Supprian T, et al: Association of serotonin transporter promoter gene polymorphism with violence: relation with personality disorders, impulsivity, and childhood ADHD psychopathology. Behav Sci Law 22:415–425, 2004

Rosenthal MZ, Gratz KL, Kosson DS, et al: Borderline personality disorder and emotional responding: a review of the research literature. Clin Psychol Rev 28:75–91, 2008

Rubia K, Lee F, Cleare AJ, et al: Tryptophan depletion reduces right inferior prefrontal activation during response inhibition in fast, event-related fMRI. Psychopharmacology (Berl) 179:791–803, 2005

Ruchsow M, Walter H, Buchheim A, et al: Electrophysiological correlates of error processing in borderline personality disorder. Biol Psychol 72:133–140, 2006

Ruchsow M, Groen G, Kiefer M, et al: Response inhibition in borderline personality disorder: event-related potentials in a Go/Nogo task. J Neural Transm 115:127–133, 2008

Rujescu D, Giegling I, Sato T, et al: Genetic variations in tryptophan hydroxylase in suicidal behavior: analysis and meta-analysis. Biol Psychiatry 54:465–473, 2003

Rusch N, van Elst LT, Ludaescher P, et al: A voxel-based morphometric MRI study in female patients with borderline personality disorder. Neuroimage 20:385–392, 2003

Russ MJ, Campbell SS, Kakuma T, et al: EEG theta activity and pain insensitivity in self-injurious borderline patients. Psychiatry Res 89:201–214, 1999

Schmahl C, Greffrath W, Baumgartner U, et al: Differential nociceptive deficits in patients with borderline personality disorder and self-injurious behavior: laser-evoked potentials, spatial discrimination of noxious stimuli, and pain ratings. Pain 110:470–479, 2004

Schneider F, Habel U, Kessler C, et al: Functional imaging of conditioned aversive emotional responses in antisocial personality disorder. Neuropsychobiology 42:192–201, 2000

Schnell K, Dietrich T, Schnitker R, et al: Processing of autobiographical memory retrieval cues in borderline personality disorder. J Affect Disord 97:253–259, 2007

Silbersweig D, Clarkin JF, Goldstein M, et al: Failure of frontolimbic inhibitory function in the context of negative emotion in borderline personality disorder. Am J Psychiatry 164:1832–1841, 2007

Soloff PH, Lynch KG, Moss HG: Serotonin, impulsivity and alcohol use disorders in the older adolescent: a psychobiological study. Alcohol Clin Exp Res 24:1609–1619, 2000

Soloff PH, Meltzer CC, Becker C, et al: Impulsivity and prefrontal hypometabolism in borderline personality disorder. Psychiatry Res 123:153–163, 2003

Staner L, Uyanik G, Correa H, et al: A dimensional impulsive-aggressive phenotype is associated with the A218C polymorphism of the tryptophan hydroxylase gene: a pilot study in well-characterized impulsive inpatients. Am J Med Genet 114:553–557, 2002

Stanley B, Molcho A, Stanley M, et al: Association of aggressive behavior with altered serotonergic function in patients who are not suicidal. Am J Psychiatry 157:609–614, 2000

Sterzer P, Stadler C, Krebs A, et al: Abnormal neural responses to emotional visual stimuli in adolescents with conduct disorder. Biol Psychiatry 57:7–15, 2005

Tebartz van Elst LT, Thiel T, Hesslinger B, et al: Subtle prefrontal neuropathology in a pilot magnetic resonance spectroscopy study in patients with borderline personality disorder. J Neuropsychiatry Clin Neurosci 13:511–514, 2001

Tebartz van Elst L, Hesslinger B, Thiel T, et al: Frontolimbic brain abnormalities in patients with borderline personality disorder: a volumetric magnetic resonance imaging study. Biol Psychiatry 54:163–171, 2003

Veit R, Flor H, Erb M, et al: Brain circuits involved in emotional learning in antisocial behavior and social phobia in humans. Neurosci Lett 328:233–236, 2002

Völlm B, Richardson P, Stirling J, et al: Neurobiological substrates of antisocial and borderline personality disorder: preliminary results of a functional fMRI study. Crim Behav Ment Health 14:39–54, 2004

Watson S, Chilton R, Fairchild H, et al: Association between childhood trauma and dissociation among patients with borderline personality disorder. Aust N Z J Psychiatry 40:478–481, 2006

World Health Organization: International Statistical Classification of Diseases and Related Health Problems, 10th Revision. Geneva, World Health Organization, 1992

Yang Y, Raine A: Functional neuroanatomy of psychopathy. Psychiatry 7:133–136, 2008

Yang Y, Raine A, Lencz T, et al: Volume reduction in prefrontal gray matter in unsuccessful criminal psychopaths. Biol Psychiatry 57:1103–1108, 2005

Zalsman G, Frisch A, Bromberg M, et al: Family based association study of serotonin transporter promoter in suicidal adolescents: no association with suicidality but possible role in violence traits. Am J Med Genet 105:239–245, 2001

Zetzsche T, Preuss UW, Bondy B, et al: 5-HT1A receptor gene C –1019 G polymorphism and amygdala volume in borderline personality disorder. Genes Brain Behav 7:306–313, 2008

Zill P, Büttner A, Eisenmenger W, et al: Single nucleotide polymorphism and haplotype analysis of a novel tryptophan hydroxylase isoform (TPH2) gene in suicide victims. Biol Psychiatry 56:581–586, 2004

CHAPTER 4

The Shedler-Westen Assessment Procedure

Making Personality Diagnosis
Clinically Meaningful

Jonathan Shedler, Ph.D.
Drew Westen, Ph.D.

One of the greatest challenges facing psychiatry and psychology is the growing schism between science and practice. The schism is especially pronounced in conceptualizing and assessing personality. For most clinical practitioners, personality diagnosis is a task requiring

This chapter is adapted, with permission, from previously published material: Shedler J, Westen D: "Personality Diagnosis With the Shedler-Westen Assessment Procedure (SWAP): Bridging the Gulf Between Science and Practice," in *Psychodynamic Diagnostic Manual (PDM)*. Edited by PDM Task Force. Silver Spring, MD, Alliance of Psychoanalytic Organizations, 2006, pp. 17–69; Shedler J, Westen D: "The Shedler-Westen Assessment Procedure (SWAP): Making Personality Diagnosis Clinically Meaningful." *Journal of Personality Assessment* 89:41–55, 2007.

judgment and expertise. Expert clinicians consider a wide range of psychological data, attending not only to *what* patients say but also to *how* they say it, and drawing complexly determined inferences from patients' accounts of their lives and relationships, from their manner of interacting with the clinician, and from their own emotional reactions to the patient (Westen and Arkowitz-Westen 1998).

For example, clinicians tend *not* to assess lack of empathy, a diagnostic criterion for narcissistic personality disorder, by administering self-report questionnaires or asking patients direct questions (Westen 1997). Not only are narcissistic patients unlikely to report their own lack of empathy, they may well describe themselves as caring people and wonderful friends. An initial sign of lack of empathy on the part of the patient is often a subtle sense on the part of the clinician of being interchangeable or replaceable—of being treated as a sounding board rather than as a fellow human being (for empirical evidence, see Betan et al. 2005; for clinical discussions, see Kernberg 1975; McWilliams 1994). The clinician might go on to consider whether she consistently feels this way with this particular patient and whether such feelings are characteristic for her in her role as therapist. She might then become aware that the patient tends to describe others more in terms of the functions they serve or the needs they fulfill than in terms of who they are as people. She might further consider whether and how these issues dovetail with the facts the patient has provided about his life, with the problems that led him to treatment, with information gleaned from family members or other collateral contacts, and so on. This type of thinking, reasoning, and inference lies at the heart of psychodynamic approaches to understanding people.

It is just such clinical judgment and inference that many researchers eschew. As successive editions of the *Diagnostic and Statistical Manual of Mental Disorders* (DSM) have minimized the role of clinical inference, investigators have increasingly treated personality diagnosis as a technical task of tabulating signs and symptoms, with relatively little consideration for how the signs and symptoms fit together, the psychological functions they serve, their meanings, the developmental trajectory that gave rise to them, or the present-day factors that serve to maintain them. Indeed, the diagnostic "gold standard" in personality disorder (PD) research is the structured interview. Such assessment methods are designed to achieve interrater reliability by minimizing the role of clinical judgment and substituting standardized questions and decision rules. Indeed, the interviews are typically administered by research assistants or trainees, not by experienced clinicians.

DSM and structured assessment procedures evolved as they did for good reason. Prior to DSM-III (American Psychiatric Association 1980), psychiatric diagnosis was unsystematic, overly subjective, and of questionable scientific merit. It sometimes revealed more about the clinician's background and theoretical predilections than it did about the patient's personality dispositions. Structured assessment methods evolved in the service of science and in reaction against the unsystematic diagnostic methods of the past. In the evolution of personality diagnosis from a largely subjective, clinical enterprise to a largely technical, research-driven enterprise, much has been gained and much has been lost. The solution to the science–practice schism cannot be to turn back the clock and abandon the scientific advances of the past decades. Nor can it be to disregard the cumulative insights of generations of clinical observers. The solution, rather, may be a marriage of the best aspects of clinical observation and empirical rigor.

This chapter describes the Shedler-Westen Assessment Procedure (SWAP), an approach to personality assessment designed to *harness* clinical judgment and inference rather than eliminate it, and to combine the best features of the clinical and empirical traditions. It provides a means of assessing personality that is both clinically relevant and empirically rigorous.

In this chapter we 1) review problems with the DSM diagnostic system for personality disorders, 2) discuss the challenges of using clinical observation and inference in research, 3) describe the development of the SWAP as a method for systematizing clinical observation and insight, 4) illustrate its use for diagnosis and clinical case conceptualization, 5) review evidence for reliability and validity, and 6) discuss recommendations for revising Axis II for DSM-5.

Why Revise Axis II?

The approach to PD diagnosis codified by DSM now finds little favor with either clinicians or researchers. There is consensus that DSM Axis II requires reconfiguration (Skodol and Bender 2009). Problems with Axis II include the following (see also Clark 1992; Grove and Tellegen 1991; Jackson and Livesley 1995; Livesley 1995; Livesley and Jackson 1992; Westen and Shedler 1999a, 2000; Widiger and Frances 1985):

1. The diagnostic categories do not rest on a sound empirical foundation and often disagree with findings from cluster and factor analyses (Blais and Norman 1997; Clark 1992; Harkness 1992; Livesley and Jackson 1992; Morey 1988).

2. Axis II commits arbitrarily to a categorical diagnostic system. For example, it may be more useful to conceptualize borderline pathology on a continuum from none through moderate to severe, rather than as present or absent. This same consideration applies to individual diagnostic criteria. For example, just how little empathy constitutes "lack of empathy"?

3. Axis II lacks the capacity to weight criteria that differ in diagnostic importance (Davis et al. 1993).

4. Comorbidity between PD diagnoses is unacceptably high. Patients who meet criteria for any PD often meet criteria for four to six PDs (Blais and Norman 1997; Grilo et al. 2002; Oldham et al. 1992; Pilkonis et al. 1995; Watson and Sinha 1998). This suggests lack of discriminant validity of the diagnostic constructs, the assessment methods, or both.

5. In attempting to reduce comorbidity, DSM work groups have gerrymandered diagnostic categories and criteria, sometimes in ways faithful neither to clinical observation nor to empirical data. For example, they excluded lack of empathy and grandiosity from the diagnostic criteria for antisocial PD to minimize comorbidity with narcissistic PD, even though the traits apply to *both* PDs (Westen and Shedler 1999a, 1999b; Widiger and Corbitt 1995).

6. Efforts to define PDs more precisely have led to narrower criterion sets over time, progressively eroding the distinction between personality *disorders* (multifaceted syndromes encompassing cognition, affectivity, motivation, interpersonal functioning, and so on) and simple personality *traits*. The diagnostic criteria for paranoid PD, for example, are essentially redundant indicators of one trait, chronic suspiciousness. The diagnostic criteria no longer describe the multifaceted personality syndrome recognized by most experienced clinicians (Millon 1990; Millon and Davis 1997).

7. Axis II does not consider personality strengths that might rule out PD diagnoses for some patients. For example, differentiating between a patient with narcissistic PD and a much healthier person with narcissistic personality dynamics may not be a matter of counting symptoms, but of noting whether the patient has such positive qualities as the capacity to love and sustain meaningful relationships characterized by mutual caring and understanding.

8. Axis II does not encompass the spectrum of personality pathology that clinicians see in practice. Among patients receiving treatment for personality pathology, fewer than 40% can be diagnosed on Axis II (Westen and Arkowitz-Westen 1998).

9. Axis II diagnoses are not as clinically useful as they might be. For example, knowing whether a patient meets criteria for avoidant PD or dependent PD tells us little about the function of the person's symptoms, the personality processes to target for treatment, or how to treat them.

10. The algorithm used for diagnostic decisions (symptom counting) diverges from the methods clinicians use—or could plausibly be expected to use—in real-world practice. Cognitive research suggests that clinicians do *not* make diagnoses by tabulating symptoms. Rather, they gauge the overall "match" between a patient and a cognitive template or prototype of the disorder (i.e., they consider the features of a disorder as a configuration or gestalt), or they apply causal theories that make sense of the interrelations between symptoms (Blashfield 1985; Cantor and Genero 1986; Kim and Ahn 2002; Westen et al. 2002).

11. PD assessment instruments do not meet standards for reliability and validity normally expected in psychological research. Questionnaires and structured interviews show relatively weak convergence with one another and with the LEAD (longitudinal evaluation using all available data) standard (Perry 1992; Pilkonis et al. 1995; Skodol et al. 1991; Spitzer 1983; Westen 1997). They also show poor test-retest reliability at intervals greater than 6 weeks (First et al. 1995; Zimmerman 1994). Poor test-retest reliability is especially problematic given that PDs are by definition enduring and stable over time.[1]

Most of the proposed solutions to these problems share the assumption that progress lies in further minimizing the role of the clinician, either by developing increasingly behavioral and less inferential diagnostic criteria or by bypassing the clinician altogether through the use of

---

[1]Poor test-retest reliability has led some researchers to suggest that PDs are less stable than previously believed. Such an interpretation of the data seems inconsistent with the observations of virtually all clinical theorists. A more viable hypothesis may be that the assessment instruments do not capture core features of personality that are salient to clinicians who treat patients with PDs and know them well. Specifically, the instruments may overemphasize transient behavioral symptoms (e.g., self-cutting and suicidality in borderline patients, which may emerge only when an attachment relationship is threatened) and underemphasize underlying personality processes that endure over time (such as affect dysregulation and feelings of emptiness and self-loathing in borderline patients) (cf. Zanarini et al. 2000).

self-report instruments. These attempted solutions may, however, be part of the problem. By eliminating clinical observation and inference, we may inadvertently be eliminating crucial psychological phenomena from consideration (Cousineau and Shedler 2006; Shedler et al. 1993). An alternative to eliminating clinical inference is to harness it for scientific use.

The Challenge of Clinical Data

The problem with clinical observation and inference is not that it is inherently unreliable, as some researchers have assumed (for a discussion and literature review, see Westen and Weinberger 2004). The problem is that it tends to come in a form that is difficult to study systematically. Rulers measure in inches and scales measure in pounds, but what metric do psychotherapists share? Imagine three clinicians, all psychodynamically oriented, reviewing the same case material. One might speak of conflict and compromise formation, another of projected and introjected self and object representations, and the third, perhaps, of self defects and fragmentation. It is not readily apparent whether the hypothetical clinicians can or cannot make the same observations. There are three possibilities: 1) they may be observing the same thing but using different language and metaphor systems to describe it; 2) they may be attending to different aspects of the clinical material, as in the parable of the elephant and the blind men; and 3) they may not be able to make the same observations at all. To determine whether clinicians can make the same observations and inferences, we must ensure that they speak the same language and attend to the same spectrum of clinical phenomena.

A Standard Vocabulary for Case Description

The SWAP is an assessment instrument designed to provide clinicians of all theoretical orientations with a standard vocabulary for case description (Shedler and Westen 1998, 2004a, 2004b; Westen and Shedler 1999a, 1999b). The "vocabulary" consists of 200 statements, each of which may describe a given patient very well, somewhat, or not at all. The clinician describes a patient by ranking or ordering the statements into eight categories, from those that are most descriptive (assigned a value of 7) to those that are not descriptive (assigned a value of 0). Thus, the SWAP yields a score ranging from 0 to 7 for each of 200 personality-descriptive variables. (The SWAP instrument is available online at www.SWAPassessment.org.)

The "standard vocabulary" of the SWAP allows clinicians to provide in-depth psychological descriptions of patients in a systematic and quantifiable form and ensures that all clinicians attend to the same spectrum of clinical phenomena (cf. Block 1961/1978). SWAP statements are written in a manner close to the data (e.g., "Tends to get into power struggles" or "Is capable of sustaining meaningful relationships characterized by genuine intimacy and caring"), and statements that require inference about internal processes are written in clear, unambiguous language (e.g., "Tends to see own unacceptable feelings or impulses in other people instead of in him/herself"). Writing items in this jargon-free manner minimizes unreliable interpretive leaps and makes the item set useful to clinicians of all theoretical perspectives.

The SWAP is based on the Q-Sort method, which requires clinicians to assign each score a specified number of times (i.e., there is a "fixed distribution" of scores). The SWAP distribution is asymmetric, with many items receiving scores of 0 (not descriptive) and progressively fewer items receiving higher scores. The use of a fixed distribution has psychometric advantages and eliminates much of the measurement error or "noise" inherent in standard rating scales.[2] The method maximizes the opportunity to observe statistical relations where they exist but does not, as some incorrectly believe, artifactually inflate reliability or validity coefficients. Block (1961/1978) described the psychometric rationale for the Q-Sort method in detail; his psychometric conclusions remain unchallenged, and we refer the interested reader to his classic text.

The SWAP item set was drawn from a wide range of sources, including the clinical literature on PDs written over the past 50 years (e.g., Kernberg 1975, 1984; Kohut 1971; Linehan 1993); Axis II diagnostic criteria included in DSM-III through DSM-IV (American Psychiatric Association 1994); selected DSM Axis I items that could reflect aspects of personality (e.g., depression and anxiety); research on coping, defense, and affect-regulatory mechanisms (e.g., Perry and Cooper 1987; Shedler

---

[2] One way it does so is by ensuring that raters are "calibrated" with one another. Consider the situation with rating scales, in which raters can use any value as often as they wish. Inevitably, certain raters will tend toward extreme values (e.g., values of 0 and 7 on a 0–7 scale), and others will tend toward middle values (e.g., values of 4 and 5). Thus, the scores reflect not only the characteristics of the patients but also the calibration of the raters. The Q-Sort method, with its fixed distribution, eliminates this kind of measurement error, because all clinicians must assign each score the same number of times. If use of a standard item set gives clinicians a common vocabulary, use of a fixed distribution can be said to give them a "common grammar" (Block 1961/1978).

et al. 1993; Vaillant 1992; Westen et al. 1997); research on interpersonal pathology in patients with PDs (Westen 1991; Westen et al. 1990); research on personality traits in nonclinical populations (e.g., Block 1971; John 1990; McCrae and Costa 1990); research on PDs conducted since the development of Axis II (see Livesley 1995); pilot interviews in which observers watched videotaped interviews of patients with PDs and, using earlier versions of the item set, described the patients; and the clinical experience of the authors.

Most important, the SWAP-200 (the first major edition of the SWAP item set) was the product of a 7-year iterative item revision process that incorporated the feedback of hundreds of clinician-consultants who used earlier versions of the instrument (Shedler and Westen 1998) to describe their patients. We asked each clinician-consultant one crucial question: "Were you able to describe the things you consider psychologically important about your patient?" We added, rewrote, and revised items based on this feedback, then asked new clinician-consultants to describe new patients. We repeated this process over many iterations until most clinicians could answer "yes" most of the time. A new, revised version of the SWAP item set, the SWAP-II, incorporates the additional feedback of more than 2,000 clinicians of all theoretical orientations (Westen and Shedler 2007a). The iterative item revision process was designed to ensure the comprehensiveness and clinical relevance of the SWAP item set.

Because the SWAP is jargon free and clinically comprehensive, it has the potential to serve as a language for describing personality pathology that can be used by any skilled clinical observer. Our studies demonstrate that experienced clinicians of all theoretical orientations understand the items and score them reliably. In one study, a nationwide sample of 797 experienced psychologists and psychiatrists of diverse theoretical orientations, who had an average of 18 years' practice experience post training, used the SWAP-200 to describe patients with personality pathology (Westen and Shedler 1999a). These experienced clinicians provided similar SWAP-200 descriptions of patients with specific PDs regardless of their theoretical commitments, and fully 72.7% agreed with the statement "I was able to express most of the things I consider important about this patient" (the highest rating category). In a subsequent sample of 1,201 psychologists and psychiatrists who used the SWAP-II, 84% "agreed" or "strongly agreed" with the statement "The SWAP-II allowed me to express the things I consider important about my patient's personality" (fewer than 5% disagreed). Again, the ratings were unrelated to clinicians' theoretical orientation. Virtually identical findings were obtained in a national sample of 950 clinicians who used the adolescent version of the instrument, the SWAP-II-A. We are unaware of other personality item sets that have been evaluated in this manner for *clinical* relevance and comprehensiveness.

Clinicians using the SWAP for the first time can complete the scoring procedure in 30–45 minutes. Clinicians familiar with the SWAP may be able to complete the procedure in 20 minutes or less. The SWAP can be scored after six or more clinical contact hours with a patient (the lower limit we specify in our research protocols). Additionally, we have developed a systematic interview, the Clinical Diagnostic Interview (Westen 2002; Westen and Weinberger 2004), that can be administered in approximately 2½ hours and yields sufficient patient information to score the SWAP reliably and validly. The interview can be used in either clinical or research settings and is designed to mirror but systematize the kind of interviewing approach used by experienced clinicians of all theoretical orientations to assess personality (Westen 1997).

Psychodynamics Without Jargon

Some investigators have assumed that clinical concepts, especially psychodynamic constructs, are too vague, theoretical, or hypothetical to study empirically. The following SWAP-II items illustrate how the instrument operationalizes some psychodynamic concepts (focusing, for purposes of illustration, on defenses). Note that the constructs—rinsed of theoretical jargon—are relevant to a wide range of clinicians, irrespective of theoretical commitments. Traditional psychoanalytic terms for the concepts (which are not part of the SWAP items) are indicated in brackets:

SWAP item #	SWAP item
116	Tends to see own unacceptable feelings or impulses in other people instead of in him/herself. [projection]
144	Tends to see self as logical and rational, uninfluenced by emotion; prefers to operate as if emotions were irrelevant or inconsequential. [intellectualization]
78	Tends to express anger in passive and indirect ways (e.g., may make mistakes, procrastinate, forget, become sulky, etc.). [passive aggression]

(continues)

SWAP item #	SWAP item
14	Tends to blame own failures or shortcomings on other people or circumstances; attributes his/her difficulties to external factors rather than accepting responsibility for own conduct or choices. [externalization]
45	Is prone to idealizing people; may see admired others as perfect, larger than life, all wise, etc. [idealization]
165	Tends to distort unacceptable wishes or feelings by transforming them into their opposite (e.g., may express excessive concern while showing signs of unacknowledged hostility, disgust about sexual matters while showing signs of unacknowledged excitement, etc.). [reaction formation]
9	When upset, has trouble perceiving both positive and negative qualities in the same person at the same time (e.g., may see others in black or white terms, shift suddenly from seeing someone as caring to seeing him/her as malevolent and intentionally hurtful, etc.). [splitting]

Capturing Clinical Nuance

Just as researchers tend to be skeptical regarding the scientific usefulness of clinical observation, many clinicians express skepticism that a structured assessment instrument can do justice to the richness and complexity of clinical case description. However, SWAP statements can be combined in patterns to capture a wide range of subtle clinical phenomena and convey meanings that transcend the content of the individual items.

Consider, for example, the SWAP-II item "Tends to be sexually seductive or provocative." If a patient receives a high score on this item along with high scores on the items "Has an exaggerated sense of self-importance (e.g., feels special, superior, grand, or envied)" and "Seems to treat others primarily as an audience to witness own importance, brilliance, beauty, etc.," the portrait that begins to emerge is one of a narcissistically organized individual who seeks sexual attention to bolster a sense of being special and uniquely desirable. If the same patient also receives high scores on the items "Tends to feel s/he is not his/her true self with others; may feel false or fraudulent" and "Tends to feel s/he is inadequate, inferior, or a failure," then a more complex psychological portrait begins to emerge. The SWAP items in combination indicate that feelings of grandiosity and inadequacy coexist in the same person, and suggest the hypothesis that grandiosity may serve the function of masking painful feelings of inadequacy. Indeed, this duality may lie at the very heart of narcissistic PD for many patients (for empirical evidence, see Russ et al. 2008). The ability to describe and quantify psychological conflict and contradiction is a key feature of the SWAP, one that distinguishes it from other dimensional models (which assume that a person can be high or low on a trait, but not both).

If the SWAP-II item describing sexual seductiveness is instead combined with the items "Tends to fear s/he will be rejected or abandoned," "Appears to fear being alone; may go to great lengths to avoid being alone," and "Tends to be ingratiating or submissive (e.g., consents to things s/he does not want to do, in the hope of getting support or approval)," the portrait that begins to emerge is one of a dependent individual who relies on sexuality as a desperate means of maintaining attachments in the face of feared abandonment.

If the SWAP-II item describing sexual seductiveness is combined with the items "Tends to act impulsively (e.g., acts without forethought or concern for consequences)," "Takes advantage of others; has little investment in moral values (e.g., puts own needs first, uses or exploits people with little regard for their feelings or welfare, etc.)," and "Experiences little or no remorse for harm or injury caused to others," the portrait that begins to emerge is one of an antisocial individual who exploits others sexually and whose primary concern is gratifying immediate needs.

If the item describing sexual seductiveness is combined with the items "Has a deep sense of inner badness; sees self as damaged, evil, or rotten to the core" and "Appears to want to 'punish' self; creates situations that lead to unhappiness, or actively avoids opportunities for pleasure and gratification," we could plausibly infer that sexuality plays a role in a larger pattern of self-devaluation and self-abasement (such a person might well become the victim of the antisocial individual described above).

These brief examples illustrate how SWAP items can be combined to communicate subtle clinical concepts, and how the same item can convey different meanings depending on the items that surround and contextualize it. We will further illustrate this in a later section with a clinical case example.

Treatment Implications

DSM diagnostic criteria are largely descriptive, providing little guidance for clinicians trying to understand the meaning and function of the symptoms or how to intervene. For example, DSM tells us that borderline patients are characterized by "a pattern of unstable and intense interpersonal relationships." The statement may be descriptively accurate, but *why* does the patient have unstable relationships and how can the clinician help? Because the SWAP addresses underlying personality processes that give rise to these characteristics, it suggests some answers.

Consider the following personality process (item 9 in the SWAP-II):

> When upset, has trouble perceiving both positive and negative qualities in the same person at the same time (e.g., may see others in black or white terms, shift suddenly from seeing someone as caring to seeing him/her as malevolent and intentionally hurtful, etc.).

The item describes the phenomenon known to psychodynamic clinicians as *splitting* and to cognitive-behavioral clinicians as *dichotomous thinking*. If the patient's perceptions of others gyrate between contradictory extremes, it follows that his relationships will be unstable. This implies a specific treatment strategy: the therapist will intervene effectively if he can help the patient recognize the extremes of thinking and perceive others in a more balanced light. For example, the therapist may observe, "When you are angry with your partner, it is hard to keep in mind that there is anything you like about him. When you are feeling close, it seems hard for you to recognize that he has flaws." Such interventions are designed to develop the patient's capacity to integrate contradictory perceptions and perceive self and others in more complex, modulated, and balanced ways. A recent clinical trial has demonstrated the efficacy of a treatment for borderline PD based on just this type of intervention (Clarkin et al. 2007; Levy et al. 2006).

DSM also tells us that borderline patients may have "transient, stress-related paranoid ideation" but leaves us in the dark about why this occurs or how to intervene. Suppose the patient has high scores on the following SWAP-II items: "Is prone to intense anger, out of proportion to the situation at hand" (item 185) and "Tends to see own unacceptable feelings or impulses in other people instead of in him/herself" (item 116). The items, considered in combination, suggest a hypothesis about the meaning and function of paranoid ideation: the patient may become paranoid (i.e., see the world as dangerous and hostile) because, in times of intense agitation, he sees his own hostility wherever he looks. (Empirically, these items *do* emerge in combination for paranoid patients; see section "Toward DSM-5: An Improved Classification of Personality Disorders" later in this chapter). The treatment implications are clear: the therapist must help the patient to recognize his own aggression and develop more adaptive ways of regulating it.

SWAP Dimensional Diagnosis

The SWAP scoring algorithms generate a dimensional score for each PD included in DSM-IV (as well as for factor-analytically derived traits, and for an alternative set of diagnostic syndromes that we identified empirically; see section "Toward DSM-5: An Improved Classification of Personality Disorders"). Additionally, the SWAP generates richly detailed narrative case descriptions relevant to clinical case conceptualization and treatment planning.

Dimensional PD scores measure the similarity or "match" between a patient and *prototype* SWAP descriptions representing each personality syndrome in its typical or "ideal" form (e.g., a prototypical patient with paranoid PD). Dimensional PD scores can be expressed as T-scores and graphed to create a PD score profile resembling a Minnesota Multiphasic Personality Inventory profile, as shown in Figure 4–1 (see p. 138). Thus, each personality syndrome is assessed on a continuum rather than diagnosed categorically as present or absent. Low PD scores indicate that the patient does not resemble or match the PD prototype, and high scores indicate that the patient matches it well, with intermediate scores indicating varying degrees of resemblance (for descriptions of the PD prototypes and scale construction methods, see Shedler and Westen 2004b; Westen and Shedler 1999a, 1999b).

Note that this dimensional approach preserves a *syndromal* understanding of personality styles and disorders. That is, it treats personality as a *configuration of functionally interrelated psychological processes* encompassing affectivity, cognition, motivation, interpersonal functioning, coping strategies and defenses, and so on. By *functionally related*, we mean that the personality processes are interdependent and have causal relations to one another. (For example, in the example of paranoid ideation given above, intense anger and the propensity to project unacceptable feelings onto others are functionally related.) The approach does not deconstruct personality configurations into separate trait dimensions such as those derived from factor analysis of questionnaire data (the approach taken by, e.g., the Five Factor Model).

A syndromal approach is consistent with research showing that clinicians view psychopathology in terms of functionally interrelated psychological processes (just as human judgment about category membership more generally relies on implicit causal theories linking component parts into coherent gestalts [Kim and Ahn 2002]). It is also consistent with empirical and conceptual recognitions that personality syndromes fall on continua from relatively healthy through severely disturbed (e.g., from neurotic through borderline). For example, a relatively healthy person with an obsessional personality style might be precise, orderly, logical, more comfortable with ideas than feelings, a bit more concerned than most with issues of authority and control, and somewhat rigid in certain areas of thought and behavior. Such a person may excel in fields where such attributes are adaptive, such as finance, engineering, or, perhaps, the development of dimensional diagnostic systems. Toward the more disturbed end of the obsessional spectrum, we find individuals who are rigidly dogmatic, oblivious to affect, and preoccupied with control, and who misapply logic in ways that lead them to miss the forest for the trees.

Although we are emphasizing here the utility of a syndromal approach, we do not discount the utility of trait approaches derived from conventional factor analysis. Indeed, factor analysis of the SWAP has identified clinically and empirically coherent trait dimensions (Shedler and Westen 2004a; Westen et al. 2005; D. Westen, N. Waller, J. Shedler, and P. Blagov, unpublished manuscript, Emory University, 2010), some of which map readily onto trait dimensions included in other dimensional trait models (Widiger and Simonsen 2005) and some of which do not (e.g., thought disorder, sexual conflict). Both syndromal and trait approaches have advantages for different assessment purposes. A combined approach may well prove most informative—for example, by describing patients syndromally, then adding trait dimensions that are not redundant with the syndromes (e.g., hostility, thought disorder) to create fine-grained psychological portraits.

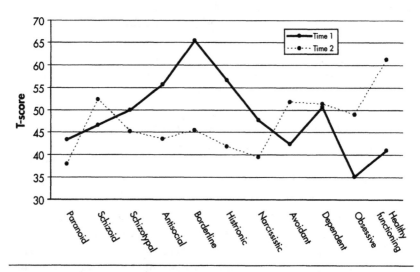

FIGURE 4–1.   Personality disorder score profile for "Melanie".

Case Illustration[3]

BACKGROUND

Melanie is a 30-year-old white woman with presenting complaints of substance abuse and inability to extricate herself from an emotionally and physically abusive relationship. Assessment with the Structured Clinical Interview for DSM-IV (SCID and SCID-II) yielded an Axis I diagnosis of substance abuse and an Axis II diagnosis of borderline PD with histrionic traits, with a Global Assessment of Functioning (GAF) score of 45.

Melanie's early family environment was marked by neglect and parental strife. A recurring family scenario is illustrative: the mother would scream at her husband, telling him he was a failure and that she was going to leave him; she would then slam the door and lock herself in her room, leaving Melanie frightened and in tears. Both parents would then ignore Melanie, often forgetting to feed her. By adolescence, Melanie was often skipping school, spending her days sleeping or wandering the streets. At age 18, she left home and began a "life on the streets," entering a series of impulsive and chaotic sexual relationships, abusing street drugs, and engaging in petty theft. In her mid-twenties, Melanie moved in with her boyfriend, a small-time drug dealer. Melanie periodically prostituted herself to obtain money or drugs for her boyfriend, who sometimes beat her when she did not bring home enough.

Melanie began psychoanalytic psychotherapy at a frequency of three sessions per week. The first 10 sessions were tape-recorded and transcribed. Two clinicians (blind to all other data) reviewed the transcripts and scored the SWAP-200 on the basis of the information contained in the transcripts. The SWAP-200 scores were then averaged across the two clinical judges to enhance reliability and obtain a single SWAP-200 description. After 2 years of psychotherapy, 10 consecutive psychotherapy sessions were again recorded and transcribed, and the SWAP assessment procedure was repeated.

PERSONALITY DISORDER DIAGNOSIS

The solid line in Figure 4–1 shows Melanie's PD scores at the beginning of treatment for the 10 PDs included in DSM-IV. A "healthy functioning"

---

[3]The material in this section is adapted from Lingiardi et al. 2006. Please see the original publication for a more complete description of the case, treatment methods, and findings.

index (rightmost data points) is graphed as well to reflect clinicians' consensual understanding of healthy personality functioning (Westen and Shedler 1999a). For ease of interpretation, the PD scores have been converted to T-scores based on norms established in a psychiatric sample of patients with Axis II diagnoses (Westen and Shedler 1999a).

Although the SWAP assesses PDs dimensionally and treats personality syndromes as continua, we have also established cutoff scores for "backward compatibility" with the categorical approach of DSM-IV. We have suggested T=60 as a threshold for making a categorical Axis II diagnosis, and T=55 as a threshold for diagnosing "features."[4]

Melanie's PD profile shows a marked elevation for borderline PD (T=65.4, approximately 1.5 standard deviations above the sample mean), with secondary elevations for histrionic PD (T=56.6) and antisocial PD (T=55.7). With application of the recommended cutoff scores, Melanie's DSM-IV Axis II diagnosis is borderline PD with histrionic and antisocial features. Also noteworthy is the T-score of 41 for the healthy functioning index, nearly a standard deviation below the mean in a reference sample of patients with Axis II diagnoses. The low score indicates significant impairment in functioning and parallels the low GAF score assigned at intake.

NARRATIVE CASE DESCRIPTION

We can generate a narrative case description by listing the SWAP items with the highest scores in the patient's SWAP description (e.g., items with scores of 5, 6, and 7). The narrative description below is based on the top 30 most descriptive SWAP-200 items. We have grouped together conceptually related items. To aid the flow of the text, we have made some minor grammatical changes and added some summary statements and connecting text (italicized). However, the SWAP-200 items are reproduced essentially verbatim.

> *Melanie experiences severe depression and dysphoria.* She tends to feel unhappy, depressed, or despondent, appears to find little or no pleasure or satisfaction in life's activities, feels life is without meaning, and tends to feel like an outcast or outsider. She tends to feel guilty, and to feel inadequate, inferior, or like a failure. Her behavior is often self-defeating and

---

[4]The relatively low thresholds reflect the fact that the reference sample consisted of patients with PD diagnoses. Thus, a T-score of 50 indicates average functioning among patients with PD diagnoses, and a T-score of 60 represents an elevation of one standard deviation relative to other patients with PD diagnoses.

self-destructive. She appears inhibited about pursuing goals or successes, is insufficiently concerned with meeting her own needs, and seems not to feel entitled to get or ask for things she deserves. She appears to want to "punish" herself by creating situations that lead to unhappiness, or actively avoiding opportunities for pleasure and gratification. *Specific self-destructive tendencies include* getting drawn into and remaining in relationships in which she is emotionally or physically abused, abusing illicit drugs, and acting impulsively and without regard for consequences. She shows little concern for consequences in general.

Melanie shows many personality traits associated specifically with borderline PD. Her relationships are unstable, chaotic, and rapidly changing. She has little empathy and seems unable to understand or respond to others' needs and feelings unless they coincide with her own. Moreover, she tends to confuse her own thoughts, feelings, and personality traits with those of others, and she often acts in such a way as to elicit her own feelings in other people (for example, provoking anger when she herself is angry, or inducing anxiety in others when she herself is anxious).[5]

Melanie expresses contradictory feelings without being disturbed by the inconsistency, and she seems to have little need to reconcile or resolve contradictory ideas. She is prone to see certain others as "all bad," losing the capacity to perceive any positive qualities they may have. She lacks a stable image of who she is or would like to become (e.g., her attitudes, values, goals, and feelings about self are unstable and changing) and she tends to feel empty. *Affect regulation is poor:* She tends to become irrational when strong emotions are stirred up and shows a noticeable decline from her customary level of functioning. She also seems unable to soothe or comfort herself when distressed and requires the involvement of another person to help her regulate affect. Both her living arrangements and her work life tend to be chaotic and unstable.

Finally, Melanie's attitudes toward men and sexuality are problematic and conflictual. She tends to be hostile toward members of the opposite sex (whether consciously or unconsciously) and she associates sexual activity with danger (e.g., injury or punishment). She appears afraid of commitment to a long-term love relationship, instead choosing partners who seem inappropriate in terms of age, status (e.g., social, economic, intellectual), or other factors.

The narrative provides a detailed psychological portrait of a severely troubled patient with borderline personality pathology. It captures psychodynamic processes characteristic of borderline personality

---

[5]Psychoanalytically informed readers will recognize these SWAP items as capturing aspects of borderline personality organization as conceptualized by Kernberg (1984) and his associates (see Chapter 1 of this volume).

(e.g., splitting, identity diffusion, projective identification) in plain, jargon-free language (cf. Schafer 1976). The description helps illustrate the difference between *descriptive psychiatry* (aimed at establishing a diagnosis) and *clinical case formulation* (aimed at understanding an individual person). In this instance, however, all findings are derived from the same quantitative assessment data.

ASSESSING CHANGE IN PSYCHOTHERAPY

The case of Melanie has a happy ending. After 2 years of psychodynamic psychotherapy, the SWAP revealed significant personality changes. The dotted line in Figure 4–1 shows Melanie's PD scores after 2 years of treatment. Her scores on the borderline, histrionic, and antisocial dimensions had dropped below T = 50, and she no longer warranted a DSM-IV PD diagnosis. Her score on the healthy functioning index had increased by two standard deviations, from 41.0 to 61.2. These personality changes paralleled concrete changes in Melanie's life circumstances, such as ending her drug abuse, getting and keeping a good job, ending her involvement with her abusive boyfriend, and no longer engaging in theft, promiscuous sex, or prostitution.

To assess change in an idiographic, more fine-grained manner, we created a change score for each SWAP item by subtracting the item score at Time 1 from the score at Time 2. The narrative description of change, below, comprises the SWAP items with change scores >4. Again, we have made some minor grammatical changes and added connecting text to aid the flow of the text (italicized), but the SWAP-200 items are reproduced essentially verbatim.

> *Melanie has developed strengths and inner resources that were not evident at the Time 1 assessment.* She has come to terms with painful experiences from the past, finding meaning in, and growing from, these experiences; she has become more articulate and better able to express herself in words; she has a newfound ability to appreciate and respond to humor; she is more capable of recognizing alternative viewpoints, even in matters that stir up strong feelings; she is more empathic and sensitive to others' needs and feelings; and she is more likeable.
>
> *There is marked improvement in many areas associated specifically with borderline psychopathology.* With respect to affect regulation, Melanie is less prone to become irrational when strong emotions are stirred up, is more likely to express affect appropriate in quality and intensity to the situation at hand, and is better able to soothe or comfort herself when distressed. She is less prone to confuse her own thoughts and feelings with those of others, less manipulative, and less likely to devalue others

and see them as "all bad." She has come to terms with negative feelings toward her parents.

Melanie is also less impulsive, more conscientious and responsible, and more aware of the consequences of her actions. Her living arrangements are more stable, as is her work life. Melanie's use of illicit drugs has decreased significantly, and she is no longer drawn to abusive relationships.

As the more severe aspects of borderline personality pathology have receded, other conflicts and symptoms have moved to the fore. For example, Melanie appears to have developed somewhat obsessional defenses against painful affect. She adheres more rigidly to daily routines and becomes anxious or uncomfortable when they are altered. She is more prone to think in an abstract and intellectualized manner and tries to see herself as more logical and rational, less influenced by emotion.

Despite her wish to act more logically and rationally, Melanie seems engaged in an active struggle to control her affect and impulses. She tends to oscillate between undercontrol and overcontrol of needs and wishes, either expressing them impulsively or disavowing them entirely. She has more difficulty allowing herself to experience strong pleasurable emotions (e.g., excitement, joy). She is more prone to repress, "forget," or otherwise distort distressing events.

Finally, there are changes in Melanie's relationships and orientation toward sexuality. Whereas before she presented in a histrionic manner (i.e., with exaggerated feminine traits), she is now more disparaging of traditionally feminine traits, instead emphasizing independence and achievement. Whereas previously she engaged in multiple chaotic sexual relationships, she now seems conflicted about her intimacy needs. She craves intimacy but tends to reject it when offered. She has more difficulty directing both sexual and tender feelings toward the same person, seeing men as either respectable and virtuous or sexy and exciting, but not both. She is more likely to hold grudges.

Reliability and Validity

Psychological and psychiatric researchers often assume that clinical observation and judgment are unreliable; a well-established research literature documents the limitations of "clinical judgment." Unfortunately, studies of "clinical judgment" have too often asked clinicians to make predictions about things that fall outside their legitimate area of expertise (and just as unfortunately, some clinicians have been all too willing to offer such prognostications). More problematically, the studies have typically conflated clinicians' ability to make accurate observations and inferences (which they do well) with their ability to combine and weight variables to derive optimal predictions (a task *necessarily* performed better by statistical methods such as regression equations). In fact, a substantial literature documents the reliability and validity of clinical observation and inference *when it is quantified and utilized appropriately* (Westen and Weinberger 2004).

The SWAP differs from other assessment approaches in that it harnesses clinical judgment, using psychometric methods developed specifically for this purpose, and then applies statistical and actuarial methods to the resulting data. In short, it relies on clinicians to do what they do best—namely, making specific behavioral observations and inferences about individual patients they treat and know well. It relies on statistical algorithms to do what they do best—namely, combining data optimally to derive reliable and valid diagnostic scales and indices.

Interrater reliability of SWAP-200 PD scale scores and other diagnostic scales is above 0.80 for all scales in all studies to date and is often above 0.90 (Marin-Avellan et al. 2005; Westen and Muderrisoglu 2003, 2006; Westen and Shedler 2007a). It is noteworthy that high reliability coefficients have been reported by independent investigators unaffiliated with our own laboratory. The reliability coefficients compare favorably with those typically reported for structured interviews that avoid clinical inference and "stick to the facts" (e.g., DSM-IV criteria). Additionally, the SWAP diagnostic scales correlate highly with a wide range of external criterion measures in both adult and adolescent samples, including genetic history variables such as psychosis in first- and second-degree relatives, substance abuse in first- and second-degree relatives, developmental history variables such as childhood physical and sexual abuse, life events including psychiatric hospitalizations and suicide attempts, violent criminal behavior, and ratings of adaptive functioning (Marin-Avellan et al. 2005; Shedler and Westen 2004a; Westen and Muderrisoglu 2003; Westen and Shedler 1999a, 2007b; Westen and Weinberger 2004; Westen et al. 2003).

Toward DSM-5: An Improved Classification of Personality Disorders[6]

It is an empirical question whether DSM-IV includes the optimal diagnostic categories and criteria. It is also an empirical question whether a diagnostic system based on personality *types* or *syndromes* is consistent with the available data (as opposed to being a mere convenience that

---

[6]The material presented here is adapted from Westen and Shedler (1999b).

facilitates clinical communication). To address these questions, we examined SWAP-200 personality descriptions provided by the treating psychologist or psychiatrist from a national sample of patients ($N=496$) diagnosed with Axis II disorders (Westen and Shedler 1999b). We used the technique of Q-factor analysis (or simply Q-analysis) to answer the following questions:

1. Are there clear, empirically identifiable diagnostic groupings among PD patients treated in the community? That is, are there groupings of patients who share common psychological features that distinguish them from other patients?
2. Do the current DSM-IV diagnostic categories adequately "fit" the data? That is, are there empirically identifiable personality syndromes that are not included in DSM-IV, or vice versa?
3. What are the most defining psychological features (diagnostic criteria) for each personality syndrome?

Q-analysis is computationally equivalent to the familiar technique of factor analysis. The difference is that factor analysis identifies groupings of similar *variables* (i.e., columns in a data matrix) that are assumed to be markers of a common underlying factor. In contrast, Q-analysis identifies groupings of similar *people* (i.e., cases or rows in a data matrix) who are assumed to represent a common diagnostic syndrome or type. The former approach is *variable-centered*; the latter is *person-centered* (for a description of computational methods, see Westen and Shedler 1999b). Q-analysis has been used by biologists conducting taxonomic research to aid in classifying species and has been used successfully in research on normal personality (Block 1971).[7]

The Q-analysis analysis demonstrated that there are empirically distinguishable personality syndromes among patients treated in the community, and that a syndromal or person-centered approach is consistent with the data. Note that the personality syndromes are best understood dimensionally, not as mutually exclusive categories (see section "SWAP Dimensional Diagnosis" earlier in this chapter). This is an important clarification, because some researchers mistakenly conflate "dimensional" with *trait* (variable-centered) models, and conflate "categorical" approaches with *syndromal* (person-centered) models. In fact, these issues are separate and independent (Westen et al. 2006a). The dimensional/categorical distinction refers to whether people are assumed to fall into discrete categories or to vary along a continuum; the syndromal/trait distinction refers to whether the unit of diagnosis is a constellation of interrelated personality characteristics or separate characteristics.

The analysis identified 11 conceptually coherent diagnostic group-ings or personality syndromes, many of which resembled DSM-IV di-agnostic categories and some of which did not. We created a *prototype personality description* for each empirically identified diagnostic syn-drome by listing the SWAP items in descending order by Q-factor score. The SWAP-200 items with the highest Q-factor scores indicate the cen-tral or defining psychological features for each diagnostic group (i.e., the diagnostic "criteria"). This represents a purely empirical approach to identifying optimal diagnostic categories and criteria.

We will use the examples of paranoid PD and depressive PD to illus-trate this approach to identifying PD syndromes and criteria (for de-scriptions of all 11 empirically identified diagnostic groupings, see Shedler and Westen 2004b; Westen and Shedler 1999b). Table 4–1 lists the SWAP-200 items most defining of patients in the paranoid person-ality diagnostic grouping, along with their associated factor scores (in-dicating their diagnostic importance). A number of findings are noteworthy. First, the empirical identification of this diagnostic group-ing validates the inclusion of paranoid PD as a diagnostic category in DSM-IV. Second, the items are clinically richer than the DSM-IV diag-nostic criteria, addressing inner experience and intrapsychic processes as well as behavior. Third, the description differs in important ways from the description provided by DSM-IV and offers crucial insights into the meaning and function of paranoid symptoms.

---

[7]A discussion of person-centered versus variable-centered assessment is be-yond the scope of this chapter and merits a chapter in its own right. We believe the distinction underlies much misunderstanding between clinicians and researchers, because clinicians tend to think in person-centered terms and re-searchers tend to think in variable-centered terms. The choice of a person- or variable-centered approach, which can profoundly affect how we think about psychological issues, is often not even recognized as a choice. Instead, one or the other approach is accepted by convention and without consideration of what is at stake. (The fact that statistical data analysis programs are designed to operate on variables rather than cases may have shaped academic psychology in ways we can barely fathom.) It is not that one approach is "right" and one is "wrong," but rather that they serve different purposes and draw our attention to different matters. Good assessment systems are like good maps, in that they must accu-rately depict the territory. But sometimes one wants a road map, sometimes a map of elevations, and sometimes a political map. A motorist navigating the interstate will have little interest in a map of elevations, no matter how many studies document its validity.

TABLE 4–1.   SWAP-200 prototype description of patients in the paranoid personality disorder diagnostic category

Item	Factor score
Tends to hold grudges; may dwell on insults or slights for long periods.	3.61
Tends to feel misunderstood, mistreated, or victimized.	3.23
Is quick to assume that others wish to harm or take advantage of him/her; tends to perceive malevolent intentions in others' words and actions.	3.08
Tends to express intense and inappropriate anger, out of proportion to the situation at hand.	2.77
Tends to be critical of others.	2.59
Tends to get into power struggles.	2.43
Tends to be angry or hostile (whether consciously or unconsciously).	2.40
Tends to see certain others as "all bad," and loses the capacity to perceive any positive qualities the person may have.	2.38
Tends to be self-righteous or moralistic.	2.25
Tends to react to criticism with feelings of rage or humiliation.	2.19
Tends to blame others for own failures or shortcomings; tends to believe his/her problems are caused by external factors.	2.15
Tends to be oppositional, contrary, or quick to disagree.	2.08
Tends to see own unacceptable feelings or impulses in other people instead of in him/herself.	2.08
Tends to become irrational when strong emotions are stirred up; may show a noticeable decline from customary level of functioning.	1.94
Tends to "catastrophize"; is prone to see problems as disastrous, unsolvable, etc.	1.82
Tends to elicit dislike or animosity in others.	1.78
Emotions tend to spiral out of control, leading to extremes of anxiety, sadness, rage, excitement, etc.	1.73
Has difficulty making sense of other people's behavior; often misunderstands, misinterprets, or is confused by others' actions and reactions.	1.53
Tends to be controlling.	1.49
Tends to elicit extreme reactions or stir up strong feelings in others.	1.44
Tends to avoid confiding in others for fear of betrayal; expects things s/he says or does will be used against him/her.	1.41
Reasoning processes or perceptual experiences seem odd and idiosyncratic (e.g., may make seemingly arbitrary inferences; may see hidden messages or special meanings in ordinary events).	1.39
Perception of reality can become grossly impaired under stress (e.g., may become delusional).	1.37

For example, the item list (Table 4–1) emphasizes paranoid patients' cognitive confusion in ways that DSM-IV does not (e.g., "tends to become irrational when strong emotions are stirred up"; "has difficulty making sense of other people's behavior"; "reasoning processes or perceptual experiences seem odd and idiosyncratic"). It also emphasizes paranoid patients' anger and aggression in ways that DSM-IV does not (e.g., "tends to hold grudges"; "tends to be angry or hostile"; "tends to express intense and inappropriate anger"), as well as their tendency to rely on projection as a defense ("tends to see own unacceptable feelings or impulses in other people instead of in him- or herself"). The findings are consistent with psychoanalytic thought, which recognizes projection as a central dynamic in paranoid patients. (Stated differently, the paranoid patient perceives the world as hostile because he sees his own hostility everywhere he looks.) The personality description has clear implications for treatment, unlike the description in DSM-IV. It tells us that a clinician treating a patient with paranoid PD will need to assist the patient with reality testing, for example, by examining his reasoning processes and helping him consider alternative constructions and interpretations of events. It also tells us that the clinician will be dealing with intense anger and aggression and that successful treatment will have to address the patient's aggression and help him to find more adaptive ways of regulating it.

The findings cannot be explained away as artifacts of clinicians' theoretical beliefs or expectations. They emerged repeatedly when we stratified the sample by the theoretical orientation of the reporting clinicians, and the personality characteristics described above were ranked just as highly by cognitive-behavioral therapists as by psychoanalysts. The SWAP-200 provides a common language for all clinicians, and the PD prototypes reflect only those personality traits that clinicians of all orientations observe consistently and reliably.

Table 4–2 lists the SWAP-200 items most defining of another personality syndrome, one absent from DSM-IV, which we have labeled "depressive (or dysphoric) personality." Despite its omission from DSM-IV, our data indicate that it is the most prevalent personality syndrome seen in the community (Westen and Shedler 1999b). Its absence from DSM-IV appears to be a significant omission. Note that the SWAP description encompasses the *multiple domains of functioning* described in DSM-IV as defining of a PD, including cognition (e.g., tends to blame self; tends to be self-critical), affectivity (e.g., tends to feel unhappy, depressed, despondent; tends to feel ashamed or embarrassed), interpersonal relations (tends to fear s/he will be rejected or abandoned; tends to be overly needy or dependent), and impulse regulation (e.g., has difficulty

TABLE 4–2. SWAP-200 prototype description of patients in the depressive (dysphoric) personality disorder diagnostic category

Item	Factor score
Tends to feel s/he is inadequate, inferior, or a failure.	3.63
Tends to feel unhappy, depressed, or despondent.	3.11
Tends to feel ashamed or embarrassed.	2.76
Tends to blame self or feel responsible for bad things that happen.	2.71
Tends to feel guilty.	2.67
Tends to fear s/he will be rejected or abandoned by those who are emotionally significant.	2.66
Tends to feel helpless, powerless, or at the mercy of forces outside his/her control.	2.52
Tends to be overly needy or dependent; requires excessive reassurance or approval.	2.30
Tends to be ingratiating or submissive (e.g., may consent to things s/he does not agree with or does not want to do, in the hope of getting support or approval).	2.12
Tends to be passive and unassertive.	2.12
Tends to be self-critical; sets unrealistically high standards for self and is intolerant of own human defects.	2.02
Tends to feel like an outcast or outsider; feels as if s/he does not truly belong.	1.94
Tends to be anxious.	1.91
Tends feel listless, fatigued, or lacking in energy.	1.79
Tends to feel empty or bored.	1.77
Appears to want to "punish" self; creates situations that lead to unhappiness, or actively avoids opportunities for pleasure and gratification.	1.71
Appears to find little or no pleasure, satisfaction, or enjoyment in life's activities.	1.71
Tends to be insufficiently concerned with meeting own needs; appears not to feel entitled to get or ask for things s/he deserves.	1.70
Is unable to soothe or comfort self when distressed; requires involvement of another person to help regulate affect.	1.60
Lacks a stable image of who s/he is or would like to become (e.g., attitudes, values, goals, and feelings about self may be unstable and changing).	1.55
Tends to feel life has no meaning.	1.49
Tends to avoid social situations because of fear of embarrassment or humiliation.	1.43
Has difficulty acknowledging or expressing anger.	1.34

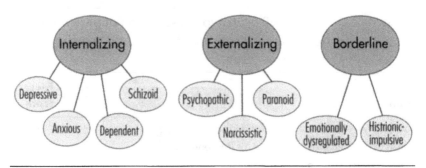

FIGURE 4–2.   Hierarchical structure of personality syndromes.

acknowledging or expressing anger). The depressive (or dysphoric) personality syndrome appears to have its origin in late childhood or early adolescence (Westen et al. 2005) and appears to be stable and enduring over time. In short, it is a *personality disorder* by every definition of the term (cf. Huprich 2003, 2005; Huprich and Frisch 2004; McDermut et al. 2003; Ryder et al. 2001).

Analysis of SWAP-II data from our most recent subject samples (N=1,201 adult patients studied with the SWAP-II, and N=950 adolescent patients with the SWAP-II-A) revealed a hierarchical structure of PD syndromes, as illustrated in Figure 4–2 (Westen and Shedler 2007a). At the superordinate level are three broad diagnostic groupings (Q-factors) that can be described as *internalizing, externalizing,* and *borderline.* The results map onto the internalizing and externalizing spectra identified in research on Axis I syndromes (Krueger 2002) and may provide a basis for an integrated understanding of Axis I and Axis II pathology. The borderline personality constellation contains elements of both internalizing and externalizing pathology and is characterized by emotional instability that is not evident in either stable internalizers or externalizers. The hierarchical structure of PD syndromes will be described in greater detail in future publications.

Dimensional Diagnosis: The Prototype Matching Approach

For research purposes, for situations in which maximum psychometric precision is required (e.g., forensic assessment), or for clarifying challenging diagnostic dilemmas, clinicians can, using the SWAP, describe patients and obtain dimensional diagnosis scores such as those graphed in Figure 4–1. (Investigators will soon be able to enter SWAP data and

Patients who match this prototype tend to be deceitful, to lie and mislead people. They take advantage of others, have minimal investment in moral values, and appear to experience no remorse for harm or injury caused to others. They tend to manipulate others' emotions to get what they want; to be unconcerned with the consequences of their actions, appearing to feel immune or invulnerable; and to show reckless disregard for the rights, property, or safety of others. They have little empathy and seem unable to understand or respond to others' needs and feelings unless they coincide with their own. Individuals who match this prototype tend to act impulsively, without regard for consequences; to be unreliable and irresponsible (e.g., failing to meet work obligations or honor financial commitments); to engage in unlawful or criminal behavior; and to abuse alcohol. They tend to be angry or hostile; to get into power struggles; and to gain pleasure or satisfaction by being sadistic or aggressive toward others. Patients who match this prototype tend to blame others for their own failures or shortcomings and to believe their problems are caused by external factors. They have little psychological insight into their own motives, behavior, etc. They may repeatedly convince others of their commitment to change but then revert to previous maladaptive behavior, often convincing others that "this time is really different."

Please form an overall impression of the type of person described, then rate the extent to which your patient matches or resembles this prototype.

5 Very good match (patient *exemplifies* this disorder; prototypical case)	**Diagnosis**
4 Good match (patient *has* this disorder; diagnosis applies)	
3 Moderate match (patient has *significant features* of this disorder)	**Features**
2 Slight match (patient has minor features of this disorder)	
1 No match (description does not apply)	

FIGURE 4–3. Antisocial-psychopathic personality disorder prototype.

receive diagnostic reports via the Internet; for information, visit www .SWAPassessment.org.) When routine use of the SWAP-200 would be impractical, we advocate a "prototype matching" approach to personality diagnosis, and we have proposed this approach for DSM-5.

Figure 4–3 illustrates the prototype matching approach. The figure shows the prototype description for one personality syndrome, identified empirically through Q-analysis, which we have labeled *antisocial-psychopathic personality* (Westen and Shedler 1999b). The description is made up of the SWAP-200 statements that are most empirically defining of the syndrome. The SWAP items are reproduced essentially verbatim but have been arranged in paragraph (rather than list) form.

The clinician's task is to consider the prototype description as a whole—that is, as a configuration or gestalt—and to rate the overall similarity or match between the prototype and the patient being assessed. The resulting diagnosis is dimensional (a 1–5 rating), but the scale can be dichotomized for convenience when a present/absent classification is desired to facilitate clinical communication (with a rating of 4 indicating "caseness"). Thus, the approach offers the advantages of dimensional diagnosis while maintaining "backward compatibility" with the categorical approach of DSM-IV.

Our research indicates that the prototype matching method has advantages over the current DSM-IV approach to personality diagnosis. In a series of studies of Cluster B disorders (antisocial, borderline, histrionic, and narcissistic), we compared prototype matching and DSM-IV diagnosis with respect to validity, diagnostic comorbidity, and clinical utility (Westen et al. 2006b). Clinicians diagnosed patients using the prototype matching method (as illustrated in Figure 4–3) and the DSM-IV diagnostic system. We compared the prototype matching method to both categorical DSM-IV diagnoses and "dimensionalized" DSM-IV diagnoses obtained by summing the number of criteria met per disorder (a method commonly used in PD research).

The prototype matching method substantially reduced diagnostic comorbidity relative to both DSM-IV diagnostic methods. For example, the median correlation between the four Cluster B disorders was 0.47 for dimensionalized DSM-IV diagnoses and 0.14 for prototype diagnoses based on empirically identified diagnostic groupings (as described in the preceding section). At the same time, the prototype diagnoses appeared to have higher validity, yielding higher correlations with ratings of adaptive functioning and developmental history variables known to be associated with antisocial PD and borderline PD. The advantages of the prototype matching approach were not only statistically significant but also clinically meaningful: prototype diagnoses predicted treatment outcomes better than either categorical or dimensionalized DSM-IV diagnoses, for both psychotherapy and antidepressant medication.

Finally, we examined clinical utility by asking clinicians to compare the prototype matching method to the DSM-IV diagnostic system with respect to ease of use, usefulness for communicating with other clinicians, ability to capture the important information about the patient, and so on. The clinicians strongly preferred prototype diagnosis to DSM-IV diagnosis on every dimension assessed, despite the fact that they had no prior experience with either the prototype matching method or the empirically derived prototype personality descriptions.

Spitzer et al. (2008) also found that clinicians prefer prototype matching both to DSM-IV diagnosis and to dimensional trait models such as the Five Factor Model, and rate the prototype method as more clinically relevant and useful.

Whether or not items from the SWAP are directly incorporated into future editions of DSM, SWAP research leads to two clear recommendations for revision of the manual. First, existing DSM-IV diagnostic criteria are too narrow, emphasizing behavioral signs and symptoms to the relative exclusion of inner experience and underlying psychological processes. Such underlying psychological processes (e.g., motives, conflicts, defenses, self and object representations) are centrally defining features of personality syndromes and crucial to their understanding (Shedler and Westen 2004b). SWAP research also makes clear that clinicians can assess underlying psychological processes far more reliably than many investigators had previously believed. Second, prototype matching has advantages over the present symptom-counting approach to diagnosis. It combines the advantages of a syndromal or configural approach to personality assessment with the advantages of dimensional diagnosis. Moreover, clinical practitioners have consistently shown a strong preference for prototype matching approaches over the present DSM-IV diagnostic system and over dimensional trait models such as the Five Factor Model (Rottman et al. 2009; Spitzer et al. 2008; Westen et al. 2006b).

Conclusion: Integrating Science and Practice

A clinically useful diagnostic system should encompass the spectrum of personality pathology seen in clinical practice and have meaningful implications for treatment. An empirically sound diagnostic system should facilitate reliable and valid diagnoses: independent clinicians should be able to arrive at the same diagnosis, the diagnoses should be relatively distinct from one another, and each diagnosis should be associated with unique and theoretically meaningful correlates, antecedents, and sequelae (Livesley and Jackson 1992; Millon 1991; Robins and Guze 1970).

One obstacle to achieving this ideal has been an unfortunate schism in the mental health professions between science and practice. Too often, research has been conducted in isolation from the crucial data of clinical observation. The results often strike clinicians as naive and of dubious clinical relevance. Ultimately, the most empirically elegant diagnostic system will have little impact if clinicians do not find it helpful for understanding their patients (First et al. 2004; Shedler and Westen 2005). On the other hand, clinical theory has too often developed without sufficient regard for questions of falsifiability and empirical credibility. The results have often struck researchers as scientifically naive.

The Shedler-Westen Assessment Procedure represents an effort to bridge the schism between science and practice by quantifying clinical observation and expertise, making clinical constructs accessible to empirical study. It relies on clinicians to do what they do best—namely, making observations and inferences about the individual patients they know and treat. It relies on quantitative methods to do what they do best—namely, aggregating observations to reveal relationships and commonalities, and combining data to yield optimal predictions (Sawyer 1966). It provides a "language" for clinical case description that is at once psychometrically sound and clinically rich enough to describe the complexities of real patients. There remains a sizeable schism between science and practice. Perhaps the SWAP will provide a language all parties can speak.

Key Clinical Concepts

- ◆ The diagnostic system provided by Axis II of DSM-IV has significant limitations for understanding personality, from both clinical and empirical perspectives. An important clinical limitation is that the DSM-IV Axis II system does not address the meaning and function of personality processes and therefore offers little guidance with respect to treatment.
- ◆ Meaningful assessment of personality requires clinical judgment and inferences about underlying psychological processes. The Shedler-Westen Assessment Procedure (SWAP) is a personality assessment instrument that harnesses clinical judgment, allowing clinicians to describe their observations and inferences systematically and reliably.
- ◆ The standard vocabulary of the SWAP captures complex intrapsychic processes (e.g., splitting, identity diffusion, and projective identification in borderline patients) in jargon-free English. Combinations of items express clinical case formulations that imply specific treatment strategies and interventions (e.g., integrating contradictory peceptions of self and others in borderline patients).
- ◆ The SWAP approach integrates descriptive psychiatric diagnosis and clinical case formulation. It preserves a syndromal approach to personality diagnosis (i.e., recognizing functional relations among multiple areas of functioning) while allowing dimensional diagnosis. Despite (or because of) its

reliance on clinical inference, the SWAP shows high reliability and validity.

◆ SWAP research has empirically identified 11 personality syndromes or groupings that provide an alternative to DSM-IV diagnostic categories. The syndromes are defined by items or criteria that address inner experience and intrapsychic processes (e.g., projection of aggression in paranoid patients) as well as overt behaviors. They also include diagnostic syndromes, such as depressive personality, that are prevalent in the community but absent from DSM.

◆ A "prototype matching" approach to diagnosis is a practical alternative to the current DSM diagnostic system and addresses many of its limitations. The resulting diagnoses are both empirically based and clinically meaningful. Clinicians judged this diagnostic system to be preferable to the existing DSM diagnostic system and also preferable to alternative dimensional trait models.

Suggested Readings

Psychodynamic Case Formulation

PDM Task Force (ed): Personality patterns and disorders: P Axis, in Psychodynamic Diagnostic Manual (PDM). Silver Spring, MD, Alliance of Psychoanalytic Organizations, 2006, pp 17–69. [A concise overview of contemporary psychoanalytic thought on personality styles and disorders, with jargon-free descriptions of the major personality syndromes and references to relevant empirical research.]

McWilliams N: Psychoanalytic Diagnosis: Understanding Personality Structure in the Clinical Process. New York, Guilford, 1994. [A more in-depth discussion of the personality syndromes recognized by psychoanalytic practitioners. A contemporary classic.]

Peebles-Kleiger MJ: Beginnings: The Art and Science of Planning Psychotherapy. Hillsdale, NJ, Analytic Press, 2002. [An elegant introduction to case formulation and treatment planning, useful to practitioners of all theoretical orientations.]

The Shedler-Westen Assessment Procedure (SWAP)

Westen D, Shedler J: Revising and assessing Axis II, part 1: developing a clinically and empirically valid assessment method. Am J Psychiatry 156:258–272, 1999a

Westen D, Shedler J: Revising and assessing Axis II, part 2: toward an empirically based and clinically useful classification of personality disorders. Am J Psychiatry 156:273–285, 1999b. [These are the seminal publications on the SWAP, describing its development and rationale.]

Lingiardi V, Shedler J, Gazillo F: Assessing personality change in psychotherapy with the SWAP-200: a case study. J Pers Assess 86:23–32, 2006. [A more thorough discussion of the case of Melanie, described briefly in this chapter. The paper illustrates the use of the SWAP as a method for assessing personality change (i.e., intrapsychic change) in psychotherapy.]

Shedler J: A new language for psychoanalytic research. Psychologist-Psychoanalyst 20:30–37, 2000. [On the relevance of SWAP research for psychoanalytic theory, practice, and training.]

Shedler J, Westen D: Refining personality disorder diagnosis: integrating science and practice. Am J Psychiatry 161:1350–1365, 2004. [Descriptions of the major personality syndromes as they are conceptualized by experienced clinicians and observed in clinical practice, with recommendations for revision of DSM.]

Spitzer RL, First MB, Shedler J, et al: Clinical utility of five dimensional systems for personality diagnosis: a "consumer preference" study. J Nerv Ment Dis 196:356–374, 2008

Westen D, Shedler J, Bradley R: A prototype approach to personality diagnosis. Am J Psychiatry 163:846–856, 2006. [Discussion of the "prototype matching" approach to personality diagnosis.]

References

American Psychiatric Association: Diagnostic and Statistical Manual of Mental Disorders, 3rd Edition. Washington, DC, American Psychiatric Association, 1980

American Psychiatric Association: Diagnostic and Statistical Manual of Mental Disorders, 4th Edition. Washington, DC, American Psychiatric Association, 1994

Betan E, Heim AK, Conklin CZ, et al: Countertransference phenomena and personality pathology in clinical practice: an empirical investigation. Am J Psychiatry 162:890–898, 2005

Blais M, Norman D: A psychometric evaluation of the DSM-IV personality disorder criteria. J Pers Disord 11:168–176, 1997

Blashfield R: Exemplar prototypes of personality disorder diagnoses. Compr Psychiatry 26:11–21, 1985

Block J: Lives Through Time. Berkeley, CA, Bancroft, 1971

Block J: The Q-Sort Method in Personality Assessment and Psychiatric Research (1961). Palo Alto, CA, Consulting Psychologists Press, 1978

Cantor N, Genero N: Psychiatric diagnosis and natural categorization: a close analogy, in Contemporary Directions in Psychopathology: Toward the DSM-IV. Edited by Klerman GL. New York, Guilford, 1986, pp 233–256

Clark L: Resolving taxonomic issues in personality disorders: the value of larger scale analyses of symptom data. J Pers Disord 6:360–376, 1992

Clarkin JF, Levy KN, Lenzenweger MF, et al: Evaluating three treatments for borderline personality disorder: a multiwave study. Am J Psychiatry 164:922–928, 2007

Cousineau TM, Shedler J: Predicting physical health: implicit mental health measures versus self report scales. J Nerv Ment Dis 194:427–432, 2006

Davis R, Blashfield R, McElroy R: Weighting criteria in the diagnosis of a personality disorder: a demonstration. J Abnorm Psychol 102:319–322, 1993

First M, Spitzer R, Gibbon M, et al: The Structured Clinical Interview for DSM-III-R Personality Disorders (SCID-II). Part II: multi-site test-retest reliability study. J Pers Disord 9:92–104, 1995

First MB, Pincus HA, Levine JB, et al: Clinical utility as a criterion for revising psychiatric diagnoses. Am J Psychiatry 161:946–954, 2004

Grilo CM, Sanislow CA, McGlashan TH: Co-occurrence of DSM-IV personality disorders with borderline personality disorder. J Nerv Ment Dis 190:552–553, 2002

Grove WM, Tellegen A: Problems in the classification of personality disorders. J Pers Disord 5:31–41, 1991

Harkness A: Fundamental topics in the personality disorders: candidate trait dimensions from lower regions of the hierarchy. J Consult Clin Psychol 4:251–259, 1992

Huprich SK: Depressive personality and its relationship to depressed mood, interpersonal loss, negative parental perceptions, and perfectionism. J Nerv Ment Dis 191:1–7, 2003

Huprich SK: Differentiating avoidant and depressive personalities. J Pers Disord 19:659–673, 2005

Huprich SK, Frisch MB: Depressive personality and its relationship to quality of life, hope, and optimism. J Pers Assess 83:22–28, 2004

Jackson DN, Livesley WJ: Possible contributions from personality assessment to the classification of personality disorders, in The DSM-IV Personality Disorders. Edited by Livesley WJ. New York, Guilford, 1995, pp 459–481

John O: The "big five" factor taxonomy: dimensions of personality in the natural language and in questionnaires, in Handbook of Personality: Theory and Research. Edited by Pervin L. New York, Guilford, 1990, pp 66–100

Kernberg O: Borderline Conditions and Pathological Narcissism. New York, Jason Aronson, 1975

Kernberg O: Severe Personality Disorders. New Haven, CT, Yale University Press, 1984

Kim NS, Ahn W: Clinical psychologists' theory-based representations of mental disorders predict their diagnostic reasoning and memory. J Exp Psychol 131:451–476, 2002

Kohut H: The Analysis of the Self. New York, International Universities Press, 1971

Krueger RF: The structure of common mental disorders. Arch Gen Psychiatry 59:570–571, 2002

Levy KN, Kelly KM, Meehan KB, et al: Change in attachment patterns and reflective function in a randomized control trial of transference-focused psychotherapy for borderline personality disorder. J Consult Clin Psychol 74:1027–1040, 2006

Linehan MM: Cognitive-Behavioral Treatment of Borderline Personality Disorder. New York, Guilford, 1993

Lingiardi V, Shedler J, Gazillo F: Assessing personality change in psychotherapy with the SWAP-200: a case study. J Pers Assess 86:23–32, 2006

Livesley WJ (ed): The DSM-IV Personality Disorders. New York, Guilford, 1995

Livesley WJ, Jackson DN: Guidelines for developing, evaluating, and revising the classification of personality disorders. J Nerv Ment Dis 180:609–618, 1992

Marin-Avellan L, McGauley G, Campbell C, et al: Using the SWAP-200 in a personality-disordered forensic population: is it valid, reliable and useful? J Crim Behav Ment Health 15:28–45, 2005

McCrae R, Costa P: Personality in Adulthood. New York, Guilford, 1990

McDermut W, Zimmerman M, Chelminski I: The construct validity of depressive personality disorder. J Abnorm Psychol 112:49–60, 2003

McWilliams N: Psychoanalytic Diagnosis: Understanding Personality Structure in the Clinical Process. New York, Guilford, 1994

Millon T: Toward a New Psychology. New York, Wiley, 1990

Millon T: Classification in psychopathology: rationale, alternatives and standards. J Abnorm Psychol 100:245–261, 1991

Millon T, Davis RD: The place of assessment in clinical science, in The Millon Inventories: Clinical and Personality Assessment. Edited by Millon T. New York, Guilford, 1997, pp 3–20

Morey LC: Personality disorders in DSM-III and DSM-III-R: convergence, coverage, and internal consistency. Am J Psychiatry 145:573–577, 1988

Oldham J, Skodol A, Kellman HD, et al: Diagnosis of DSM-III-R personality disorders by two semistructured interviews: patterns of comorbidity. Am J Psychiatry 149:213–220, 1992

Perry JC: Problems and considerations in the valid assessment of personality disorders. Am J Psychiatry 149:1645–1653, 1992

Perry JC, Cooper SH: Empirical studies of psychological defense mechanisms, in Psychiatry. Edited by Cavenar J, Michels R. Philadelphia, PA, JB Lippincott, 1987, pp 1–19

Pilkonis PA, Heape CL, Proietti JM, et al: The reliability and validity of two structured diagnostic interviews for personality disorders. Arch Gen Psychiatry 52:1025–1033, 1995

Robins E, Guze S: The establishment of diagnostic validity in psychiatric illness: its application to schizophrenia. Am J Psychiatry 126:983–987, 1970

Rottman BM, Ahn WK, Sanislow CA: Can clinicians recognize DSM-IV personality disorders from five-factor model descriptions of patient cases? Am J Psychiatry 166:427–433, 2009

Russ E, Bradley R, Shedler J, et al: Refining the construct of narcissistic personality disorder: diagnostic criteria and subtypes. Am J Psychiatry 165:1473–1481, 2008

Ryder AG, Bagby RM, Dion KL: Chronic low-grade depression in a nonclinical sample: depressive personality or dysthymia? J Pers Disord 15:84–93, 2001

Sawyer J: Measurement and prediction, clinical and statistical. Psychol Bull 66:178–200, 1966

Schafer R: A New Language for Psychoanalysis. New Haven, CT, Yale University Press, 1976

Shedler J, Westen D: Refining the measurement of Axis II: a Q-sort procedure for assessing personality pathology. Assessment 5:333–353, 1998

Shedler J, Westen D: Dimensions of personality pathology: an alternative to the five-factor model. Am J Psychiatry 161:1743–1754, 2004a

Shedler J, Westen D: Refining personality disorder diagnosis: integrating science and practice. Am J Psychiatry 161:1350–1365, 2004b

Shedler J, Westen D: A simplistic view of the five-factor model: Drs. Shedler and Westen reply (letter). Am J Psychiatry 162:1551, 2005

Shedler J, Westen D: Personality diagnosis with the Shedler-Westen Assessment Procedure (SWAP): bridging the gulf between science and practice, in Psychodynamic Diagnostic Manual (PDM). Edited by PDM Task Force. Silver Spring, MD, Alliance of Psychoanalytic Organizations, 2006, pp 476–513

Shedler J, Westen D: The Shedler-Westen Assessment Procedure (SWAP): making personality diagnosis clinically meaningful. J Pers Assess 89:41–55, 2007

Shedler J, Mayman M, Manis M: The illusion of mental health. Am Psychol 48:1117–1131, 1993

Skodol A, Bender D: The future of personality disorders in DSM-V? Am J Psychiatry 164:4:1–2, 2009

Skodol A, Oldham J, Rosnick L, et al: Diagnosis of DSM-III-R personality disorders: a comparison of two structured interviews. Int J Methods Psychiatr Res 1:13–26, 1991

Spitzer RL: Psychiatric diagnosis: are clinicians still necessary? Compr Psychiatry 24:399–411, 1983

Spitzer RL, First MB, Shedler J, et al: Clinical utility of five dimensional systems for personality diagnosis: a "consumer preference" study. J Nerv Ment Dis 196:356–374, 2008

Vaillant GE (ed): Ego Mechanisms of Defense: A Guide for Clinicians and Researchers. Washington, DC, American Psychiatric Press, 1992

Watson D, Sinha BK: Comorbidity of DSM-IV personality disorders in a nonclinical sample. J Clin Psychol 54:773–780, 1998

Westen D: Social cognition and object relations. Psychol Bull 109:429–455, 1991

Westen D: Divergences between clinical and research methods for assessing personality disorders: implications for research and the evolution of Axis II. Am J Psychiatry 154:895–903, 1997

Westen D: Clinical Diagnostic Interview. 2002. Available at: http://www.psychsystems.net/lab. Accessed October 3, 2009.

Westen D, Arkowitz-Westen L: Limitations of Axis II in diagnosing personality pathology in clinical practice. Am J Psychiatry 155:1767–1771, 1998

Westen D, Muderrisoglu S: Reliability and validity of personality disorder assessment using a systematic clinical interview: evaluating an alternative to structured interviews. J Pers Disord 17:350–368, 2003

Westen D, Muderrisoglu S: Clinical assessment of pathological personality traits. Am J Psychiatry 163:1285–1287, 2006

Westen D, Shedler J: Revising and assessing Axis II, part 1: developing a clinically and empirically valid assessment method. Am J Psychiatry 156:258–272, 1999a

Westen D, Shedler J: Revising and assessing Axis II, part 2: toward an empirically based and clinically useful classification of personality disorders. Am J Psychiatry 156:273–285, 1999b

Westen D, Shedler J: A prototype matching approach to diagnosing personality disorders: toward DSM-V. J Pers Disord 14:109–126, 2000

Westen D, Shedler J: Personality diagnosis with the Shedler-Westen Assessment Procedure (SWAP): integrating clinical and statistical measurement and prediction. J Abnorm Psychol 116:810–822, 2007a

Westen D, Shedler J: The Shedler-Westen Assessment Procedure (SWAP): making personality diagnosis clinically meaningful. J Pers Assess 89:42–55, 2007b

Westen D, Weinberger J: When clinical description becomes statistical prediction. Am Psychol 59:595–613, 2004

Westen D, Lohr N, Silk K, et al: Object relations and social cognition in borderlines, major depressives, and normals: a TAT analysis. J Consult Clin Psychol 2:355–364, 1990

Westen D, Muderrisoglu S, Fowler C, et al: Affect regulation and affective experience: individual differences, group differences, and measurement using a Q-sort procedure. J Consult Clin Psychol 65:429–439, 1997

Westen D, Heim AK, Morrison K, et al: Classifying and diagnosing psychopathology: a prototype matching approach, in Rethinking the DSM: Psychological Perspectives. Edited by Beutler LE, Malik M. Washington, DC, American Psychological Association, 2002, pp 221–250

Westen D, Shedler J, Durrett C, et al: Personality diagnosis in adolescence: DSM-IV Axis II diagnoses and an empirically derived alternative. Am J Psychiatry 160:952–966, 2003

Westen D, Dutra L, Shedler J: Assessing adolescent personality pathology. Br J Psychiatry 186:227–238, 2005

Westen D, Gabbard G, Blagov P: Back to the future: personality structure as a context for psychopathology, in Personality and Psychopathology. Edited by Krueger RF, Tackett JL. New York, Guilford, 2006a, pp 335–384

Westen D, Shedler J, Bradley R: A prototype approach to personality diagnosis. Am J Psychiatry 163:846–856, 2006b

Widiger TA, Corbitt EM: Antisocial personality disorder, in The DSM-IV Personality Disorders. Edited by Livesley WJ. New York, Guilford, 1995, pp 103–126

Widiger T, Frances A: The DSM-III personality disorders: perspectives from psychology. Arch Gen Psychiatry 42:615–623, 1985

Widiger TA, Simonsen ES: Alternative dimensional models of personality disorders: finding common ground. J Pers Disord 19:110–130, 2005

Zanarini MC, Skodol AE, Bender D, et al: The Collaborative Longitudinal Personality Disorders Study: reliability of Axis I and II diagnoses. J Pers Disord 14:291–299, 2000

Zimmerman M: Diagnosing personality disorders: a review of issues and research methods. Arch Gen Psychiatry 51:225–245, 1994

PART II

PSYCHODYNAMIC TREATMENT APPROACHES

CHAPTER 5

Psychotherapeutic Treatment of Cluster A Personality Disorders

Paul Williams, Ph.D.

Cluster A personality disorders comprise paranoid personality disorder (PPD), schizoid personality disorder (SPD), and schizotypal personality disorder (StPD). Patients who fall within these diagnostic categories are the least likely to present for individual psychotherapy because of the inflexibility and severity of the conditions, the comparatively poor response to treatment, and, not infrequently, inaccurate diagnosis. However, the growth in public expectation from the talking therapies and the slow but steady progress made by researchers into the origins and prevalence of these disorders have led more Cluster A patients to seek out psychotherapeutic help than was the case in the past, although the number remains small relative to the number of patients with borderline personality disorder (BPD) seeking treatment.

Demographically, Cluster A disorders affect 0.5%–2.5% (PPD), slightly less than 1% (SPD), and approximately 3% (StPD) of the U.S. population, with comparable rates in Europe, and the consequences for individuals affected can be highly disabling (Elkin 1999). The incidence of each category appears to be higher in men than in women, and in describing this cluster of conditions emphasis has tended to be placed on odd, eccentric, or "cold" behavior. These characteristics are most evident in SPD and StPD. It is thought that a biological relationship may exist between the disorders and the schizophrenias, although of the three Cluster A personality disorders, StPD can be more demonstrably linked to schizophrenia phenomenologically and genetically (McGlashan 1983). SPD and StPD are sometimes grouped as part of a continuum, given the similarity of certain symptoms.

There remains no distinctive set of psychotherapeutic theories applicable to these conditions. More research is required into the developmental and psychic structural aspects of the illnesses before generally accepted psychological theories for the conditions can be established. There is, in fact, strikingly little research into Cluster A disorders compared with other personality disorders (notably BPD), and more is needed if the conditions are to become better understood. Psychodynamic researchers have noted the stability of diagnosis and treatment outcomes (see, e.g., McGlashan 1986; Sandell et al. 1997; Stone 1985, 1993). Clinical investigation into Cluster A type personalities tends to focus on the nature of internal object relationships, defenses, psychotic anxieties, and transference–countertransference phenomena (reports on these phenomena include Gabbard 2000; Grotstein 1995; Jackson 2000; Jackson and Williams 1994; Lucas 1992; Meissner 1986; Rey 1994; Robbins 2002; Rosenfeld 1964, 1969; Segal 1978; Sohn 1997; Target and Fonagy 1996a).

Attention to psychotic anxieties is of particular importance to those who study and treat Cluster A disorders. Psychotic elements occur in severe neuroses, psychosomatic disorders, sexual perversions, and personality disorders *alongside* neurotic constellations, and this is particularly the case with Cluster A personality disorders. Patients with these disorders are not psychotic per se, but they are vulnerable to psychotic thinking and compromised ego functioning that create confusion between internal and external realities.

In undertaking the treatment of Cluster A patients, the psychodynamic psychotherapist is faced with a series of theoretical, clinical, and technical challenges that will draw upon his or her resources to the full. The prevalence of psychotic anxieties in parallel to neurotic anxieties has led these individuals to fall out of the orbit of normal human relations. They display defenses that are sometimes seen in psychosis and will not respond to a therapist who does not take seriously their loss of faith in people. This lost capacity leaves a profound imprint on their internal world: failed internalization of trusting relationships generates chronic mistrust and anxiety. Difficulty in the management of affects is one area, among many, that causes particular problems. These individuals tend to "globalize" their affective experience because of chronic *splitting*, swinging from one set of powerful feelings to another with little capacity to integrate gradations of feeling or different and contradictory experiences. This, in turn, can be linked in some cases to the violent, coercive activity of an overdeveloped superego whose task it is to control affect storms and strong instinctual impulses with extreme rigidity. The guilt, shame, and despair in this seemingly irresolvable psychic conflict has been well documented (for a recent review of these conflicts in serious disturbance, see Wurmser 2007). Whereas these affective crises tend to be more obviously and openly expressed in Cluster B personality disorders, they are more muted and internally directed in Cluster A (Gunderson 2008). However, they are no less powerful for this, and they demand the steady attentiveness of the clinician if opaque internal crises are not to ferment into eruptions of acting out that may threaten the treatment.

Once the patient is in treatment, a capacity in the therapist for flexibility and careful attention to fluctuating countertransference experiences will improve treatment prospects. Research into the role of countertransference factors has confirmed the centrality to effective treatment of the therapist's responsiveness (particularly to the patient's psychotic anxieties) as well as the hazards of inattention to countertransference phenomena (Hinshelwood 1994; Lieberz and Porsch 1997). Potential transference difficulties may be obvious or may only be hinted at by the patient, sometimes evolving inaudibly, and the therapist may be required to use occasional unobtrusive questions or to proffer provisional ideas based on countertransferential indicators that serve as much to illuminate the penumbra of object relations difficulties that beset the patient as they do to interpret psychic reality. Many psychotherapists find it important to obtain psychiatric backup during therapy to act as a support for both patient and therapist, often in times of extreme transference intensity when psychotic anxieties may threaten to overwhelm the patient's beleaguered ego (for a useful summary of guidelines regarding the psychiatric treatment of patients with Cluster A personality disorders, see "Treatment Outlines for Paranoid, Schizotypal, and Schizoid Personality Disorders" 1990). Despite their cold, hostile, or bizarre behavior, Cluster A patients suffer painful, highly confusing experiences deriving from major problems of self-esteem linked to a fragmented personality structure and reliance on primitive self representations. Therapeutic gains in these areas, although sometimes limited and usually the outcome of painstaking effort on both sides, can make a significant difference to the quality of their lives.

Paranoid Personality Disorder

The main characteristic of paranoid personality disorder is distrust and suspiciousness. The motives of other people are construed as hostile and exploitative. The PPD patient's thoughts and feelings are preoccupied by conflicts and threats *felt to emanate from the outside*. Such individuals suffer doubts about the loyalty of others and anticipate betrayal as a "given" consequence of human engagement. As a result of their preoccupation with external threats, they are vigilant and seek to keep a safe distance from others. Relationships, where these are allowed to occur, may be conducted on an apparently polite, formal, and controlling basis in order to sustain disconnection from disturbing affects, ultimately of a hostile nature. Negative stereotyping may be a feature of relations with others, and this may lead to a search for security through contact with people who share the patient's paranoid beliefs. Individuals can express PPD through hostility, sarcasm, stubbornness, or a cynical worldview. However, the beleaguered, self-righteous attitude characteristic of PPD conceals a deep sensitivity to the ordinary struggles of life (especially setbacks), an unwillingness to forgive, inflation of subjective judgment, and great difficulty in accepting another's viewpoint. An example of this negativity is conveyed in the following typical type of exchange in psychotherapy with a PPD patient. The vignette is taken from the twice-weekly psychotherapy of an isolated man in his 30s who entered therapy (with a male therapist) as a result of fears regarding self-harming and suicidal thoughts. In this session he had been complaining at length, not for the first time and without appropriate affect, about his boss's overbearing behavior:

> **Patient:** …that guy in the office behaves as though he knows everything. He's got a problem. Nobody gets on with him. Only last week he told one of the clerks that unless she got her act together she'd be out—in front of everyone! Somebody should blow the whistle on that sort of behavior…it's offensive. [*pause*]
>
> **Therapist:** It sounds like you are very angry today with your boss because of the crass, insensitive way you feel he deals with people and that you are struggling to control these feelings.…I am wondering whether a similar struggle takes place here when you sometimes feel talked down to as a result of the things we discuss, which are often difficult and painful.
>
> **Patient:** What's that got to do with it? Why say that? It has nothing to do with you. Are you accusing me of blaming him when it's all in me? He IS offensive.…You've got a professional job to do…you aren't allowed to behave like that… And anyway, I'd tell you if you did.

Here, the patient succeeds in communicating his anger (via splitting and projective identification) while denying its felt reality and a connection in the transference to his psychotherapist. This need to control affects and interpersonal contact is common in PPD. Such defenses serve to conceal feelings of inferiority based on low self-esteem. Humiliation, shame, and depressive feelings are the underlying characteristics of PPD, and these persistently threaten the ego. Sensitivity by the therapist to these threats to the personality is a priority. So great is the power of projective processes in PPD that it may take years for the patient to establish sufficient trust in the motives of his psychotherapist to be able to talk about himself openly. The pressures on the therapist's capacity to bear countertransference experiences of being misunderstood, misinterpreted, and devalued are high.

Encounters with PPD may leave other people disoriented, offended, or even provoked into conflict, sometimes without any proper understanding of how conflict arose in the first place. Initial history taking by the clinician may point to a withdrawal from relationships in childhood and a long-standing preoccupation with ruminative, conflict-based fantasies. PPD can be differentiated from formal psychotic illness by an absence of delusions or hallucinations (Sperry 1995), although the scale of projective mechanisms used can sometimes resemble delusional thinking. Medication—usually neuroleptics or selective serotonin reuptake inhibitor (SSRI) antidepressants—may be given, often in combination with psychotherapy; however, PPD patients struggle with any treatment regime because of their distrust.

Freud (1911/1958) saw paranoia as the consequence of projecting (predominately sexual) ideas that are incompatible with the ego into the external world, and the subsequent delusional elaborations as representing a "patch over the ego"—an attempt to recover meaning in a world that had become disintegrated and meaningless. Although paranoia is still regarded as deriving from defensive projective systems, and an unconscious fear of being drawn into a homosexual relationship may be discerned in PPD, Freud's focus on homosexuality as the central pathogenic factor in paranoia has given way to wider consideration of the role of primitive emotional conflicts and modes of thought (Bell 2003). These developmental processes involve difficulties in the acquisition of a stable sense of self; the management of powerful, primitive affects, particularly aggression (whether of innate or of a psychosocial origin, or both); and ways in which the personality negotiates psychosensory and enactive modes of function and the processes of separation, self-object discrimination and individuation (Mahler et al. 1975). There is a widespread view today that the perceived threat of the consequences of aggression for the subject's ego gives rise to pervasive splitting and the chronic use of projective identification, probably beginning early in life. Rycroft, in one of the few articles on the treatment of paranoia in the extensive PEP electronic archive, notes this use of splitting and projective identification and how Freud, given his concern at the time with establishing fixation points for psychopathology, omitted to mention, in his considerations of paranoia, the concept of denial—a defense that nowadays is commonly coupled with projection and projective identification and is seen as providing the basis of paranoid disorders (Rycroft 1960, p. 68).

Many clinicians today pay particular attention to the object relations crisis in PPD, in which the individual feels unable to surrender or yield to the experience of dependence upon the primary object for fear of unmanageable conflict leading to destruction. Melanie Klein contributed significantly to this understanding, having located the paranoid phase within Abraham's first anal stage and subsequently conceiving of this state of mind as the earliest object relationship of the oral stage, from which she evolved her concept of the *paranoid-schizoid position*. This concept is useful in understanding all Cluster A disorders and, in particular, the functional role of paranoia. The initial object in Klein's view is partial (the earliest representation being the breast, followed by the mother) and is subject to splitting into "good" and "bad" aspects—idealized and denigrated, respectively. The ego attempts to rid itself of "bad" object experiences, using projective mechanisms. Introjection of the "bad" part-object threatens the infant with a fear of destruction. Splitting, idealization, disavowal, and denial contribute to a defensive, omnipotent attempt to ward off the "bad" object, and the ensuing interplay of projective and introjective mechanisms is today accepted by many as pivotal in the understanding of paranoid conditions such as PPD. Kernberg (1975), Rosenfeld (1969), Stone (1993), and Gabbard (2000), among others, have also noted how the PPD patient persistently and violently splits the object, leading to separated "good" and "bad" aspects, reflecting a developmental failure of mentalization in infancy (Target and Fonagy 1996b). *Object constancy* (the internalization of a reliably available, caring other) is not established. The PPD patient succumbs, probably early in life, to chronic expulsion of aggressive impulses by projection. *Projective identification* locates these impulses in mental representations of others as a means of controlling fears of annihilating the object and of being annihilated in turn. Beneath this defensive strategy lie feelings of helplessness, worthlessness, inadequacy, and depression (Meissner 1988; Rosenfeld 1969). Environmental failure to contain disturbing infantile feelings, above all aggression and hatred, plays a fundamental paranoiagenic role in paranoid thinking (cf. Balint 1969; Kohut and Wolf 1978; Winnicott 1962).

The psychotherapy of PPD demands exceptional tact and patience on the part of the psychotherapist, because premature interpretation of aggression or of underlying depression and feelings of rejection and humiliation can lead to negative therapeutic reactions, acting out, and even termination of treatment. At the same time, these states of mind are precisely those that require psychotherapeutic attention. The scale of superego dominance of the ego, through extreme, harsh, and intransigent injunctions purporting to provide protective advice and safety, is a particular focus for many therapists. Judicious use of transference and countertransference understanding of part-object experiences can lead to a deepening appreciation of the subjugation and humiliation of the ego by the superego and the incarceration of the patient's sense of self. The compulsive, irrational, globalizing but constricted activity of the overdeveloped superego may, with enough time and insight, come to be differentiated from the patient's genuine wishes to trust the therapist, leading to the acquisition of a "third" position from which both participants become able to reflect together on this crippling intrapsychic conflict (Ogden 1999). The beginnings of emotional dependence on the therapist as a distinct, trustworthy object may be deeply disconcerting for the patient, because this can be felt to be an unprecedented and threatening experience. The separation anxieties, feelings of loss, and confusion that can accompany the development of a genuine object-relating stance testify to a state of deep regression that may have prevailed throughout the course of the patient's life. A vulnerability to suspiciousness about others may remain with the PPD patient even after therapy. However, many therapists consider that with sufficient "psychic disinvestment" in the values and activities of the overdeveloped superego, and increased investment in grasping the libidinal and aggressive vicissitudes that accompany relations with objects, the PPD patient can achieve an impressive level of stability.

Schizoid Personality Disorder

Schizoid personality disorder is characterized by emotional detachment from social and personal relationships. Expressions of feeling toward others are limited because emotional contact is both painful and felt to lack personal meaning. Compelling interpersonal experiences seem to pass the SPD individual by, but at the same time they have an impact on him in ways that can seem outwardly muted but that are internally powerful. The schizoid person can feel isolated and in great pain if left alone for too long. Forced to seek out contact with others to relieve this pain, he may in turn become oppressed and persecuted if the contact is felt to be too prolonged or too intimate. Close association with others can lead to feeling overwhelmed by anxiety and a fear of loss of personal identity (sense of self). Hostility is rare; passive resistance and withdrawal predominate. Poor social skills and limited emotional range compound the "mechanical" characteristics of SPD behavior. When under threat, SPD individuals detach themselves still further. Confrontational therapy techniques are inadvisable, because these heighten already severe anxieties. The fantasy life of SPD individuals can be intense: the difficulty for the psychotherapist lies in accessing it, but if this is achieved, SPD patients can do well.

Psychoanalytic theory considers the schizoid person to be essentially someone who craves love but who cannot love for fear that love (not only hate) will destroy the object (Fairbairn 1952). Fairbairn was one of the first psychoanalysts to depict in detail the mental processes involved in this extreme condition. In a summary of his work, Khan noted the main observations made by Fairbairn:

i. Schizoid conditions constitute the most deep seated of all psycho-pathological states.

ii. The therapeutic analysis of the schizoid provides an opportunity for the study of the widest range of psycho-pathological processes in a single individual; for in such cases it is usual for the final state to be reached only after all available methods of defending the personality have been exploited.

iii. Contrary to common belief, schizoid individuals who have not regressed too far are capable of greater psychological insight than any other class of person, normal or abnormal.

iv. Again contrary to common belief, schizoid individuals "show themselves capable of transference to a remarkable degree, and present unexpectedly favourable therapeutic possibilities." Fairbairn went on to show the presence and importance of depersonalization, derealisation, disturbances of reality-sense, e.g., feelings of artificiality, experiences such as the "plate-glass feeling," feelings of unfamiliarity with familiar persons or environmental settings and feelings of familiarity with the unfamiliar ones; déjà vu also features significantly in their experience. In their social extension of behaviour such persons can become fanatics, agitators, criminals, revolutionaries, etc. Fairbairn singled out three prominent characteristics of individuals in the schizoid category: an attitude of omnipotence, an attitude of isolation and detachment and a preoccupation with inner reality. (Khan 1960, p. 428)

For Fairbairn, the fundamental splits in the ego seen in the schizoid individual create a concomitant oral-incorporative libidinal attitude that accounts for the tendency to treat other people as persons with less than inherent value (Khan 1960, p. 429). This regressive stance toward objects Fairbairn connected to an experience of the maternal object as either indifferent or possessive. The schizoid person has little experience of spontaneous and genuine expressions of love and affection that convince him that he is lovable in his own right, and depersonalization and de-emotionalization of relationships come to characterize contact with people (Khan 1960, p. 430). Additionally, the fact that the schizoid person cannot give emotionally means that he relates by playing a role and/or by employing exhibitionistic attitudes. "Giving" is replaced by "showing." This superior attitude derives from overvaluation of his own mental contents and personal capacities, the use of intellectualized defenses, and a narcissistic inflation of the ego arising out of secret possession of, and identification with, internal libidinized objects. Fairbairn's view is that in early life such individuals were afflicted by a sense of deprivation and inferiority and remained fixated on their mothers. The libidinal cathexis of an already internalized "breast-mother" is intensified and extended to relationships with other objects, resulting in, among other things, an overvaluation of the internal at the expense of the external world. Such a person must neither love nor be loved and must keep his libidinal objects at a distance (Khan 1960, p. 430).

The following clinical extract illustrates some of the qualities just described and the particular problems faced by the therapist in dealing with SPD:

> The patient, a middle-aged man in psychoanalytic psychotherapy three times weekly, began his session by complaining that he had felt bad after the session the previous day. He said he had had to drive to an appointment at lunchtime to see an acquaintance but got to a certain point on the journey and realized he could either branch off and go home or continue on the road to his meeting. He went to the meeting. He then said he had had thoughts in his mind about his psychotherapy session and had wanted to stop and write them down but that he was on a busy road and so couldn't do that. He had now forgotten what the thoughts were. He got to his destination but felt too tired to go up to the house and ring the bell. He had no energy left and thought of turning back. He turned the car around, pulled off the road, and went to sleep for about an hour. Then he went home. It was early, he realized, but he was still tired, and when he got in he went to sleep for several hours—for 3 hours, he thought.

> **Therapist:** You said you felt bad after our session yesterday.
> **Patient:** Bad?…bad…[*silence*]…I thought I hadn't been eating properly. Physically I am not entirely well, I still have a cough, maybe I am not entirely well yet….[*silence*] Tiredness…heaviness. I can feel it in my body…[*silence*]
> [*pause*]
> **Therapist:** You seemed a little surprised when I reminded you of what you said about feeling bad after the session yesterday.
> **Patient:** I don't recall saying that. I am not saying I did not, but if I did I am surprised that I did…[*silence*]…I don't remember what happened in the session. It feels a very long time ago…as if it were a long time ago.

In this brief vignette, typical of the type of interaction this man sustains with others (and which is also characteristic of many schizoid individuals), it is possible to see how the patient is "at a crossroads" with regard to his internal and external worlds. He attempts to engage with the external world, with his friend and with his psychotherapist, but is pulled back by anxiety regressively into his internal world, away from objects and toward a world of infantile orality that he experiences as less painful and conflicted.

A sense of latent hostility toward objects is also evident in the transference in the patient's references to falling asleep for "an hour" and "3 hours," although the patient has no conscious awareness of this. Many psychotherapists elect to use a "two-step" model of intervention and interpretation so as to allow the SPD patient to better tolerate the impact of references to the transference. Transference interpretations always draw the patient sharply into the analytic relationship, and this can prove traumatic for SPD patients.

The following vignette is from a session with a different patient and demonstrates how a supportive interpretation is followed by a more traditional interpretation of transference content:

> The patient, a woman in her 40s, finds that the separation anxiety evoked by gaps in the therapy (e.g., between sessions, during breaks) is so painful that it makes her want to quit. She finds it difficult to "hear" interpretations of her mental pain as being linked to the separations, so focused is she on the pain itself and the action of quitting in order to relieve it. In this session she reiterated that her only option was to quit the therapy. The therapist was able to say:
> "I understand your wish to stop your therapy and, of course, I have no power to stop you: to do what we are doing would be a difficult undertaking for anyone and I think that recently you have been finding it especially painful [*supportive intervention*].

"I think you feel frustrated and hurt by the comings and goings to and from our sessions and are often left having to cope with a great deal on your own. I think this makes you feel resentful and you feel like quitting to stop the upset and pain. It must be very hard to talk about these feelings. I suspect that you are worried that I might not be able to stand it if you talk about them" [*interpretation of underlying anxieties*].

By working through the crisis on these lines, the patient gained more insight into her fantasy of the destructiveness of her feelings that was behind her wish to quit, and she became able to begin to use object-related thinking and speech more, as opposed to making plans for direct action, to deal with her distress.

Clinical complications in treating schizoid individuals psychodynamically include the fact that they tend to provoke or seduce the analyst into a tantalizing relation to their material (e.g., in past history or internal reality), giving rise to the danger of overinterpretation. There is self-engrossment in relation to which the analyst is a spectator. The pseudo-enthusiasm of these patients masks a dread of their sense of inner emptiness being found out. Affects have a discharge urgency about them. The ego of the patient either inhibits or facilitates this discharge but is not related to it. These patients need new objects and new experiences to enable them to experience themselves personally. They lean on the hopefulness of others, which they mobilize and around which they can integrate their ego functioning for short periods. In the end they reduce the hopefulness to futility, and the persons involved feel defeated. Patients repeat this, with compulsion, in the analytic situation to test the psychotherapist, and the burden this puts on the clinician's counter-transference can be enormous and exhausting (Khan 1960, p. 431). Schizoid patients tend to "act out" their past experiences and current tensions in the analytic situation. They are terrified of ego regression and dependency needs, and require the clinician's readiness to cooperate in a controlled and limited involvement. They have, however, a deep need for help and seek to use the clinician to bear their affective crises in order for the ego to integrate very slowly through identification so that they can begin to experience themselves as persons.

Anxiety is the greatest obstacle to treatment of SPD; it creates impasses, as the analytic situation, through its very nature, mobilizes large quantities of affects and aims at their containment and assimilation. Two techniques are used by schizoid patients to combat their anxiety states: The first is the translation of anxiety into psychic pain as seen in the vignette above, and some patients can become almost addicted to such pain (Khan 1960, p. 432). The second technique is the translation of anxiety into diffuse and excessive tension states. These tension states can become a source of opposition to the analytic process, because the patient's intellectual defences are fed from this source. Genetically speaking, anxiety in these patients is not so much a reaction to strong and powerful libidinal impulses or to a primitive, sadistic superego as it is a sense of acute threat to the intactness and survival of the ego from the inner experience of utter emptiness and desolation. Any means of producing and maintaining psychic tension reassures them against the threat of anxiety deriving from this sense of emptiness. Psychic pain and masochism are used regularly to ward off this primary inner predicament. Masochistic pain raises the threshold of cathexes and so sponsors a sense of self (Khan 1960, p. 433).

Fairbairn, Khan, Balint, Klein, Rosenfeld, Kernberg, and others have noted that the principal internal strategies of defense employed by schizoid individuals are splitting, devaluation of objects and emotional experiences, excessive projective identifications, and idealization (Khan 1960, p. 434). Regarding idealization, Khan makes the point that schizoid patients often give the impression of being psychopathic or amoral, and one is tempted to relate this either to defective superego formation or to a primitively sadistic superego. Scrutiny of intrapsychic functioning often reveals a highly organized *ego-ideal* not built from introjection of idealized primary parental objects but assembled *in lieu of* adequate primary figures. This way of dealing with deprivation derives from magical thinking. The idealized, magically acquired internal object that resembles an ego-ideal is used to fend off hopelessness, emptiness, and futility. In the transference the patient will idealize the psychotherapist and the analytic process to offset disillusionment and hopelessness, which the patient feels certain will be the outcome in a real relationship (Khan 1960, p. 435).

SPD can be differentiated from PPD by a reduced level of suspiciousness of others and greater, chronic withdrawal. SPD is distinguishable from StPD by its less odd, eccentric, or obviously disturbed presentation, withdrawal again being its hallmark. Similarities of presentation of SPD with autism or Asperger's syndrome can sometimes make diagnosis complicated. Psychotic illness or severe depression may occur within SPD but can in some cases be linked to an accompanying personality disorder (such as avoidant personality disorder or PPD). Despite their detachment, many SPD individuals become very concerned about the unfulfilled lives they lead. Many do not marry or form sexual relationships, and if they do, they settle for nondemanding partners. Enough contact to offset loneliness may be found in the workplace or through limited socializing.

There is no generally accepted treatment for SPD. Group psycho-therapy may be used to help with socialization. Psychotherapy (which is usually individual but may be a combination of group and individual), perhaps with some medication, is sometimes recommended. Pharmacological treatments alone seem to have little impact on these patients, as their problems lie fundamentally in establishing relationships. Psychodynamic psychotherapy, although a potentially painful and confusing undertaking for schizoid individuals, probably offers the best hope for change. If the patient can become able to engage affectively with the therapist, even to a modest degree, the prospect of acquisition of insight and the promise of growth of the personality are genuine ones.

As with PPD, the psychotherapy of SPD requires tact and patience on the part of the psychotherapist. Perhaps the principal area of challenge in SPD lies in the primitive translation of anxiety (often pervasive) into psychic and physiological pain, which acts as a deterrent to dependency and trust. It can be of therapeutic and developmental value to the SPD patient to grasp emotionally, cognitively, and relationally the "impossibility" of the dilemma of claustro-agoraphobic anxiety in which they find themselves (cf. Rey 1994) and how this contributes to their heightened anxiety, and thus mental pain. By addressing ways of relating that are less dependent on the terms of reference of these psychotically based anxieties, many SPD patients become much better able to manage their extreme "suffocation–isolation" preoccupation and, over time, reduce the levels of omniscience and idealization that sustain it. This permits reflection on the fundamental fear of loss of the object that drives the patient's anxiety and mistrust. Eventually, the acquisition of a more modest but sincere dependence on the therapist and the analytic relationship can have the enduring effect of moderating extreme anxieties, as the patient feels more connected to the actual world and to others. Depressive anxieties may arise, bringing with them a new order of painful experiences such as acute fears of loss and grief with regard to the past. These anxieties are associated primarily with neurosis rather than psychosis.

Schizotypal Personality Disorder

StPD is characterized by a "pervasive pattern of social and interpersonal deficits marked by acute discomfort with, and reduced capacity for, close relationships as well as by cognitive or perceptual distortions and eccentricities of behavior" (American Psychiatric Association 2000, p. 697; see also World Health Organization 1992). "Schizotypal personality" is a category that derives from the term *schizotype*, first employed by Rado in 1953 to bring together schizophrenic and genotype into one category. *Schizotypal* refers to a disordered personality in which there are constitutional defects similar to those underlying schizophrenia. Brief psychotic episodes due to stress may arise in StPD, but these are usually transient. Some individuals with StPD may go on to develop schizophrenia, but they are a small minority.

The principal characteristics of StPD are distortions in cognition and perception, including a disturbed view of the body, and the presence of odd, magical, or eccentric beliefs or ideas. StPD (and SPD) individuals have considerable difficulty in experiencing pleasure (anhedonia). They may show ideas of reference and superstitions, and they experience chronic social anxiety. Close relationships are felt to be threatening, and social isolation is not uncommon. StPD individuals feel themselves to be at odds with, rather than part of, the world. They feel excluded—that they do not fit—and are resentful of feeling this way, often appearing agitated, frustrated, or disgruntled, while being unable to specify their complaint or the extent of their prevailing feelings. Withdrawal and avoidance are used to counter confusion and conflict. Strong feelings evoke intense anxiety because of a fear both of becoming engulfed by feelings and of being immersed in conflict, and this can threaten the patient's hold on reality. The need to avoid strong feelings leads to a tendency to overfocus on tangential issues (hence the characteristic of eccentricity). The patient may not be aware of the oddness of his or her beliefs and behavior and feels threatened if confronted. The patient's illusions and preoccupations defend against fragmented ego functioning and a precarious sense of self. Social contacts, support from family and friends, and engagement in therapeutic relationships are necessary to counter the tendency to remain withdrawn and thus become increasingly susceptible to psychotic thinking.

The chaotic and eccentric thinking that is characteristic of StPD may at times be mixed with paranoid and manic ideation. Ongoing assessment of the StPD patient's ego strength is therefore required. Containing the patient's multifarious anxieties and interpreting the meaning of his or her fixed ideas (which sometimes resemble delusions) are prerequisites for effective psychodynamic psychotherapy.

Despite the genetic link with schizophrenia and the susceptibility to ego fragmentation, StPD patients who enter psychotherapy may do better than SPD patients because of their greater affective availability. StPD patients may reveal areas of reasonable ego strength: this, combined with less rigid defenses than those of SPD patients, may enable them to respond more readily to analytic interpretations and to tolerate depressive affects. Progress may be slow and erratic, and results rarely approximate to a normal life. Gradual personality integration is possible, however, and can lead to a marked improvement in daily living. Treatment, especially in severe cases, may involve low dosages of the kinds of medications used in schizophrenia. As well, SSRIs can improve obsessive, compulsive, and depressive symptoms in StPD.

What follows is a description, rather than a clinical extract, of the psychotherapy of a 55-year-old woman with StPD. Its purpose is to give some indication of the range of complexities that confront the psychotherapist when treating StPD.

This particular patient is the sixth of seven children and was brought up in affluent but dysfunctional circumstances. As a child, she saw more of her rather austere nanny than she did of her mother. Her authoritarian but available father assumed the status of "rescuer" in the patient's mind, and she has turned to him throughout her life when in difficulty, despite feeling intimidated and humiliated when she does so. She has been able to talk to men with more ease than to women. Intimacy of any kind leads her to feel agitation, fear of conflict, and incipient guilt and shame. She complains of feeling unlike other people, feeling excluded, and being jealous of people who seem to have close relationships, while at the same time she can idealize her own background and upbringing. She blames herself for her feelings of ingratitude. Periodically she can feel depressed and hopeless, and she takes a low dosage of antidepressant medication to ease these feelings. The patient displays the troubled and tangential thinking typical of the StPD patient when faced with dependent feelings. For example, she can move from one subject to a completely different subject in a disconnected way, with little or no awareness of the incongruity. Conversely, she can fall silent, becoming prey to ruminative and persecuting thoughts. Her superego is overactive, often cautioning her about the multitude of dangers she faces if she trusts her psychotherapist or anyone else. This leads to recurrent confusion, as she often experiences her intense need for her trustworthy psychotherapist and her wish to violently reject her "dangerous" psychotherapist simultaneously. When she can no longer bear this exhausting internal conflict, she sometimes takes to her bed and can remain there for days. When withdrawn in this way she can disconnect almost entirely from others: her immediate family reported one occasion when she did not speak for a week and ate very little. During such crises, her psychotherapist reports sessions in which the patient is completely silent. The silence often contains an aggressive determination.

Her three-times-weekly psychotherapy has had a containing and stabilizing effect, and she has come to value her relationship with her therapist. At the same time, her growing dependency has aroused levels of psychotic anxiety that in the past she kept at bay by remaining distant from others. The support of her family has been helpful in containing her many anxieties. The split and fragmented nature of her mental functioning, typical of StPD patients and reminiscent of schizophrenic thinking, presents the therapist with the challenge of helping the patient to integrate into an already fragile ego potentially overwhelming, disparate thoughts and feelings that seem disconnected from one another and that are felt by the patient to be incompatible. The patient's internal object relations world reflects parallel fractures, with objects being experienced partially and usually in conflict with one another. Compelling aspects of objects intrude into her mind and are made even more threatening by the projective activity of the patient, which heightens the intensity of part-objects (Williams 2004). One clear feature in this patient is an underlying paranoid quality to her relationships that is similar to the primitive, threatening anxieties seen in paranoid schizophrenia. Her dread of disintegration seems to be connected to dissociated feelings of narcissistically derived rage that threaten to emerge when her capacity for idealization and withdrawal feels threatened. At these times she can feel terror that she will be annihilated.

It has required considerable containing activity on the part of the therapist in order for the patient to begin to be able to talk about her feelings, as she was consumed by a delusional conviction that the therapist could not bear her, and that this was the reason why (customary) breaks in the therapy occurred. Containment and interpretation of her feelings of rejection and the associated paranoid anxieties were the principal therapeutic tasks. When the patient did talk of her feelings, she was impeded by thought blocking, retching (inside and outside the sessions, although she did not vomit), and a tendency to refute, in a histrionic manner, what she had said moments earlier. She occasionally brought with her a utensil/container as a source of comfort, and sometimes when she experienced fear of dying or of committing suicide, she experienced physical symptoms such as shaking and rocking. The therapist's countertransference experience was decisive in understanding the patient's confusing behavior and thoughts. A particular set of repeated countertransference feelings was anxiety that therapy was hopeless and the patient would quit or, worse, not survive, alongside frustration at her inability and unwillingness to speak openly about what troubled her. These countertransference responses enabled the therapist to reflect on what feelings the patient was likely holding at bay and to speculate on why it would be these feelings in particular. Eventually, when ideas derived from these countertransference feelings were carefully introduced, the patient was able to speak, little by little, of a lifelong tendency to be compliant, tremendous frustration at feeling "different" and misunderstood, and an internal hatred and bitterness at feeling neglected that gave rise to fantasies of murder and dismemberment—thoughts that she felt were unforgivable. This case, thought somewhat severe, is nonetheless typical of an StPD patient's responses to psychodynamic psychotherapy and underscores the need in the psychotherapist for patience, sensitivity, and an understanding of complex axes of transference and countertransference experience that encompass conflict, deficit, compromised and failed developmental milestones, and, above all, the intrusion of psychotic thinking that fragments ego functioning.

Conceptualization of StPD stresses early fragmentation of the ego and damage to the sense of self of a type associated with schizophrenic states. As a consequence, low self-esteem accompanies and fuels difficulties in personal relationships. Psychological functioning reveals primitive, part-object relationships; impoverished mental representations; developmental deficits (in terms of the capacity to mentalize); and a potential for psychotic thinking under stress. The StPD patient's failure to internalize adequate representations of the object means that he or she remains fixated at the paranoid-schizoid level of development (Klein 1946). Because trauma (externally and/or internally derived) is held to have occurred at the oral stage, StPD anxieties are viewed as extremely primitive, requiring thoroughgoing containment followed by interpretation at points when the ego is neither overwhelmed by anxiety nor paralyzed by defenses. Both StPD and SPD patients fit the "philobatic" profile described by Balint (1969). He proposed two internal solutions to the failure of the relationship between mother and baby. The "basic fault" in the infant's personality may be expressed as either the "ocnophilic" or the "philobatic" tendency in later life. The former is a response to a chronic "emptiness inside" and seeks to fill it by compulsively demanding more and more from others. The latter involves giving up on others and retreating into a world of fantasy. Bowlby's "avoidantly attached" category is a similar characterization of these individuals who are too afraid of aversive contact to seek out relationships (Bowlby 1969, 1988).

Key Clinical Concepts

◆ Cluster A personality disorders are characterized by a prevalence of psychotic anxieties in parallel to the patient's neurotic anxieties. The expressive forms of these different levels of anxiety vary according to the condition, but all have in common a need for the clinician to pay particular attention to the impact of psychotic thinking on the therapeutic alliance, the transference, and the patient's ego functioning.

- The therapist needs to be aware of how he or she is being experienced by the Cluster A patient in object relations terms—as part or whole ("Who or what am I currently representing for the patient, and in what way?"). Sufficient engagement with the Cluster A patient is only possible if this awareness is acquired. At one moment the therapist may be experienced positively, even as an idealized figure, but a dramatic change can occur and the therapist may be seen as a persecuting critic or tyrant. This change can take place without the therapist's saying anything controversial and signifies the radical disjuncture in the patient's capacity for affective control and the extent of splitting of the ego and objects.

- A nondefensive, nonconfrontational approach and willingness on the part of the therapist to tolerate being a "bad" (i.e., inadequate) object, as well as a "good" object, is essential to establishing basic trust and a reduction in splitting.

- Countertransference monitoring of how the patient is making the therapist feel (e.g., "I am now experiencing strong feelings [these may be boredom, sexual or aggressive feelings, etc.]: to what extent do these feelings originate in me or is the patient inducing me to feel these?") is a critical component in understanding the use of splitting, projective identification, and the part-object functioning that characterizes Cluster A mental representations. It is likely that the patient's core pathogenic relationships will become discernible first in the countertransference.

- All Cluster A patients have suffered significant damage to their self-esteem. An awareness in the psychotherapist of the patient's propensity for deep feelings of shame and humiliation will help in the weathering of bouts of acting out and negative therapeutic reactions. The latter are stubborn resistances to improvement, usually following some improvement. They are to be expected, as are actings-out by patients over money, timings, holidays, and so forth, and need to be responded to by reality-based, firm but supportive interventions, together with interpretation of the anxieties being defended against.

♦ Avoiding malignant regression is important. Regression is a defensive reversion, under stress, to earlier forms of thinking and object-relating and is often inevitable in therapy. *Benign* regression signifies a healthy satisfying of certain infantile needs by working these through collaboratively in the therapy. *Malignant* regression denotes a situation is which the patient tries but fails to have these needs met and the situation yields a vicious cycle of demanding, addiction-like states. The therapist, if he or she is to achieve the trust of a Cluster A patient, must avoid reacting to the patient in an overemotional way that fuels malignant regression but remain rooted in analytic work, keeping in mind the compromised ego of the infant in the patient.

♦ Awareness of deficit as well as conflict models is useful in understanding the quality of patients' attachments, as these can be highly primitive and confused.

♦ Therapeutic goals require realistic assessment and regular monitoring: progress may be slow and erratic with setbacks and perhaps ultimately limited eventual gains. These gains may translate into improvements in daily living that are of inestimable value.

Suggested Readings

Bell D: Paranoia: Ideas in Psychoanalysis. New York, Totem Books, 2003

Fairbairn WRD: Psychoanalytic Studies of the Personality. London, Tavistock, 1952

Hinshelwood RD: Clinical Klein: From Theory to Practice. New York, HarperCollins, 1994

Khan MR: Clinical aspects of the schizoid personality: affects and technique. Int J Psychoanal 41:430–436, 1960

Rey H: Universals of Psychoanalysis in the Treatment of Psychotic and Borderline States. London, Free Association Books, 1994

Stone M: Schizotypal personality: psychotherapeutic aspects. Schizophr Bull 11:576–589, 1985

Treatment outlines for paranoid, schizotypal and schizoid personality disorders. The Quality Assurance Project. Aust N Z J Psychiatry 24:339–350, 1990

Wurmser L: Torment Me But Don't Abandon Me: Psychoanalysis of the Severe Neuroses in a New Key. Lanham, MD, Rowman & Littlefield Publishers, 2007

References

American Psychiatric Association: Diagnostic and Statistical Manual of Mental Disorders, 4th Edition, Text Revision. Washington, DC, American Psychiatric Association, 2000

Balint M: The Basic Fault: Therapeutic Aspects of Regression. New York, Brunner/Mazel, 1969

Bell D: Paranoia: Ideas in Psychoanalysis. New York, Totem Books, 2003

Bowlby J: Attachment and Loss. Harmondsworth, UK, Penguin, 1969

Bowlby J: A Secure Base: Clinical Applications of Attachment Theory. London, Routledge, 1988

Elkin GD: Introduction to Clinical Psychiatry. New York, McGraw-Hill, 1999

Fairbairn WRD: Psychoanalytic Studies of the Personality. London, Tavistock, 1952

Freud S: Psycho-analytic notes on an autobiographical account of a case of paranoia (dementia paranoides) (1911), in The Standard Edition of the Complete Psychological Works of Sigmund Freud, Vol 12. Translated and edited by Strachey J. London, Hogarth Press, 1958, pp 1–82

Gabbard GO: Psychodynamic Psychiatry in Clinical Practice, 3rd Edition. Washington, DC, American Psychiatric Press, 2000

Grotstein JS: Object relations theory in the treatment of the psychoses. Bull Menninger Clin 59:312–332, 1995

Gunderson J: Borderline Personality Disorder: A Clinical Guide. Washington, DC, American Psychiatric Publishing, 2008

Hinshelwood RD: Clinical Klein: From Theory to Practice. New York, HarperCollins, 1994

Jackson M: Weathering the Storms. London, Karnac Books, 2000

Jackson M, Williams P: Unimaginable Storms: A Search for Meaning in Psychosis. London, Karnac Books, 1994

Kernberg O: Borderline Personality and Pathological Narcissism. Northvale, NJ, Jason Aronson, 1975

Khan MR: Clinical aspects of the schizoid personality: affects and technique. Int J Psychoanal 41:430–436, 1960

Klein M: Notes on some schizoid mechanisms. Int J Psychoanal 27:99–110, 1946

Kohut H, Wolf ES: The disorders of the self and their treatment: an outline. Int J Psychoanal 59:413–426, 1978

Lieberz K, Porsch U: Countertransference in schizoid disorders. Psychother Psychosom Med Psychol 47:46–51, 1997

Lucas RN: The psychotic personality: a psychoanalytic theory and its application in clinical practice. Psychoanalytic Psychotherapy 6:73–79, 1992

Mahler MS, Pine F, Bergman A: The Psychological Birth of the Human Infant. London, Karnac Books, 1975

McGlashan T: The Chestnut Lodge follow-up study, III: long-term outcome of borderline personalities. Arch Gen Psychiatry 43:20–30, 1986

Meissner WW: The Paranoid Process. Northvale, NJ, Jason Aronson, 1986

Meissner WW: Treatment of Patients in the Borderline Spectrum. Northvale, NJ, Jason Aronson, 1988

Ogden T: Reverie and Interpretation: Sensing Something Human. London, Karnac Books, 1999

Rey H: Universals of Psychoanalysis in the Treatment of Psychotic and Borderline States. London, Free Association Books, 1994

Robbins M: The language of schizophrenia and the world of delusion. Int J Psychoanal 83:383–405, 2002

Rosenfeld H: On the psychopathology of narcissism: a clinical approach. Int J Psychoanal 45:332–337, 1964

Rosenfeld HA: On the treatment of psychotic states by psychoanalysis: an historical approach. Int J Psychoanal 50:615–631, 1969

Rycroft C: The analysis of a paranoid personality. Int J Psychoanal 41:59–69, 1960

Sandell R, Blomberg J, Lazar A, et al: Findings of the Stockholm Outcome of Psychotherapy and Psychoanalysis Project (STOPPP). Paper presented at the annual meeting of the Society for Psychotherapy Research, Geilo, Norway, 1997

Segal H: On symbolism. Int J Psychoanal 59:315–319, 1978

Sohn L: Unprovoked assaults: making sense of apparently random violence, in Reason and Passion: A Celebration of the Work of Hanna Segal. Edited by Bell D. London, Tavistock, 1997, pp 57–74

Sperry L: Diagnosis and Treatment of DSM-IV Personality Disorders. New York, Brunner-Routledge, 1995

Stone M: Schizotypal personality: psychotherapeutic aspects. Schizophr Bull 11:576–589, 1985

Stone M: Long-term outcome in personality disorders. Br J Psychiatry 162:299–313, 1993

Target M, Fonagy P: An Outcome Study of Psychotherapy for Patients With Borderline Personality Disorder. New York, International Universities Press, 1996ba

Target M, Fonagy P: Playing with reality, II: the development of psychic reality from a theoretical perspective. Int J Psychoanal 77:459–479, 1996b

Treatment outlines for paranoid, schizotypal, and schizoid personality disorders. The Quality Assurance Project. Aust N Z J Psychiatry 24:339–350, 1990

Williams P: Incorporation of an invasive object. Int J Psychoanal 85:1–15, 2004

Winnicott DW: The aims of psychoanalytic treatment, in The Maturational Processes and the Facilitating Environment. London, Hogarth Press, 1962, pp 166–170

World Health Organization: International Statistical Classification of Diseases and Related Health Problems, 10th Revision. Geneva, World Health Organization, 1992

Wurmser L: Torment Me But Don't Abandon Me: Psychoanalysis of the Severe Neuroses in a New Key. Lanham, MD, Rowman & Littlefield Publishers, 2007

CHAPTER 6

Mentalization-Based Treatment and Borderline Personality Disorder

Anthony Bateman, M.A., F.R.C.Psych.
Peter Fonagy, Ph.D., F.B.A.

Mentalization-based treatment (MBT) of borderline personality disorder developed from within the psychoanalytic tradition. Since Stern (1938, 1945) reported that patients with borderline personality disorder (BPD) did not respond as anticipated to standard psychoanalytic therapy, practitioners have been adapting techniques to accommodate the particular difficulties presented in therapy by these patients. Kazdin (2004) suggested that effective therapy has to be tailored to an understanding of what we know about the processes that directly bear on the onset and course of a clinical problem. MBT developed in the spirit of this principle. We drew on evidence from the study of child development to formulate a theoretical model of the core pathology of BPD. We tailored our therapy to address the problems in adulthood arising from these central developmental difficulties. In this chapter we outline our developmental view of borderline personality disorder and summarize key aspects of MBT that we consider to be crucial in treating BPD.

Mental States and Mentalizing

Our mental states may be either internally determined, as when we feel guilty about something we feel or think, or externally activated, as when someone criticizes us and provokes a sense of failure. Of course, many of our mental states rely on both external and internal determinants. We respond by forming a mental representation of what is going on in our mind. This mental representation may determine our subsequent behavior: as we feel nervous and realize that we are in danger from someone who threatens us, we start to ready ourselves to move out of the way or we avoid their gaze. But if we are in a situation in which we cannot understand mental states, or alternatively we have a compromised capacity to accurately recognize our own and others' motivations, we are likely to become easily confused and, as a consequence, we may behave inappropriately or seemingly randomly.

The ability to understand mental states is called *mentalization* (Fonagy 1989). Mentalization is the capacity to make sense of ourselves and others, implicitly and explicitly, in terms of subjective states and mental processes (Table 6–1). Understanding other people's behavior and our own in terms of thoughts, feelings, wishes, and desires is a major developmental achievement that originates in the context of the attachment relationship. Our understanding of others and ourselves critically depends on whether as infants our own mental states were adequately understood by caring, attentive, nonthreatening adults (Fonagy et al. 2002).

While the idea that we understand ourselves and others in terms of what is going on in the mind appeals immediately to our common sense about how we function in everyday life, the process by which we actually do it is complex. It is very easy to make mistakes, and feeling misunderstood or not understanding something or someone makes us feel uncomfortable. Our reaction to this feeling will depend on the extent to which we are able to continue the process of mentalizing. A number of factors will determine the degree to which we are able to retain our

---

TABLE 6–1.   Key aspects of mentalizing

Mentalizing is the ability to understand ourselves and others in terms of mental states

Mental states are opaque

We use internal and external cues to recognize underlying mental states

Arousal undermines our mentalizing capacity

---

capacity to mentalize in such circumstances. The most important factor, as we have mentioned, is our developmentally determined competence in managing emotional states. But the ability to mentalize is determined not solely by our developmental experience but also by our current competence. Even everyday experiences such as feeling tired can influence how we manage our feelings. Further, the relationship or context we are in may itself have a direct bearing on our ability to maintain mentalizing. In some contexts we will be able to continue reflecting; in others, we are unable to do so. So, although to some extent a capacity to mentalize has the qualities of a trait and we all start with a baseline ability, our mentalizing capacity may fluctuate over time and with current circumstances, especially current interpersonal context and level of emotional arousal.

Components of Mentalizing

Mentalizing is a multidimensional construct, and breaking it down into dimensional components is helpful for understanding mentalization-based treatment. Broadly speaking, mentalization can be considered according to four intersecting dimensions: automatic/controlled or implicit/explicit, internally/externally based, self/other oriented, and cognitive/affective process (Table 6–2). Each of these dimensions possibly relates to a different neurobiological system (for further discussion of this, see P. Luyten, P. Fonagy, L. Mayes, R. Vermote, B. Lowyck, A. Bateman, and M. Target, "Mentalization as a Multidimensional Concept," 2009, submitted). But although separating out the different dimensions of mentalizing may help clarity, the key to successful mentalizing is the integration of all the dimensions into a coherent whole.

IMPLICIT AND EXPLICIT MENTALIZING

Most of us mentalize automatically in our everyday lives—not to do so would be exhausting. Automatic or implicit mentalizing allows us to rapidly form mental representations based on previous experience and

TABLE 6–2.   Dimensions of mentalizing

Self and other

Cognitive and affective

Automatic/implicit and controlled/explicit

Internal and external

to use those as a reference point as we gather further information to confirm or disconfirm our tentative understanding of motivations. This is reflexive, requires little attention, and is beneath the level of our awareness (Satpute and Lieberman 2006). If it does not seem to be working we move to more explicit or controlled mentalizing (Table 6–3). Explicit mentalizing requires effort and attention; it is therefore slower and more time-consuming and most commonly done verbally. Our capacity to manage this controlled mentalizing varies considerably, and the threshold at which we return to automatic mentalizing is, in part, determined by the response we receive to our explicit attempts to understand someone in relation to ourselves and the secondary attachment strategies we deploy when aroused and under stress. Behavioral, neurobiological, and neuroimaging studies suggest that the move from controlled to automatic mentalizing and thence to nonmentalizing modes is determined by a "switch" between cortical and subcortical brain systems (Arnsten 1998; Lieberman 2007) and that the point at which we switch is determined by our attachment patterns.

Different attachment histories are associated with attachment styles that differ in the associated background level of activation of the attachment system and in the point at which the switch from more prefrontal, controlled to more automatic mentalizing occurs (Luyten et al., 2009, submitted). Dismissing individuals tend to deny attachment needs, asserting autonomy, independence, and strength in the face of stress by using attachment deactivation strategies. In contrast, a preoccupied attachment classification or an anxious attachment style is generally thought to be linked with the use of attachment hyperactivating strategies (Mikulincer and Shaver 2008). Attachment hyperactivating strategies have been consistently associated with the tendency to exaggerate both the presence and the seriousness of threats, with frantic efforts to find support and relief often expressed in demanding, clinging behavior. Both Adult Attachment Interview and self-report studies have found a predominance of anxious-preoccupied attachment strategies in BPD patients (e.g., Fonagy et al. 1996; Levy et al. 2005). In borderline patients we and others have noted a characteristic pattern of fearful attachment (attachment-anxiety and relational avoidance), painful intolerance of aloneness, hypersensitivity to social environment, expectation of hostility from others, and greatly reduced positive memories of dyadic interactions (e.g., Critchfield et al. 2008; Fonagy et al. 1996; Gunderson and Lyons-Ruth 2008).

An important cause of anxious attachment in BPD patients is the commonly observed trauma history of these individuals. Attachment theorists, in particular Mary Main and Erik Hesse, have suggested that

TABLE 6–3.   Implicit and explicit mentalizing

Implicit/Automatic	Explicit/Controlled
Reflexive	Involves effort
Fast	Slow
Requires little attention	Requires attention
Beneath the level of our awareness	Aware and often verbal

maltreatment leads to the disorganization of the child's attachment to the caregiver because of the irresolvable internal conflict created by the need for reassurance from the very person who also (by association perhaps) generates an experience of lack of safety. The activation of the attachment system by the threat of maltreatment is followed by proximity seeking, which drives the child closer to an experience of threat and thus leads to further (hyper)activation of the attachment system (Hesse 2008). This irresolvable conflict leaves the child with an overwhelming sense of helplessness and hopelessness. Congruent with these assumptions, there is compelling evidence for problematic family conditions in the development of BPD, including physical and sexual abuse, prolonged separations, and neglect and emotional abuse, although their specificity and etiological import have often been questioned (e.g., New et al. 2008; Zweig-Frank et al. 2006). Probably a quarter of BPD patients have no maltreatment histories (Goodman and Yehuda 2002), and the vast majority of individuals with abuse histories show a high rate of resilience and no personality pathology (McGloin and Widom 2001; Paris 1998). Early neglect may be an underestimated risk factor (Kantojarvi et al. 2008; Watson et al. 2006), as there is some evidence from adoption and other studies to suggest that early neglect interferes with emotion understanding (e.g., Shipman et al. 2005) and this effect plays a role in the emergence of emotional difficulties in preschool (Vorria et al. 2006) and even in adolescence (Colvert et al. 2008). One developmental path to impairments in mentalizing in BPD may be a combination of early neglect, which might undermine the infant's developing capacity for affect regulation, with later maltreatment or other environmental circumstances, including adult experience of verbal, emotional, physical, and sexual abuse (Zanarini et al. 2005), that are likely to activate the attachment system chronically (Fonagy and Bateman 2008).

BPD patients who mix deactivating and hyperactivating strategies, as is characteristic of disorganized attachment, show a tendency for *both* hypermentalization *and* a failure of mentalization. On the one hand, because attachment deactivating strategies are typically associated with minimizing and avoiding affective contents, BPD patients often have a tendency for hypermentalization—that is, continuing attempts to mentalize, but without integrating cognition and affect. At the same time, because the use of hyperactivating strategies is associated with a decoupling of controlled mentalization, this leads to failures of mentalization as a result of an overreliance on models of social cognition that antedate full mentalizing (Bateman and Fonagy 2006).

This dual tendency has important clinical implications for mentalization-based treatment. The therapist needs to develop strategies related to excessive demand and dependent behavior, as well as ensure an ability to manage sudden therapeutic ruptures often characterized by dismissive statements about the therapist's inadequacies, with the accompanying danger of leaving treatment.

INTERNAL AND EXTERNAL MENTALIZING

The dimension of internal and external mentalizing refers to the predominant focus of mentalizing (Lieberman 2007) (Table 6–4). Internal mentalizing refers to a focus on one's own or others' internal states—that is, thoughts, feelings, desires; external mentalizing implies a reliance on external features such as facial expression and behavior. This is not the same as the self/other dimension, which relates to the actual object of focus. Mentalization focused on a psychological interior may be self or other oriented. Again, this distinction has important consequences for MBT. Patients with BPD have a problem with internal mentalizing, but they also have difficulties with externally focused mentalizing. Inevitably both components of mentalizing inform each other, so borderline patients are doubly disadvantaged. The difficulty is not so much that patients with BPD necessarily misinterpret facial expression, although they might sometimes do so, but more that they are highly sensitive to facial expressions and so tend to react rapidly and without warning (Lynch et al. 2006; Wagner and Linehan 1999). Any

---

TABLE 6–4.   Internal and external mentalizing

Internal mentalizing refers to a focus on one's own or others' internal states such as thoughts

External mentalizing relies on external features such as facial expression and behavior

Patients with borderline personality disorder have problems with both internal and external mentalizing

---

movement of the therapist might trigger a response—glancing out of the window, for example, might lead to a statement that the therapist obviously is not listening and so the patient might feel compelled to leave; a nonreactive face is equally disturbing, as patients continuously attempt to deduce the therapist's internal state by using information derived from external monitoring. Anything that disrupts this process will create anxiety, which leads to a loss of mentalizing and the reemergence of developmentally earlier ways of relating to the world.

A reduced ability to arrive at an emotional understanding of others by reading their facial expressions accurately exaggerates a compromised ability in BPD to infer mental states from a focus on internal states. To maintain or repair cooperation during social/interpersonal exchange and interaction, we have to understand social gestures and the likely interpersonal consequences when shared expectations about fair exchange or social norms are violated by accident or intent. To do this we have to integrate external mentalizing with an assessment of the underlying internal state of mind of the other person. The importance of this interactional process in the pathology of BPD has been creatively demonstrated experimentally. Using a multi-round economic exchange game played between patients with BPD and mentally healthy partners, King-Casas et al. (2008) showed that behaviorally, individuals with BPD showed a profound incapacity to maintain cooperation and were impaired in their ability to repair broken cooperation on the basis of a quantitative measure of coaxing. They failed at understanding the intentions of others—an internally based task. They expected their partners to be mean to them and they were unable to change this understanding even when evidence suggested it was incorrect—for example, when their partner was generous. In other words, they were unable to read the intentions of their partner and to alter their own behavior reciprocally. This gradually led their partner in the game to become mean, suggesting that the partner was provoked to become the very person he was being seen as. Analogously, therapists working with patients with BPD must bear in mind the risk of being provoked into becoming the very therapist that their patient accuses them of being.

SELF AND OTHER MENTALIZING

Impairments and imbalances in the capacity to reflect about oneself and others are common, and it is only when they become more extreme that they begin to cause problems (Table 6–5). Some people become experts at "reading" other people's minds, and if they misuse this ability or exploit it for their own gain, we tend to think they have antisocial charac-

TABLE 6–5.   Self and other mentalizing

Patients with borderline personality disorder are vulnerable to losing self and other mentalizing, particularly in interpersonal interactions

Patients with antisocial personality disorder are good at reading other people's minds but misuse this ability and exploit it for their own gain

Patients with narcissistic personality disorder focus on themselves and their own internal states. They become experts in what others can do for them to meet their needs.

teristics; others focus on themselves and their own internal states and become experts in what others can do for them to meet their requirements, and we then suggest they are narcissistic. Thus excessive concentration on either the self or other leads to one-sided relationships and distortions in social interaction. Inevitably this will be reflected in how patients present for treatment and interact with their therapists. Patients with BPD may be oversensitive, carefully monitoring the therapist's mind at the expense of their own needs and being what they think the therapist wants them to be. They may even take on the mind of the therapist and make it their own. Therapists should be wary of patients who eagerly comply with everything said to them. Such compliance may alternate with a tendency to become preoccupied with and overly concerned about internal states of mind, with the result that the therapist feels left out of the relationship and unable to participate effectively.

COGNITIVE AND AFFECTIVE MENTALIZING

The final dimension to consider relates to cognitive and emotional processing—belief, reasoning, and perspective taking on the one hand and emotional empathy, subjective self-experience, and mentalized affectivity on the other (Jurist 2005) (Table 6–6). A high level of mentalizing requires integration of both cognitive and affective processes. But some people are able to manage one aspect to a greater degree than the other.

TABLE 6–6.   Cognitive and affective mentalizing

Cognitive mentalizing involves belief, reasoning, and perspective taking

Affective mentalizing uses emotional empathy, affect experience, and subjective self experience

Patients with borderline personality disorder are overwhelmed by affective processes and cannot form representations integrating emotional and cognitive processes

Patients with BPD are overwhelmed by affective processes and cannot integrate them with their cognitive understanding—they may understand why they do something but feel unable to use their understanding to manage their feelings; they are compelled to act because they cannot form representations integrating emotional and cognitive processes. Others, such as people with antisocial personality disorder, invest considerable time in cognitive understanding of mental states, to the detriment of affective experience.

The Mentalizing Model of Borderline Personality Disorder

The capacity to understand self and others as being guided by aims and intentions is considered to be a key developmental achievement, and the disruption of this ability is a major aspect in the psychopathology of BPD (Table 6–7). Fundamentally we view BPD as a disorder of the self. The self develops in the affect-regulatory context of early relationships. Our mentalizing model of BPD is rooted in Bowlby's attachment theory and its further elaboration by developmental psychologists, paying particular attention to the ideas of contingency theory proposed by Gergely and Watson (1999). We assume that infants require their emotional signals to be accurately or contingently mirrored by an attachment figure if they are to acquire a robust sense of self. The mirroring must also be "marked" (e.g., exaggerated)—in other words, slightly distorted—if the infant is to understand that the caregiver's display is a representation of the infant's emotional experience rather than an expression of the caretaker's. In this way the infant will gradually build a representation of his own states and those of others. Absence or unreliable availability of marked contingent mirroring is associated with the later development of disorganized attachment. Infants whose attachment has been observed to be disorganized exhibit behaviors like freezing (dissociation) and self-harm (e.g., head banging) and go on to develop oppositional, highly controlling behavioral tendencies in middle childhood.

We assume that a child who does not have the opportunity to develop a representation of his own experience through mirroring will instead internalize the image of the caregiver as part of his self representation. This discontinuity within the self has been called the *alien self*. Due to the inevitability of failures of mirroring with even the most attuned caregiver, the internalization of such incongruent representations is considered to be a normal part of development. However, within disorganized attachment relationships this takes place to the extent that it

TABLE 6–7.   Mentalizing model of borderline personality
disorder

Mentalizing is vulnerable to disruption

Genetic and environmental factors are important in development of
mentalizing fragility

Poor affect regulation, low attentional control, and fragile interpersonal
understanding occur

Activating (provoking) risk factors include emotional abuse, trauma, and
nonmentalizing social systems

Attachment system is hyperreactive

is liable to fragment the self-structure. The controlling behavior of children with a history of disorganized attachment is understood as the persistence of a pattern analogous to projective identification, where the experience of incoherence within the self is reduced through externalization. The intense need for the caregiver that is characteristic of separation anxiety in middle childhood is associated with disorganized attachment, where it reflects the need for the caregiver as a vehicle for externalization of the alien part of the self rather than simply an insecure attachment relationship.

Normally, experiences of fragmentation within the self-structure are reduced by the concurrent development of mentalization, but disorganized attachment and the consequent need for massive externalization of the alien self through projective identification create a poor context for mentalizing to develop. The most important cause of disruption in the development of mentalization is psychological trauma, early or late in childhood, which undermines the capacity to think about mental states or the ability to give narrative accounts of one's past relationships. Psychological trauma may work to impair a child's capacity for mentalizing in four ways, as detailed below and listed in Table 6–8:

1. The child may defensively inhibit the capacity to think about others' thoughts and feelings in the face of the experience of others' genuinely malevolent intent.
2. Early excessive stress can distort the functioning of arousal mechanisms, resulting in the inhibition of orbitofrontal cortical activity (the location of mentalizing) at far lower levels of threat than would normally be the case—a move from controlled mentalizing to automatic mentalizing.
3. Any trauma arouses the attachment system, leading to a search for attachment security. Where the attachment relationship is itself

TABLE 6–8.   Mechanisms of impaired mentalizing after psychological trauma

Traumatic experience leads to defensive inhibition of capacity to mentalize

Early stress distorts functioning of arousal mechanisms, lowering the threshold for automatic mentalizing

Prolonged arousal of the attachment system stimulated by trauma leads to specific impairments in mentalizing

Identification with the aggressor may lead to dissociation of an internalized "alien self"

traumatizing, such arousal is exacerbated because in seeking proximity to the traumatizing attachment figure, the child may be further traumatized. Such prolonged activation of the attachment system may have specific inhibitory consequences for mentalization.

4. The child, in "identifying with the aggressor" as a way of gaining illusory control over the abuser, may internalize the intent of the aggressor in an alien (dissociated) part of the self. While this might offer temporary relief, the destructive intent of the abuser will in this way come to be experienced from within rather than outside of the self, leading to unbearable self-hatred.

The phenomenology of BPD is the consequence of the inhibition of mentalization—which may occur even without the experience of overt trauma—and the reemergence of modes of experiencing internal reality that antedate the development of mentalization. In addition, there is a constant tendency to re-externalize the self-destructive alien self through projective identification. Individuals with BPD are "normal" mentalizers, albeit sometimes with a lower base level than others, except in the context of attachment relationships; within such relationships they tend to misread minds, both their own and those of others, when emotionally aroused. As a relationship with another person moves into the sphere of attachment, the BPD patient's ability to think about the mental state of the other can rapidly disappear. When this happens, prementalistic modes of organizing subjectivity emerge, with the power to disorganize these relationships and destroy the coherence of self-experience that normal mentalization sustains through narrative. In the mode of psychic equivalence (normally described by clinicians as concreteness of thought), in which alternative perspectives cannot be considered, there is no experience of "as if" and everything appears to be "for real." This can add drama as well as risk to interpersonal experience, and the exaggerated reaction of patients to apparently small events is justified by the seriousness with which they suddenly experience their own and others' thoughts and feelings. In the pretend mode, conversely, thoughts and feelings can come to be almost dissociated to the point of near-meaninglessness. In these states patients can discuss experiences without contextualizing them in any kind of physical or material reality. Attempting psychotherapy with patients who are in this mode can lead the therapist to lengthy but inconsequential discussions of internal experience that have no link to genuine experience. Finally, early modes of conceptualizing action in terms of that which is apparent can come to dominate motivation. Within this mode there is a primacy of the physical; experience is felt to be valid only when its consequences are apparent to all. Affection, for example, is only felt to be genuine if accompanied by physical expression.

The most disruptive feature of borderline psychopathology is the apparently unstoppable tendency to create unacceptable experience within the other through the externalization of the abuser, who has been internalized by the traumatized individual as an alien part of the self. This can create a terrified alien self in the other—therapist, friend, parent—who becomes the vehicle for what is emotionally unbearable. An adhesive, addictive pseudo-attachment to the individual who becomes the recipient of the projection may develop because the alternative to such projective identification is to attack or destroy the self by self-harm and suicide.

What Is Mentalization-Based Treatment?

Mentalization-based treatment (Bateman and Fonagy 2004, 2006) places mentalizing, as discussed above, at the center of the therapeutic process. As a therapy it is not defined primarily by a clustering of specific and related techniques but rather by the process that is engendered in therapy. With this in mind, and in the context of our discussion about mentalizing itself, a number of principles become evident.

First, the therapist can use any technique as long as the primary aim is to stimulate a mentalizing process. The overall aim of treatment should be simultaneously to stimulate a patient's attachment to and involvement with treatment while helping the patient maintain mentalization. Second, competent delivery of MBT requires the therapist to avoid nonmentalizing techniques—that is, those that are likely to reduce mentalizing in the patient or inadvertently to undermine the mentalizing process; it is well known but rarely openly acknowledged that psychotherapy may induce harm. Third, good outcomes will depend on improving the mentalizing skill of the patient as therapy progresses. Fourth, effective implementation requires the clinician to focus on his or her own capacity to mentalize—mentalizing in the clinician begets mentalizing in the patient, and nonmentalizing provokes nonmentalizing. We cannot take the clinician's mentalizing skill for granted; research on psychotherapy process indicates that clinicians' mentalizing capacities vary, for example, from patient to patient (Diamond et al. 2003). This may be especially pertinent in the treatment of patients with BPD, who may be exquisitely sensitive to their therapists and who may induce strong reactive emotional states.

Finally, MBT is likely to be most effective for those patients with mentalizing deficits. But there is an important rider to add to this statement. We can conceive of most mental disorders as the mind misinterpreting its own experience of itself, thus ultimately as disorders of mentalization. Yet the key issue here is not whether a mental disorder can be redescribed in terms of the functioning of mentalization but rather whether the dysfunction of mentalization is core to the disorder and/or a focus on mentalization is heuristically valid—that is, provides an appropriate domain for therapeutic intervention. For example, mentalizing problems have been described in schizophrenia (Frith 2004), but we cannot infer from this that a mentalizing-based intervention will ultimately be useful as a treatment method itself. The same applies to conditions such as autism, in which patients have been shown to suffer more or less complete mind blindness (Baron-Cohen et al. 2000). Again, whether an emphasis on mentalizing provides an appropriate focus for interventions is currently an open question.

WHAT'S NEW?

MBT has been studied most extensively for the treatment of BPD. It is currently being adapted to treat other conditions and other personality disorders, such as antisocial personality disorder and paranoid personality disorder, although the modifications to the approach that may be necessary in working with patients with these conditions remain to be determined.

In an earlier work we described MBT as "the *least novel* therapeutic approach imaginable, simply because it revolves around a fundamental human capacity—indeed, the capacity that makes us human" (Allen et al. 2008, p. 6). MBT has produced no new psychotherapeutic techniques and, despite appearances, is not a new therapy. The most that can be claimed for MBT is that it structures treatment for BPD, organizes inter-

---

TABLE 6–9.   Mentalization-based treatment

Therapist attitude using a non-knowing stance is crucial

Interventions are tailored to the patient's mentalizing capacity

Use of the workings of the mind of the therapist in an open and authentic fashion is necessary

Mentalizing the patient/therapist relationship is important

---

ventions according to specific principles based on our understanding of the development of BPD, cautions against some therapy techniques that may be harmful given the core pathology associated with mentalizing, and has been subjected to, and continues to be subjected to, research. The aims of MBT are modest: this is not a therapy aiming to achieve major structural/personality change or alter cognitions and schemas; its aim is to enhance embryonic capacities of mentalization so that the individual is more able to solve problems and to manage emotional states, particularly within interpersonal relationships, or at least feels more confident about the ability to do so. As we have pointed out, our intentions in working with the patient are to promote a mentalizing attitude to relationships and problems, to instill doubt where there is certainty, and to enable the patient to become increasingly curious about his own mental states and those of others. We will briefly describe below (and have outlined above in Table 6–9) how we think this can be done.

Therapist Attitude

First, the attitude of the therapist is crucial. The therapist will stimulate a mentalizing process as a core aspect of interacting with others and thinking about oneself—in part through a process of identification, in which the therapist's ability to use his mind and to demonstrate delight in changing his mind when presented with alternative views and better understanding will be internalized by the patient, who gradually becomes more curious about his own and others' minds and consequently better able to reappraise himself and his understanding of others. But in addition, the continual reworking of perspectives and understanding of oneself and others in the context of stimulation of the attachment system and within different contexts is key to a change process, as is the focus of the work on current rather than past experience. The therapist's task is to maintain mentalizing and/or to reinstate it in both himself and his patient while simultaneously ensuring that emotional states are active and meaningful. Excessive emotional arousal will impair the patient's mentalizing capacity and potentially lead to acting out, whereas inadequate emphasis on the relationship with the therapist will allow avoidance of emotional states and a narrowing of contexts within which the patient can function interpersonally and socially. The addition of group therapy to individual sessions increases dramatically the contexts in which this process can take place, and so MBT is practiced in both individual and group modes.

Tailoring Interventions

Second, the therapist has to ensure that any intervention is consonant with the patient's mentalizing capacity and not the therapist's own. Many therapists overestimate the mental capacities of patients with BPD. A patient with difficulty in mentalizing self and other cannot understand complex statements related to self and other within the patient-therapist relationship—for example, "You think that I think that you…" Such interventions are likely to increase confusion when there is already perplexity about self and other, especially if the patient is currently unable to mentalize. At other times the patient may be able to distinguish self and other, and so more complex interventions become possible. In MBT therapists follow a general principle that the greater the emotional arousal of the patient, the less complex the intervention should be. Supportive comments, gentle exploration of a problem, and clarification require less mental effort on behalf of the patient than other interventions and so are considered "safe" interventions during high states of arousal. In contrast, interpretive mentalizing and mentalizing the transference heighten arousal and so carry the danger of stimulating use of secondary attachment strategies of either hyperactivation and overarousing the patient or deactivation and inducing pretend mode, both of which decrease mentalizing. We therefore suggest that these interventions be used with care. They are likely to be of most benefit when the patient is optimally aroused—that is, able to remain within a feeling while continuing to explore its context.

Therapist Mind

Third, there is a constant temptation for therapists to piece things together, to make sense of things according to their own models of mental function, in short to mentalize, and to deliver this understanding or insight to the patient. In principle this aspect of therapist activity is anti-mentalizing—the therapist takes over the mind of the patient rather than stimulating the patient to develop his own mentalizing process. This might have adverse consequences for therapy by inadvertently stimulating pretend mode. Unable to make personal sense from the therapist's understanding, or at best able to use only cognitive under-standing, the patient takes over the model of the therapist and uses it to develop meaningless representations. These have no depth, that is, are not linked with earlier representations and understanding or integrated with emotional experience, and so fail to stimulate integration of mentalizing processes. As a result the understanding becomes sealed from the external world, lacks utility outside therapy, and cannot be applied in an ever-widening range of circumstances and contexts. All therapies have the ability to stimulate pretend mode, and the MBT therapist has to be continually aware that he might be inadvertently creating this state of mind in the patient and so inducing harm. A number of strategies may be used to rekindle mentalizing if pretend mode becomes apparent.

Authenticity

This brings us to the fourth important aspect of MBT: the mental processes of the therapist must be available to the patient. Mental processes are opaque. This, combined with the BPD patient's characteristic vulnerability to loss of mentalizing within relationships and sensitivity to facial expressions, means that the mentalizing therapist needs to try to make his mental processes transparent to the patient as the therapist tries to understand him, openly deliberating while "marking" his statements carefully. This requires a directness, honesty, authenticity, and personal ownership that is problematic partly because of the dangers of boundary violations in the treatment of BPD. Our emphasis on the need for authenticity is not a license to overstep boundaries of therapy or to develop a "real" relationship; we are merely stressing that the therapist needs to make himself mentally available to the patient and must demonstrate an ability to balance uncertainty and doubt with a continued struggle to understand. This becomes particularly important when patients correctly identify feelings and thoughts experienced by the therapist. The therapist needs to be prepared for questions that put him on the defensive—"You're bored with me," "You don't like me much, either, do you," and so on. Such challenges to the therapist can arise suddenly and without warning, and the therapist needs to be able to answer with authenticity. If the therapist does not do so the patient will become more insistent and evoke the very experience he is complaining of, if indeed the therapist was not already feeling it at the time.

A patient's accurate perception of what is in the therapist's mind needs validation—"You are bored with seeing me, aren't you," is likely to be asked from a position of psychic equivalence in which the patient may himself be feeling bored. Within psychic equivalence the patient cannot distinguish self and other easily and operates from a perspective that others have the same experience.

If the therapist is indeed feeling bored, it is important that he say so in a way that stimulates exploration of what is boring within the patient-therapist interaction. An MBT therapist will take equal responsibility for creating boring therapy and move to making this a focus of therapy for that moment—"Now you mention it, I *was* feeling a bit bored, and I am unsure where that is coming from. Is it related to what you are talking about or how you are talking about it, or is it more me at the moment? You know, I'm really not sure."

If the therapist is not bored then he needs to find a way to express this that opens up the possibility of exploring what stimulated the patient's question. To do this the therapist first needs to be open about his current feeling rather than attempt to stimulate the patient's fantasies about it. We suggest that asking the patient "What makes you think I am bored?" without first clarifying whether or not you are bored is likely to induce pretend mode once again or, alternatively, simply lead to a persistence of psychic equivalent fantasy; it is better to tell the patient what the therapist is experiencing within the therapy at that moment: "As far as I am aware, I was not bored; in fact, I was trying to grasp what you were saying. I felt muddled. But now I am intrigued that you and I were having such a different experience of this at the moment." The aim here is for the therapist to stimulate exploration of alternative perspectives. If this is to occur, the different perspectives have to be clear.

Patient-Therapist Relationship

Finally, we discuss the principles the MBT therapist follows in relation to use of the transference as an aspect of the patient-therapist relationship. It has been suggested that transference is not used in MBT (Gabbard 2006). The answer to the question of whether MBT is a transference-based therapy or not probably depends on how the term *transference* is defined and how it is used. We have cautioned practitioners during training about using transference interpretation as a technique to generate insight into a borderline patient's problems, and secondly about genetic aspects such as linking current experience to the past, because of their potential iatrogenic effects (Bateman and Fonagy 2004). But equally we train MBT therapists to "mentalize the transference" as a key component of therapy and we have set out a series of steps to be followed. These are described below and outlined in Table 6–10.

Our first step is the validation of the transference feeling through the second step, exploration. The danger of the genetic approach to the

---

TABLE 6–10.   Steps in mentalizing the transference

1. Validation of the transference feeling
2. Exploring how the patient experiences the feeling
3. Acknowledging the therapist's contribution to the transference feeling
4. Collaborating to arrive at an alternative perspective
5. Presenting the alternative perspective
6. Monitoring the patient's reactions and one's own

---

transference is that it might implicitly invalidate the patient's experience. The MBT therapist spends considerable time in the not-knowing stance, verifying how the patient is experiencing what he states he is experiencing. This exploration leads to the third step. As the events that generated the transference feelings are identified and the behaviors that the thoughts or feelings are tied to are made explicit, sometimes in painful detail, the therapist's contribution to these feelings and thoughts will become apparent. The third step is for the therapist to acknowledge the ways in which he may have contributed to the patient's experience. Most of the patient's experiences in the transference are likely to have some basis in reality, even if they have only a very partial connection to it. It often turns out that the therapist has been drawn into the transference and has acted in some way consistent with the patient's perception of him. It may be easy to attribute this to the patient, but this would be completely unhelpful. On the contrary, the therapist should initially explicitly acknowledge even partial enactments of the transference as inexplicable voluntary actions that need to be explored and for which he accepts agency rather than identifying them as a distortion of the patient. Authenticity is required in order to do this well. Drawing attention to the therapist's contributions may be particularly significant in modeling to the patient that one can accept agency for involuntary acts and that such acts do not invalidate the general attitude the therapist tries to convey. Only then can distortions be explored. The fourth step is collaboration in arriving at an alternative perspective. Mentalizing alternative perspectives about the patient-therapist relationship must be arrived at in the same spirit of collaboration as any other form of mentalizing. The metaphor we use in training is that the therapist must imagine sitting beside the patient rather than opposite him or her. Patient and therapist sit side by side looking at the patient's thoughts and feelings, where possible both adopting the inquisitive stance. The fifth step is for the therapist to present an alternative perspective, and the final step is to monitor carefully the patient's reaction as well as his own.

We suggest these steps be taken in sequence, and we talk about mentalizing the transference to distinguish the process from transference interpretation, which is commonly viewed as a technique to provide insight. *Mentalizing the transference* is a shorthand term for encouraging patients to think about the relationship they are in at the current moment (the therapist relationship) with the aim of focusing the patient's attention on another mind, the mind of a therapist, and helping the patient contrast his own perception of himself with the way he is perceived by another, by the therapist, or indeed by members of a therapeutic group. Although we might point to similarities in patterns of relationships in the therapy and in childhood, or currently outside of the therapy, the aim of doing this is not to provide a patient with an explanation (insight) that he might be able to use to control his behavior patterns. Our aim is far more simply to draw the patient's attention to another puzzling phenomenon that requires thought and contemplation, as part of our general inquisitive stance aimed at facilitating the recovery of mentalization within affective states. This recovery we see as the overall aim of treatment.

Conclusion

Mentalization-based therapy remains a promising treatment for borderline personality disorder and there is growing interest in its use in other disorders. Perhaps more importantly, mentalizing may be a common factor in effective psychotherapies for BPD, where any therapy that enhances mentalizing has a good chance of effecting change. Therapists of all orientations continually construct and reconstruct in their own mind an image of the patient's mind. As long as they do not impose their constructions on the patient and they engage in a contingent process of highlighting their verbal or nonverbal interactions, such activities will be inherently mentalizing. Their training and experience further sharpens their capacity to show that their reaction is related to the patient's state of mind rather than their own. It is this nonconscious implicit process that enables the patient with BPD to identify what he feels. Finally, mentalizing in psychological therapies is prototypically a process of shared, joint attention, where the interests of patient and therapist intersect in their joint focus on the patient's mental state. The shared attentional processes entailed by all psychological therapies must serve to strengthen the interpersonal integrative function so singularly lacking in BPD. Although this is a speculative claim, an understanding of the common ground between different psychotherapies might allow a more efficacious therapy to be developed. This endeavor should be the next development in the psychotherapeutic treatment of BPD.

Key Clinical Concepts

- ◆ Mentalization is the capacity to make sense of ourselves and others, implicitly and explicitly, in terms of subjective states and mental processes.
- ◆ Mentalizing is multidimensional—automatic/controlled, external/internal, self/other, cognitive/affective.
- ◆ Mentalizing is affected by emotional states.
- ◆ Mentalization-based treatment (MBT) promotes the process of mentalizing in states of emotional arousal and within relationships, including the patient-therapist relationship.
- ◆ MBT therapists avoid nonmentalizing interventions.
- ◆ MBT therapists tailor interventions to the mentalizing capacity of the patient.

Suggested Readings

Allen JG, Fonagy P, Bateman A: Mentalizing in Clinical Practice. Washington, DC, American Psychiatric Publishing, 2008
Bateman A, Fonagy P: Mentalization-Based Treatment for Borderline Personality Disorder: A Practical Guide. Oxford, UK, Oxford University Press, 2006
Fonagy P, Bateman AW: Mechanisms of change in mentalization-based therapy of BPD. J Clin Psychol 62:411–430, 2006
Fonagy P, Bateman AW: Mentalization-based treatment of BPD. J Pers Disord 18:36–51, 2004

References

Allen JG, Fonagy P, Bateman AW: Mentalizing in Clinical Practice. Washington, DC, American Psychiatric Publishing, 2008
Arnsten AF: The biology of being frazzled. Science 280:1711–1712, 1998
Baron-Cohen S, Tager-Flusberg H, Cohen DJ: Understanding Other Minds: Perspectives From Autism and Developmental Cognitive Neuroscience. Oxford, UK, Oxford University Press, 2000
Bateman A, Fonagy P: Psychotherapy for Borderline Personality Disorder: Mentalization-Based Treatment. Oxford, UK, Oxford University Press, 2004
Bateman A, Fonagy P: Mentalization-Based Treatment for Borderline Personality Disorder: A Practical Guide. Oxford, UK, Oxford University Press, 2006
Colvert E, Rutter M, Beckett C, et al: Emotional difficulties in early adolescence following severe early deprivation: findings from the English and Romanian adoptees study. Dev Psychopathol 20:547–567, 2008

Critchfield KL, Levy KN, Clarkin JF, et al: The relational context of aggression in borderline personality disorder: using adult attachment style to predict forms of hostility. J Clin Psychol 64:67–82, 2008

Diamond D, Stovall-McClough C, Clarkin J, et al: Patient-therapist attachment in the treatment of borderline personality disorder. Bull Menninger Clin 67:227–259, 2003

Fonagy P: On tolerating mental states: theory of mind in borderline patients. Bulletin of the Anna Freud Centre 12:91–115, 1989

Fonagy P, Bateman A: The development of borderline personality disorder— a mentalizing model. J Pers Disord 22:4–21, 2008

Fonagy P, Leigh T, Steele M, et al: The relation of attachment status, psychiatric classification, and response to psychotherapy. J Consult Clin Psychol 64:22–31, 1996

Fonagy P, Target M, Gergely G, et al: Affect Regulation, Mentalization, and the Development of Self. London, Other Press, 2002

Frith CD: Schizophrenia and theory of mind. Psychol Med 34:385–389, 2004

Gabbard GO: When is transference work useful in dynamic psychotherapy? Am J Psychiatry 163:1667–1669, 2006

Gergely G, Watson J: Early social-emotional development: contingency perception and the social biofeedback model, in Early Social Cognition: Understanding Others in the First Months of Life. Edited by Rochat P. Hillsdale, NJ, Erlbaum, 1999, pp 101–137

Goodman M, Yehuda R: The relationship between psychological trauma and borderline personality disorder. Psychiatr Ann 32:268–280, 2002

Gunderson JG, Lyons-Ruth K: BPD's interpersonal hypersensitivity phenotype: a gene-environment-developmental model. J Pers Disord 22:22–41, 2008

Hesse E: The Adult Attachment Interview: protocol, method of analysis, and empirical studies, in Handbook of Attachment Theory and Research, 2nd Edition. Edited by Cassidy J, Shaver PR. New York, Guilford, 2008, pp 552–558

Jurist EJ: Mentalized affectivity. Psychoanal Psychol 22:426–444, 2005

Kantojarvi L, Joukamaa M, Miettunen J, et al: Childhood family structure and personality disorders in adulthood. Eur Psychiatry 23:205–211, 2008

Kazdin AE: Psychotherapy for children and adolescents, in Bergin and Garfield's Handbook of Psychotherapy and Behavior Change, 5th Edition. Edited by Lambert MJ. New York, Wiley, 2004, pp 543–589

King-Casas B, Sharp C, Lomax-Bream L, et al: The rupture and repair of cooperation in borderline personality disorder. Science 321:806–810, 2008

Levy KN, Meehan KB, Weber M, et al: Attachment and borderline personality disorder: implications for psychotherapy. Psychopathology 38:64–74, 2005

Lieberman MD: Social cognitive neuroscience: a review of core processes. Annu Rev Psychol 58:259–289, 2007

Lynch TR, Rosenthal MZ, Kosson DS, et al: Heightened sensitivity to facial expressions of emotion in borderline personality disorder. Emotion 6:647–655, 2006

McGloin JM, Widom CS: Resilience among abused and neglected children grown up. Dev Psychopathol 13:1021–1038, 2001

Mikulincer M, Shaver PR: Adult attachment and affect regulation, in Handbook of Attachment Theory and Research, 2nd Edition. Edited by Cassidy J, Shaver PR. New York, Guilford, 2008, pp 503–531

New AS, Triebwasser J, Charney DS: The case for shifting borderline personality disorder to Axis I. Biol Psychiatry 64:653–659, 2008

Paris J: Does childhood trauma cause personality disorders in adults? Can J Psychiatry 43:148–153, 1998

Satpute AB, Lieberman MD: Integrating automatic and controlled processes into neurocognitive models of social cognition. Brain Res 1079:86–97, 2006

Shipman K, Edwards A, Brown A, et al: Managing emotion in a maltreating context: a pilot study examining child neglect. Child Abuse Negl 29:1015–1029, 2005

Stern A: Psychoanalytic investigation of and therapy in the borderline group of neuroses. Psychoanal Q 7:467–489, 1938

Stern A: Psychoanalytic therapy in the borderline neuroses. Psychoanal Q 14:190–198, 1945

Vorria P, Papaligoura Z, Sarafidou J, et al: The development of adopted children after institutional care: a follow-up study. J Child Psychol Psychiatry 47:1246–1253, 2006

Wagner AW, Linehan MM: Facial expression recognition ability among women with borderline personality disorder: implications for emotion regulation? J Pers Disord 13:329–344, 1999

Watson S, Chilton R, Fairchild H, et al: Association between childhood trauma and dissociation among patients with borderline personality disorder. Aust N Z J Psychiatry 40:478–481, 2006

Zanarini MC, Frankenburg FR, Reich DB, et al: Adult experiences of abuse reported by borderline patients and Axis II comparison subjects over six years of prospective follow-up. J Nerv Ment Dis 193:412–416, 2005

Zweig-Frank H, Paris J, Ng Ying Kin NM, et al: Childhood sexual abuse in relation to neurobiological challenge tests in patients with borderline personality disorder and normal controls. Psychiatry Res 141:337–341, 2006

Transference-Focused Psychotherapy and Borderline Personality Disorder

Frank E. Yeomans, M.D., Ph.D.
Diana Diamond, Ph.D.

Transference-focused psychotherapy (TFP; Clarkin et al. 2006; Yeomans et al. 2002) is a manualized form of psychodynamic psychotherapy that has been developed specifically to treat borderline pathology. The characteristics of the treatment correspond to the belief that borderline conditions are rooted in disturbances of internal object relations (Kernberg 1975, 1984; Kernberg and Caligor 2005), as will be explicated

This chapter represents work from the Cornell Psychotherapy Research Project supported by grants from the National Institute of Mental Health, the International Psychoanalytic Association, and the Kohler Fund of Munich and a grant from the Borderline Personality Disorder Research Foundation. The foundation and its founder, Dr. Marco Stoffel, are gratefully acknowledged.

below. While this chapter will address applying TFP to borderline personality disorder (BPD), the core principles and techniques are also applicable with some modification to other personality disorders (Caligor et al. 2007; Diamond 2007; Diamond and Yeomans 2008).

There is growing evidence that TFP results in significant clinical improvement in both the symptomatic and the psychosocial realm (Clarkin et al. 2001, 2007; Levy et al. 2006b; Doering et al., in press). In previous papers we have presented our research data from three separate studies that show change in borderline patients in a number of dimensions, including significant decreases in suicidal and parasuicidal acts and ideation, in depression and anxiety, and in service utilization, along with improved psychosocial functioning and improvements in narrative coherence and the capacity for mentalization (the ability to comprehend mental states of self and others) after 1 year of TFP (Clarkin et al. 2001, 2007; Levy et al. 2006b). Our focus in this chapter will be on the therapy itself. We will review 1) the object relations model of the pathology, 2) the core strategies, tactics, and techniques of the treatment, and 3) proposed mechanisms of change. We will also present clinical material that illustrates the application of TFP.

TFP is a comprehensive treatment program in that it addresses a number of elements of borderline pathology in a year-long, or longer, intervention with patients who bring both general and idiosyncratic issues to the treatment situation. Although we emphasize transference interpretation as central to the therapy and therapeutic change, it is only one among many elements of the treatment, as summarized in Figure 7–1 (Levy et al. 2006a; Yeomans et al. 2008). In TFP, change is hypothesized to occur through a series of treatment interventions. This begins with a contract setting and evaluation phase that creates a secure base in which patient and therapist may address and reflect on the range of intense and often stormy affects first aroused in the treatment situation. It then proceeds through a phase of identifying the dominant object relational scenarios that emerge for the particular patient and—through the techniques of clarification, confrontation, and interpretation—linking them to the patient's fluctuating affect states and to the role reversals that occur in treatment, as each pole of the self-object dyad is lived out in the transference relationship. Addressing the transference relationship systematically is thought to increase the patient's capacity to cognitively represent and contain his affective experience, which in turn leads to improvements in reflective function or mentalization and the capacity to symbolically manage and reflect on his experience in the transference (Caligor et al. 2009; Kernberg et al. 2008).

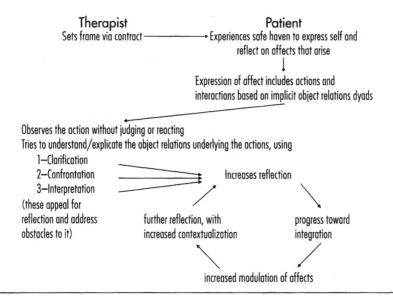

FIGURE 7–1. Transference-focused psychotherapy.

An Object Relations Model of Borderline Pathology

While this chapter focuses on BPD, the basic principles of TFP can be used for any personality disorder organized at the borderline level (see Chapter 1, "An Object Relations Model of Personality and Personality Pathology," this volume). The TFP model of borderline pathology considers psychoanalytic understandings of the structural organization of personality (Kernberg 1984, 2004; Kernberg and Caligor 2005) as they are increasingly informed by research at multiple levels, including the neural, social cognitive, neurocognitive, and interpersonal (Adolphs 2003; Depue and Lenzenweger 2005; Fertuck et al. 2009; Posner et al. 2002; Zaki and Ochsner, in press). This model posits a dynamic interaction of temperament (individual differences in affect activation and regulation and motor reactivity), environmental factors such as abuse or neglect, an absence of a coherent sense of self and others in the context of an insecure working model of attachment, deficits in mentalization, and low effortful control (Clarkin et al. 2006; Gabbard et al. 2006; Silbersweig et al. 2007). While the foregoing are among the major factors generally considered to contribute to BPD, there is currently lively debate as to which features of the disorder are at its core and therefore should be targeted as the core of treatment. Dialectical behavior therapy (DBT) sees constitutional emotional dysregulation and deficits in mindfulness as the core of the disorder (Linehan 1993; Wupperman et al. 2008). Mentalization-based treatment (MBT) sees a developmental deficit in the capacity for mentalization as its core (Bateman and Fonagy 2004). Gunderson and Lyons-Ruth (2008) consider the core to be interpersonal hypersensitivity and insecure working models of attachment.

The TFP model sees identity diffusion as the core of BPD identity disorder. Identity diffusion is the lack of continuity of experience of self and others that stems from a split, polarized internal world in which others are likely to be experienced as persecutors or idealized rescuers (Kernberg 1975, 1984). This view has been amplified by research investigations in a number of areas. Attachment research has linked borderline pathology to a range of insecure (primarily anxious/preoccupied and/or disorganized/unresolved) attachment patterns that presuppose maladaptive working models of self and attachment figures (Diamond et al. 2003; Fonagy et al. 1996; Main 1999). Studies of mentalization have shown deficits in that capacity that render the individual unable to assess accurately the contents of his or her own mind or the mind of the other (Bateman and Fonagy 2004; Fonagy et al. 1996). Neurocognitive research has found faulty information processing in borderline patients that is influenced by negative affect and impaired social cognition. More specifically, recent findings support the widely held observation that borderline patients are likely to form precipitous and negative and even hypervigilant or frankly paranoid transferences in the therapeutic situation (Gabbard et al. 2006; Kernberg 1975, 1984). Social cognitive neuroscientific investigations suggest that intense negative emotions interfere with cognitive control mechanisms in BPD (Fertuck et al. 2006; Silbersweig et al. 2007) and that there is enhanced sensitivity to social stimuli. In the social recognition realm, there is some evidence for a "paradox" (Krohn 1974) in which individuals with BPD exhibit enhanced sensitivity to the emotional and mental states of others in the moment but tend to attribute untrustworthiness to neutral human faces of strangers (Donegan et al. 2003; Fertuck et al. 2009).

At the level of neural systems, brain imaging studies have identified the neural correlates of these social and cognitive processes, which underlie the preponderance of negative affect generally and the inability to regulate aggression in particular (Silbersweig et al. 2007) and have long been hypothesized to be a crucial aspect of borderline personality disorder by Kernberg (1975, 2004). These neural correlates include the following:

1. Hyperreactivity of the amygdala, particularly in the left hemisphere, which may predispose the patient to misinterpret neutral facial expressions in or out of the treatment situation as malevolent
2. Diminished functioning and reduced volume in the prefrontal regions, which impairs the ability to regulate or modulate affect and hence to mentalize
3. Hyperresponsiveness of the hypothalamic-pituitary-adrenal axis, leading to a chronic state of hypervigilance and affective arousal (Rinne et al. 2002)
4. Reduced hippocampal volume, leading to a) the tendency to automatically recapitulate self-object-affect schemas that are encoded as implicit (unconscious) procedural memories and b) an impaired capacity to generate autobiographical narratives based on both implicit and explicit memories (Gabbard 2009)
5. Reward circuitry associated with the nucleus accumbens, which, driven by dopamine secretion, strengthens the gratification from maladaptive relational patterns and the quest to repeat them (Gabbard et al. 2006)

Although the majority of these factors are particularly evident in patients who have suffered childhood abuse, which encompasses most but not all borderline patients, Gabbard et al. (2006) make the interesting observation that distortions in the internal worlds of self and object may themselves catalyze overactivation of the amygdala. Consequently, interventions focused on the elements in the mind that determine the processing of affectively charged perceptions, especially in the social interpersonal sphere, are crucial in achieving symptom reduction, enhancing the patient's sense of self and the quality of his interpersonal relations, and improving involvement in work and other creative endeavors.

An object relations point of view emphasizes that the BPD patient's perceptions of events are strongly influenced by internal representations of self and others and by the intense affects that link them. Internalized representations of interactions with others are composed of a specific representation of the self and the other linked by the affective experience. In early development, an individual's internal representational world is conceptualized as being made up of multiple sets of such dyads, each characterized by a different representation of the self and other and linked by a different affect. These internal representations are activated by life events and in turn influence how the event is perceived or "read." One-dimensional representations interfere with accurately perceiving events. In the course of normal psychological development, these disparate one-dimensional representations of self and other become integrated into more complex, multifaceted, and modulated representations that correspond more accurately to the complexity of self, of others, and of the world. In individuals with borderline personality organization, the one-dimensional, polarized, and caricatured representations of self and others are not integrated into this more complex whole that provides a sense of coherence, continuity, and context in the individual's experience of self and others (Clarkin et al. 2006).

This model takes into account the role of mental processes such as impulse, affect, and fantasy that transform experiences so that the internalized images are not an exact reproduction of what has actually happened in the past. In this model, affects are the main vehicles that give rise to primary internal representations (Kernberg 2004; Sandler and Sandler 1987). More specifically, Kernberg's formulation of object relations theory sees affects as the primary psychophysiological dispositions that are activated by early bodily experiences in the context of the development of object relations. Affects become linked with self and object representations in elementary dyads as highly pleasurable and intensely unpleasurable experiences accrue in the course of early development, and, in their supraordinate organization, affects come to form the building blocks for libidinal and aggressive drives. In the course of normal development, the representations of self and objects evolve into the more integrated and complex tripartite structures of id, ego, and superego, forming the substrate for the unconscious as well as conscious experience.

Thus, primitive affects constitute a primary motivational system that integrates cognitive appraisal of momentary experiences of gratification or frustration with the subjective experience of pleasure or unpleasure in the context of particular object relations. Hence, although the internal images that are reactivated in the patient's responses to the therapist and others may reproduce a specific experience or relationship from the past, they may also represent an internal construction, the ultimate origin of which cannot be identified precisely. Our focus is this current psychic reality—how it is structured and how it can be modified.

The unilateral, polarized representations of self and other that constitute psychological structure are often in contradiction with one another and therefore underlie the BPD patient's inability to experience a coherent self or view of others. This fragmented, diffuse, and contradictory sense of self, which we refer to as *identity diffusion,* leaves the patient at risk for inaccurate, extreme perceptions accompanied by overwhelming affects in the experience of the moment, leading to misrepresentation of self and others and to affect dysregulation and consequent behavioral and interpersonal problems. In addition, deficits in mentalization, or the capacity to think in terms of intentional mental states of self and other (e.g., beliefs, motives, emotions, desires), leave borderline individuals without the cognitive skills to comprehend and contain the extreme affective experiences that are the legacy of their split, polarized object world. The split mental representations, which can be activated by even minor trigger events, and the failures of mentalization that accompany them are seen as the underpinnings of the discontinuity of the patient's life experience and the related inability to construct an internal narrative with the breadth and depth to accurately contextualize any experience in the moment—leaving the patient subject to brutal shifts, to be tossed by trigger events from one extreme experience of self and other to another. Especially under stress, the patient experiences affects in a primary, unsymbolized way, in contrast to an experience of affect as contained and modulated by language and symbolic function (*mentalized affectivity* [Jurist 2005]). The intensity of the immediate experiences, not grounded or modulated by a solid foundation of identity, leads to extreme emotional reactions that can be self-defeating and destructive to relations with others as the patient responds to the other as though only the momentary emotion existed in the relationship.

This view corresponds with the neurocognitive investigations summarized above that indicate that borderline patients are particularly hypervigilant and are prone to interpret interpersonal stimuli in a negative manner, leading to the immediate and sometimes drastic activation of an array of negative affects and their associated internal representations of self and others in interpersonal situations, including the therapeutic arena. Although the patient's conscious experience of such self-object dyads is typically to identify with the victim of aggression and to see another party as the aggressor, the entire negative object-relational dyad exists within the patient. Among current therapies for BPD, this point of view seems to be unique to TFP. Consequent to the internalization of the victim-persecutor dyad, otherwise normal and healthy aggressive or assertive strivings tend to crystallize around the fierce internal representation of a real or fantasized persecutory figure. This creates an internal structure where any stirring of negative affect (e.g., anger, envy, despair) activates an extreme image that is experienced as toxic, leading to a discharge of the affect through acting out or projection. The work of integration helps patients to tolerate and manage such negative affects without resorting to primitive defenses and helps to disentangle their healthy aggressive strivings from an image that is so extreme that it makes any experience of aggressive affect intolerable.

When a dyad is activated in a patient's mind, the patient's subjective experience can oscillate, or shift, from one pole of the dyad to the opposite pole. For example, the patient may react to a disappointment by experiencing herself as the victim of a cruel other and subsequently lash out at the other in a hostile way. This can be seen as the patient enacting the victim-persecutor dyad first (and consciously) as the victim and then (in action but not in awareness) as the persecutor. In our experience, in addition to oscillation within one dyad there is also a layering within the internal object world, such that negatively charged dyads often protect the patient from longings for closeness and affiliation with the therapist, whom, given the frequent deficits in social cognition, the patient often experiences as untrustworthy or harmful (Fertuck et al. 2009; Koenigsberg 2009).

The work of therapy thus includes encouraging awareness of both the double identification (with victim and with persecutor) within negative dyads and the split between negatively charged dyads and the equally extreme and unrealistic idealized positive dyads within the patient's internal world. In this way the patient's negative affects can be integrated into a more nuanced whole, with the goal of enhancing the capacity to manage rather than be at the mercy of aggressive strivings, and idealized positive affects can be modulated to more realistic expectations. The techniques of TFP, which will be further delineated below, foster the integration and modulation of split-off experiences, allowing the extreme affects to be gradually understood in terms of self and object representational dyads that can be integrated with their opposite self-object-affect constellations. This integration permits the modulation of affect, particularly the mastery and sublimation of aggressive affects, and the strengthening of cognitive functions, including the beginning of reflective function.

The integration of previously split-off negative and especially aggressive feelings is generally the greatest challenge for the patient. It entails coming to terms with aspects of the self that were denied while they were being acted out and projected. Although the process of integrating these affects can be painful and can include feelings of remorse as the patient experiences appropriate guilt for behaviors that were previously seen as justified, the process is essential in enriching the patient's experience of self and range of emotional experience. The patient learns that anger and aggression, which were previously experienced only in a caricatured and extreme form, can be mastered and used in the service of positive goals such as ambition, competitiveness, and creativity.

The fundamental split in the borderline patient is not the split between "good victim" and "bad persecutor," but rather between this victim/persecutor dyad, both poles of which are imbued with pure negative affect, and a loved-self/perfect-provider dyad, imbued with pure positive, and equally unrealistic, affect. These positive and negative affective experiences tend to defend against one another: that is, an experience of positive affect does not allow for any tinge of negative affect, and vice versa. This system attempts to defend against the anxiety that arises in the patient when opposing positive and negative affects, and their related representations, begin to be experienced simultaneously. Any incipient co-occurrence of opposed affects precipitates the return of the split internal state in order to protect the internal ideal images of self and others from the hatred and rage associated with the persecutory, aggressively laden ones. This state prevents the patient from having full awareness and appreciation of the extent of her internal world, leading often to feelings of emptiness, discontinuity of self, and affective instability. This dissociated defensive structure distorts and erases awareness and thinking—a fragmentation and disconnection of thinking by attacks on the linking of thoughts (Bion 1967). Powerful affects are then expressed in action without cognitive awareness. TFP attempts to discover what relationship dyads underlie primitive affects and impulsive behaviors so that increased understanding of the internal images can lead to mastery of the affects and control of the behaviors.

Primitive Defenses

It is this internal dissociated organization of the mind that underlies primitive defense mechanisms, based on the fundamental split between positive and negative affects and impulses. Given BPD patients' difficulty accepting and tolerating the experience of negative affects, patients tend either to act them out without conscious awareness or, given their propensity to be hyperattuned to visual and interpersonal cues, to experience them as originating in others via projection. For example, the patient may feel deeply slighted or injured if the therapist has to reschedule a session or is not able to reschedule at the patient's convenience, and consequently the patient may threaten to interrupt or even leave the treatment, behaving in hostile, rejecting ways that reveal his interpretation of the therapist's behavior and intentions. This pattern of experiencing affects and impulses through projective mechanisms, in which the patient experiences parts of his own internal world as originating in a person with whom he is interacting, leads to additional disarray in interpersonal relations; this can be in the form of instability and confusion in cases where the projection of negative affect alternates with experiencing the other as benevolent, or in the form of stable hostile relations when a stable projection of negative affect leads to a consistent relation with an other as the defined enemy-persecutor.

Variants of splitting and projecting are 1) projective identification, in which the patient induces in the other party the affect/impulse that he cannot tolerate in himself, and 2) omnipotent control, in which the patient projects hostile affect onto the other and then feels a need to control the other to avoid becoming the victim of the perceived hostility. It is because of the prominence of projective mechanisms that therapists must be carefully attuned to their countertransference (the emotions that they experience in the interaction with the patient). They must be able to reflect on their reactions and determine which reactions are provoked by the patient in a way that represents the activation within the therapist of an affect that the patient has difficulty accepting within himself (projective identification). The understanding of these reactions within the therapist can lead to valuable information about the patient's internal world.

The Core Method of Transference-Focused Psychotherapy

The BPD patient's extreme affective reactions and the related behavior are disruptive both to the patient's life and to treatment, and BPD patients also tend to discharge affects in a way that can bypass conscious awareness and the possibility to reflect on, integrate, and modify the affects. Treatment, therefore, must be structured in such a way as to control acting out and to provide a frame within which the patient can experience, observe, and reflect on his or her representations of self and others.

TFP is based on the understanding that the object relations dyads that structure the internal world of the patient will emerge in the transference to the therapist and that it is therefore most effective to focus on this arena in working with the patient. Working within the transference can initially help establish whether the patient's affective response is to an objective reality (e.g., a husband who is a monster and therefore responsible for the patient's misery) or to an internal image (e.g., an inner persecutory other that is projected onto the therapist when the latter cannot change a session time) or both. Focusing on affects as they are experienced in the immediate relationship also helps avoid intellectualized interpretive work that does not involve affect.

The foundation of the therapy is to facilitate the reactivation, under controlled circumstances, of the dissociated or projected internalized object relations that constitute the transference, in order to observe and gain awareness of the nature of the patient's internal representations and then integrate them into a fuller, richer, and more nuanced identity.

Another way to think about this process, in terms of attachment theory and research, is that the treatment situation in TFP, with its dyadic intimacy and intensity, activates the primary internal working models of attachment, which in the case of more severely disturbed patients are likely to be insecure, multiple, contradictory, and conflictual in nature (Diamond et al. 2003; Fonagy and Bateman 2005; Main 1999), with the goal of moving the patient toward increased attachment security.

The Treatment Contract

In order to achieve the goal of greater attachment security, the therapist must first create conditions that provide containment of intense affects and acting-out behaviors and that enhance the possibility for reflection. Thus, after the evaluation of the patient, the first element of the treatment is the contracting phase, which establishes a structure. The discussion of the guidelines of treatment starts by defining the nature of the patient's problem as psychological: as a core identity disturbance that has multiple manifestations, including intense and rapidly shifting affects and the acting-out behaviors that accompany them. The guidelines include a description of the responsibilities of both patient and therapist to the treatment, including recommendations for how to manage acting out (Clarkin et al. 2006; Levy et al. 2007; Yeomans et al. 1992). These guidelines create a structure that discourages the disruption of the treatment, with the goal of providing conditions of safety and stability in the therapeutic environment so that the reactivated internal dyads or working models of attachment can be experienced with an adequate level of containment to observe and reflect on. The treatment contract ultimately can function as a harbor of safety or a safe haven for both patient and therapist as the patient is buffeted by the extreme affects associated with the split, polarized internal representations or, in some cases, is deadened and rendered robot-like by the dearth of affects and thoughts resulting from systematic attacks on linking (Bion 1967)—as may occur early in treatment when the internal world has been decimated by severe splitting and seemingly irreversible projections, rendering the patient prone not only to self-destructive acting out but to destruction of the treatment itself.

The Therapeutic Process

The dyadic intimacy of the treatment setting, along with the unequal roles and relationships of patient and therapist, leads quickly to the activation of the patient's internal object relations patterns. As this occurs, the therapist tries to clarify cognitively what the patient perceives and its relation to what the patient feels. This clarification requires monitoring of three different channels of communication between patient and therapist: the content of the verbal discourse, nonverbal communication and behavior, and the countertransference reactions that are elicited in the therapist. Different dissociated aspects of the patient's internal world will be conveyed alternately through each of these channels.

TFP begins by encouraging this reactivation of primitive object relations in a context designed to help the therapist reflect on what is happening rather than react directly in the ways the patient both expects and fears. This reactivation is facilitated by the therapist's adopting a stance of neutrality (not to be confused with coldness or indifference) in relation to the forces involved in the patient's conflicts (either intrapsychic or interpersonal). That is, the therapist does not side with the patient's urges to act or with her urges to inhibit an action (keeping in mind that BPD pathology can present both as excessive action and as excessive inhibition) except in situations where to act would be unduly destructive or self-destructive. Rather, the therapist takes the position of observing the conflict the patient is in and engaging the patient to observe it as well. Conflicts could involve loving forces versus aggressive forces, urges to act on a particular force versus internal inhibition against taking action, or urges to act versus concern about the consequences of taking action. This focus on delineating the conflict as within the patient rather than between the patient and the therapist is essential, as patients often experience intense anxiety from their conflicts without a clear awareness of the internal conflict itself, owing to their tendency to project a part of them onto another person. The therapist's avoiding siding with one part of the patient's conflict helps the patient to recognize and reflect on the conflict, enhancing the ability to successfully deal with conflicts rather than to be at their mercy.

The therapist's neutrality both assists in the reactivation of the patient's characteristic object relations dyads and helps the patient to observe, see, accept, and eventually integrate parts of the self that previously were not consciously tolerated but were enacted and/or projected. With the fostering of reflection and containment through the identification of self-object dyads and their linking affects, the repetitive automatic reenactment of such internal dyads is short-circuited and there is a gradual cognitive structuring of what at first seems both rigid and chaotic.

Although it is difficult to define a psychodynamic treatment in terms of specific stages, since each patient-therapist dyad will have its own unique trajectory, TFP generally progresses along the following lines:

In the initial phase of therapy, the major task is to tolerate the affective chaos and confusion that BPD patients often bring to treatment and that often take the form of kaleidoscopic shifts between affect outbursts or storms, verbalized primitive fantasies, or primitive enactments. The second phase involves identifying the self and object representations that crystallized out of the therapist's attention to the patient's extreme affect states or affect deadness. Subsequent phases, as delineated earlier, involve exploring role reversals in the transference as the patient alternates between the self and object poles of the dyadic constellations evoked in the treatment. More advanced phases involve exploring the ways in which different dyads may defend against each other and interpreting systematically dyads as they are lived out in the transference with their multiple layerings and dissociated aspects in the interests of integration and modulation of the internal world, with interpretation of the unconscious motivations and conflicts that fuel the splitting defenses. As this work is done within the transference, patients generally begin to develop relationships outside of therapy in a more complex and realistic way as well. Having described these general phases, we caution the reader not to expect them to unfold in a purely linear fashion.

The Interpretive Process

This movement through the phases of TFP is effected partly through the steps of the interpretive process that overlap with but are not synonymous with the sequences of treatment. Clarification, confrontation, and interpretation of the patient's self and object dyads as they are experienced with the therapist and with external figures help the patient expand his reflective capacities as an instrument in working toward an integrated identity. By engaging the patient in identifying and observing these scenarios as they are experienced in the therapy setting, the therapist appeals to the patient's capacity to reflect on them as constructions rather than as veridical images of self and others, with the goal of increasing the patient's cognitive capacity to represent affect. The therapist then helps the patient understand the anxieties that make it difficult to integrate primitive positive (libidinal) and negative (aggressive) affects.

The borderline patient's capacity for sustaining a clear distinction between self and other is defective because of splitting and projective mechanisms. The ability to arrive at representations of the motivations of others uncontaminated by the motivations of the self (which may also not be clear to the individual) is severely compromised. Interpretation in the here and now begins with an effort to understand an affect, or an action related to an affect, in terms of the representations of self and other that lie beneath and motivate the affect/action. This often involves focusing attention on internal representations characterized by affects and impulses that are "unacceptable," whether they be aggressive or libidinal in nature. Bringing these underlying representations to conscious awareness helps the patient clarify the motivation behind his feeling or action and allows for further elaboration of the accuracy of the representations. When successfully carried out, this increased understanding of self and other in the momentary experience—which often involves gaining the awareness that the interaction is more benign than it was initially experienced to be, but can also involve achieving the ability to experience and tolerate affects that were previously deemed unacceptable—helps the patient tolerate affects without having to deny them, discharge them in action, or condemn himself for having them. The work then proceeds to helping the patient to integrate disparate experiences of self and others across time.

The interpretive process begins with clarification. Clarification does not involve offering the patient explanations, but rather involves inviting the patient to say more about what he is feeling in the moment: it is an effort to expand his ability to understand and express his current experience. This can involve the patient's experience of an outside event that he is describing or his experience of the immediate interaction with the therapist. The latter is particularly useful as it permits joint exploration of a shared experience where the affect is immediately accessible. In this sense, clarification is similar to MBT's tenet that a core feature of therapy is helping the patient improve his capacity to accurately perceive his internal state and that of the person with whom he is interacting.

It should be noted that Bateman and Fonagy (2004) and others have found that conventional transference interpretations are not always effective with borderline patients, and that with such patients it makes more sense to think in terms of an interpretive process that must be tailored to the specific clinical needs of the patient with this pathology. Nonetheless, our psychodynamic approach emphasizes the centrality of the interpretive process and sees the process of facilitating improvement for the BPD patient as going beyond helping the patient mentalize the moment. Since TFP sees conflict between forces/affects within the mind as fundamental to borderline pathology, it does not believe that the capacity to accurately read self states suffices to resolve those conflicts. The research of Per Høglend et al. (2008) may be relevant to this discussion. Høglend and colleagues found that the use of transference interpretation was more effective than avoidance of it in patients with low quality of object relations. Since only 22% of the study's subjects were diagnosed with BPD or multiple personality disorders, further exploration is needed with a purely borderline population.

In TFP, confrontation is the second phase of the interpretive process. This technique invites the patient to reflect on contradictions that appear as the disparate elements of the patient's internal world are revealed in therapy. Although the patient's feelings toward the therapist or toward others may be clearly articulated and noncontradictory at times, at other times these feelings may be in contradiction with what the patient has communicated on other occasions or at variance with the patient's attitude and behavior. The technique of confrontation presents the patient with these contradictions, of which he is often unaware.

The third level of the interpretive process helps the patient become aware of how the understanding of a particular affect in relation to an object could be related to other, conflicting affects that exist within the individual. The therapist might say: "It may be that you talk about dropping out of treatment after each session where we have experienced a positive contact because a part of you is convinced that the positive feeling is not real but is a trick and will lead to my hurting you. If this were true, it would make sense that you would want to leave, and it would explain that you seem to be more 'at home' in hostile relations." A later stage of interpretation might focus on the patient's split-off and projected identification with an aggressive part that makes it impossible to escape from relations that take on a negative tone. Once this projection of part of the self is understood, it can be integrated so that the awareness of the aggressive part both removes it as an obstacle to more successful libidinal fulfillment and allows for adaptive uses of aggressive affects, such as striving for higher achievement.

Interpretations in TFP are largely based on an appreciation of the psychological structure of the patient—not primarily on interpreting historical antecedents, as is sometimes considered the traditional way of interpreting in psychoanalysis. It is not wrong to offer an interpretation such as: "Your fear of allowing yourself to feel close to me is understandable, given that your early experience in life was to be humiliated by those you loved." However, the process of changing the patient's way of experiencing might be advanced more by addressing how the patient's expectation of the other may be largely determined by the makeup of her own mind: "It could also be that you are afraid of feeling close to me because you assume that I could react to you as you do to others: one false move and they are cut out of your life...."

Beyond achieving an understanding of the mental state of self and other in the moment, the patient both becomes aware of the representations of self and other involved in a momentary affective state and also can place these representations into a general context of knowledge about self and other across time—an integrated view of self and other that has coalesced. At this level, the patient can contextualize momentary feelings toward another into the broad internal sense of experience of the relationship that has developed over time. The interpretive process and the phases of TFP delineated above are overlapping but not synonymous in that at almost any point in the process of TFP, one might go through the entire interpretive process in one session or stay in one phase of interpretation for many sessions, depending on the nature of the individual patient's pathology and progress.

Empirical Research on TFP

A series of three related studies has now been conducted at the Personality Disorders Institute to investigate the impact of TFP on symptomatology, social adjustment, utilization of psychiatric and medical services, attachment organization, and mentalization in patients with BPD or borderline personality organization. These studies have been described in detail in previous publications (Clarkin et al. 2001, 2007; Levy et al. 2006b). Here we will give a brief summary of our findings to show the empirical evolution and support for our conceptualization of the interpretive process of TFP. With the assistance of a treatment development grant from the National Institute of Mental Health (John F. Clarkin, Principal Investigator), we generated initial effect sizes of the treatment over a 1-year period. In the initial study, 17 women with BPD who had had at least two incidents of suicidal or self-injurious behavior in the previous year were selected for treatment. TFP demonstrated significant changes for the 17 patients in a number of crucial areas. There was a significant decrease in the average medical risk of parasuicidal acts and improvement in the average physical condition following these acts. After 12 months of treatment, the percentage of patients who had made a suicide attempt in the prior 12 months decreased from 53% to 18%. Further, there were significantly fewer emergency room visits, hospitalizations, and days hospitalized (Clarkin et al. 2001). Finally, after 1 year of TFP there were significant changes in scores of reflective functioning (RF), an attachment-based measure of mentalization (P. Fonagy, M. Steele, H. Steele, and M. Target, "Reflective-Functioning Manual: Version 4.1. For Application to the Adult Attachment Interviews," University College, London, 1997), along with shifts from disorganized to more organized forms of attachment, both secure and insecure, for the majority of the subjects (Diamond et al. 2003).

Subsequent to this initial study, we compared the results of patients with borderline personality disorder treated with TFP to those of patients with BPD who received 1-year treatment as usual (TAU) in our own clinical setting. Psychiatric emergency room visits and hospitalizations during the treatment year were significantly lower in the TFP group as compared to TAU. Patients who completed TFP showed an increase in Global Assessment of Functioning scores, whereas those in TAU did not. All of the within-subjects and between-subjects effect sizes for the TFP treatment participants indicated significant change, whereas effect sizes for the TAU group showed either deterioration or small effect sizes.

In order to assess improvement in TFP as compared with other manualized treatments, we conducted a randomized controlled trial (Clarkin et al. 2004, 2007; Levy et al. 2006b) comparing three types of interventions in a 1-year outpatient treatment study: TFP, DBT, and a psychodynamic supportive therapy (Rockland 1992). The study included administering the Adult Attachment Interview (AAI) (C. George, N. Kaplan, M. Main, "The Berkeley Adult Attachment Interview," Department of Psychology, University of California, Berkeley, 1998) before and after the 1-year intervention to the patients in all three treatments.

Our data analysis suggests that in general the three treatments were effective to varying degrees in reducing symptoms and improving functioning from the beginning to the end of the treatment year. Patients in all three treatment groups showed significant positive change in depression, anxiety, global functioning, and social adjustment. Only TFP and DBT were significantly associated with improvement in suicidality. Only TFP and supportive psychodynamic therapy were associated with improvement in anger. TFP and supportive therapy were each associated with improvement in facets of impulsivity. Interestingly, only TFP was significantly predictive of change in irritability and verbal and direct assault (Clarkin et al. 2007).

Most relevant to this chapter, we conceptualized reflective functioning, or RF (P. Fonagy et al., 1997), as a mechanism of change in the treatment of borderline patients and hypothesized that because of the nature of the treatment, RF would improve in TFP but not in DBT or supportive psychotherapy. The RF index of mentalization is obtained from the AAI (C. George et al., 1998), which was given prior to and after 1 year of treatment for patients in all treatment conditions. The AAI data were rated for overall attachment classification by using the Adult Attachment Classification System developed by Mary Main and her colleagues (M. Main, R. Goldwyn, "Adult Attachment Scoring and Classifications System." Unpublished scoring manual. Department of

Psychology, University of California, Berkeley, 1998). In addition, the AAI data were rated for RF. Results showed that the mean RF score of the patients who had been treated with TFP increased, whereas the RF score of the patients in the other two treatments did not change significantly after 1 year of treatment (Levy et al. 2006b).

We also compared the levels of narrative coherence, or the extent to which the individual is able to relate her early attachment history in a way that is fresh, believable, and internally consistent, on the AAIs of patients in the three groups. The narrative coherence subscale of the AAI has been found to be the best predictor of attachment security ($r=0.96$, $P<0.001$) (Waters et al. 2001). As with the RF finding, patients in the TFP group showed significant increases in narrative coherence after 1 year, whereas those in the other two groups did not. For patients in TFP, narrative coherence scores improved to a level just short of indicating attachment security. In the randomized controlled trial, 31.7% were initially classified as unresolved and 18% were rated as "cannot classify" (Levy et al. 2006b). After 1 year of treatment there was a significant increase in the number of patients classified with secure states of mind with respect to attachment in TFP, but not DBT or supportive psychodynamic psychotherapy.

A first question in response to this finding is what the clinical relevance of increased RF and narrative coherence may be. A second question is what these data suggest in terms of therapeutic techniques that help in the treatment of borderline patients. With regard to clinical relevance, the increased ability to reflect on one's own and an other's mind should lead to less of the inaccurate attribution of negative intentions to others that is typical of patients with BPD. Consequently, benign or positive events will no longer be seen as malevolent and the patient will be able to avoid the downward spiral of misinterpretation and engendering of negative responses.

With regard to the relevance of significant shifts toward attachment security noted in patients in TFP, it is important to note that a number of empirical studies have now linked attachment security with optimal personality functioning, psychosocial functioning, and cognitive functioning throughout development. Domains linked with attachment security include peer relationship quality and cognitive functioning in childhood (Suess et al. 1992), attentional control (Harman et al. 1997), a more complex understanding of mixed emotions at age 6 years (Steele et al. 1999), the quality of intimate relationships in adolescence, and the degree of psychological security in romantic relationships in early adulthood (Grossmann and Grossmann 2003; Sroufe et al. 2005). Furthermore, in adulthood, secure internal working models of attachment have been associated with the sense of being worthy of help, the capacity to call on supportive figures in times of loss or distress, and the capacity to accurately evaluate challenging social and emotional situations involving partners (Grossmann and Grossmann 2003). In addition, the significant increase in the coherence subscale ratings for patients in TFP, but not DBT or supportive psychodynamic therapy, suggests increased capacity to construct a clear, lively and credible autobiographical narrative. Such narrative competence has been associated with a number of aspects of social competence and affect regulation (Fonagy and Bateman 2005; Fonagy et al. 2002; Main et al. 1985).

With regard to the relevance of findings to therapeutic techniques, the shift in RF scores strengthens our conviction that the interpretive approach in TFP leads to structural intrapsychic as well as symptomatic change. RF has been linked to a number of neurocognitive mechanisms including attentional capacities, executive functioning, and impulsivity—all of which are central to those with personality disorders (Levy et al. 2006a). The capacity for RF has also been found to be a protective factor in individuals with histories of trauma or abuse linked to insecure attachment. Fonagy et al. (1996) found that individuals who had an abuse history were less likely to have BPD if they had high RF. Furthermore, other studies have shown that mothers classified as having lack of resolution of loss or trauma were more likely to have children classified with secure attachment if they (the mothers) had high scores in RF on the AAI; their counterparts with low RF were more likely to have children classified with disorganized attachment status (Slade et al. 2005). Thus the capacity for RF may moderate the negative impact of a traumatic early attachment history and potentially guard against the transgenerational transmission of insecure attachment patterns.

Further, the data suggest that interpretation has a role in increasing the patient's RF. Our study compared TFP, in which the interpretive process is considered a mechanism of change, with DBT and a manualized supportive psychodynamic therapy that avoided the use of transference interpretation. Interestingly, DBT includes an emphasis on mindfulness, which shares certain characteristics with mentalization: the encouragement of the nonjudgmental awareness of the self in the here-and-now moment. The fact that our data do not show an increase in RF in the patients treated with DBT suggests that interpretations that expand the patient's awareness of split-off and projected parts of herself and help build the broader contextualized sense of self and other that we consider the second level of RF may be instrumental in achieving increased RF. The fact that the supportive psychodynamic treatment, which also did not lead to an increase in RF ratings, emphasized clarification of internal states without interpretation further supports the idea that interpretations have a role in increasing RF.

Clinical Illustration

We are aware that the TFP strategy of helping the patient resolve the externalization of unbearable self-states is a difficult challenge that may temporarily increase the patient's anxiety by questioning his or her defensive system. However, working actively in the transference with the internal bad persecutory object that the patient must project over and over again (Gabbard 2009; Gabbard et al. 2006; Kernberg 2004)—what Fonagy et al. (2002) call the "alien self"—and with the maladaptive defenses mobilized to cope with such negatively tinged representations, in our view ultimately modulates the negative affects associated with these representations, fosters reflection on them, and enriches the internal world with a fuller, more nuanced range of affective coloring. All of this in turn helps to diminish the influence of negative affects, particularly aggression, that interfere with the healthy experience and expression of loving affects, leading to improved interpersonal functioning in addition to symptom change. Our clinical vignette illustrates our approach and many of the key elements of TFP. The patient, whom we call Mira, is a composite with identifying details altered to protect confidentiality.

> Mira had a history of depression, anxiety, self-mutilation, alcohol abuse, bulimia, and suicide attempts since early adolescence, with repeated hospitalizations and failed outpatient treatments. She was referred to TFP with Dr. Z at age 24 after hospitalization for a serious overdose and her prior therapist's refusal to take her back. Mira was the second child born to a middle-class couple, with a father who was a theater director and a binge drinker and a mother who was an unsuccessful actress and who became severely depressed after the patient was born and continued to experience episodes of major depression with psychotic features. Mira's father was subject to angry outbursts and cruel behaviors such as hanging up a bird feeder in the back yard and shooting the birds that came to feed there. Perhaps in contrast to this, Mira developed a special interest in animals and volunteered at an animal shelter. Mira showed talent as an actress in school productions. She had several platonic affairs with her directors, one of whom was a friend of her father's. She had been in therapy a number of times since her first suicide attempt at age 15 and had been hospitalized four times. She married in her early 20s after dropping out of college and was unemployed. She wanted to become a mother but believed that she was "too sick" to care for a child.
>
> Mira's therapy began with an assessment that established the diagnosis of BPD with narcissistic and antisocial features. Her therapist dis-

cussed the diagnostic impression and its relation to the treatment recommendation for an exploratory therapy that would focus both on curbing her self-destructive behaviors and exploring the elements within her that motivated these behaviors. The treatment contract, in addition to establishing the standard treatment parameters, included attending Alcoholics Anonymous (AA) meetings, reporting to the emergency room if she felt she could not contain her self-destructive urges, and engaging in some productive activity. Mira was able to enroll in some college courses.

Mira's initial clinical course was marked by acting out that required a combination of limit setting and containment. This involved clarifying the representational states that led to her self-destructive actions. After having agreed to the treatment with some expression of gratitude that her therapist would accept her into therapy when so many previous treatments had ended badly, she began to express frustration with him, complaining that he would not accept phone calls at night as her prior therapist would, he would not offer her direct advice and encouragement, and he would not give her a hug when she was discouraged. In short, she experienced him as a "robot." She reported ongoing urges to cut herself but adhered to the treatment contract, which stipulated going to the emergency room if she felt at risk of acting out. The major interventions at this stage focused on clarifying and reflecting upon her experience of the therapist. Not surprisingly, the image of Dr. Z as a potentially fearful and dangerous object emerged quite quickly in the context of an early session where the patient talked about her parents' lack of concern for her, demonstrated most recently by the mother's telling Mira that she no longer could afford to phone or visit the patient.

> **Dr. Z:** Where do you imagine I'd fall on the concerned versus not concerned spectrum?
> **Mira:** Well, you're probably about where my parents are.
> **Dr. Z:** Your parents who don't have enough money to phone you anymore.
> **Mira:** And my dad who was wondering why I didn't just jump in front of a train cause that would work (*laughs*). But, uh, you're not that bad.
> **Dr. Z:** Well, but it feels that way.

Thus, although there is the emergence early in treatment of an object relational dyad of caretaking figures perceived as cold and abusive in relation to the helpless, abused self, the therapist does not interpret this dyad, but rather focuses initially on the patient's experience of him.

One month into therapy, Mira went to the emergency room and was hospitalized for suicidal ideation. She stabilized quickly and was discharged after 3 days. Dr. Z tried to explore what feelings motivated this event. Mira seemed indifferent to the attempt to explore her internal state and attributed her current difficulties to adjusting to the new therapy, stating that she knew it was good for her but acknowledging that she missed her previous therapist's active support. Sensing an oscillation within the dyad that was active at that time, Dr. Z described his impression that the patient was talking in a superficial and indifferent way, and wondered if these suicidal feelings might not be linked to her experience of him as indifferent to her. Mira continued in the same detached vein, saying she just needed some time to get used to him.

The following month, Dr. Z became more concerned that something important was being split off and not expressed directly in therapy. Mira announced that she had started seeing Peter, a man from her AA meeting whom she found much more fun than her "plodding" husband. Dr. Z saw this as a challenge to her marriage and also as a challenge to himself and the therapy. Attempting to maintain neutrality, he tried to help Mira explore the different aspects of what she was acting out, which he imagined to be something along the lines of someone feeling neglected who was acting dramatically to try to obtain care from the neglectful caretaker. The next week Mira reported that Peter had shown her his revolver and she talked excitedly about a murder-suicide pact, which of course alarmed Dr. Z. He was struck by Mira's change from an indifferent tone to what seemed like a dangerous and angry challenge. He asked about her level of concern. She responded with a superficially indifferent but somewhat provocative tone, saying that Dr. Z apparently did not know how to appreciate two people sharing a fantasy. Dr. Z confronted Mira with the gap between the serious and destructive message she was conveying and her indifferent tone that had a hint of provocation. He tried to engage her in reflecting on this development, but she protested that he was making a big deal about nothing. Dr. Z believed this development reflected the emergence of an angry, wrathful part of Mira that followed the experience of him as an indifferent robot. The affair with Peter and the destructive turn it was taking seemed to be the enactment of a punitive part of Mira and, at another level, an appeal for Dr. Z to become more active in relation to her. To summarize the dyads that were emerging: the first, and more accessible to Mira's awareness, was that of a needy child in relation to a neglectful caretaker; the second, more evident in her actions, was that of a vengeful victim determined to punish her persecutor. Any awareness of this dyad was limited to the role of victim, with the persecutory pole of the dyad being enacted in relation to Dr. Z.

Mira's alternating identifications with both poles of this object relational dyad were evident in the cat-and-mouse game that she had initiated by her involvement with a sadistic man; it had elements of sadism toward Dr. Z, who felt anguished by her talk of murder-suicide. She seemed to react with a sly smile to his expression of discomfort when she spoke of that. In addition, Mira's abrupt announcement of a dangerous situation had elements of control: one person forcing another to intervene on her behalf. Finally, and most subtly, there was a dyad of a person being cared for by an appropriately concerned person. This dyad was not usually visible in what the patient said but had come through in her behavior since the beginning of therapy in the form of her regular attendance and participation in the treatment.

Dr. Z's challenge was to deal with all of the above in a way that maintained safety and advanced understanding. Forced to temporarily deviate from neutrality because of the danger, Dr. Z made clear that Mira's new relationship was incompatible with therapy and explained that she would have to choose between the two. The patient became angry, saying that she felt excited about someone for the first time in ages and that Dr. Z had no right to interfere with that. While feeling the need to ensure as best he could that safety was in place by declaring his opposition to Peter, Dr. Z felt that he could also help Mira become more aware of the motivations behind her actions by addressing some of the split-off and enacted affects. He asked her thoughts about his stepping out of his usual role and taking a position. She angrily retorted that he was "covering his ass" because he did not want any "blood on his watch." Dr. Z addressed the object relational dyad on the surface at that moment by pointing out how this view of him as exclusively self-serving would explain her anger and frustration. However, he felt that the dyad that longed for a connection was close enough to the surface for him to mention it. Carrying the process of interpretation a step further, he referred to the dyad that he sensed beneath the surface and suggested that it must be especially difficult to seek care from someone whom she experienced as self-serving and indifferent.

Mira rejected this at first, saying that it was ridiculous to talk about any kind of longing in a therapy setting because it wasn't a "real" relationship. Dr. Z responded that the therapy setting did not prevent people from having the full range of human feelings and was perhaps the only place where the full range could be discussed without the danger of being acted on. He quickly added that he was aware that this particular situation could be painful. Mira's demeanor changed to sadness. She blurted out that every relationship was hopeless and that was why she might just as well "end it." Dr. Z noted the shift in affect and suggested that they had the opportunity in front of them to explore and perhaps change a system where any relationship seemed doomed.

Dr. Z's challenge then was to bring in the angry and aggressive elements that Mira, without apparent awareness, had added to the situation and that contributed to "dooming" relationships she engaged in. He asked her thoughts about her manner when she brought up the murder-suicide pact. She at first said that she was just simply reporting everything to him. He then wondered if she could recall what looked like a smile when he was listening with some distress.

> **Mira:** So, are you telling me I'm bad?
>
> **Dr. Z:** Is that what it feels like?...It sounds like it might be upsetting that I might think you're bad. I was wondering if you might judge yourself as bad if you ever felt any pleasure in hostile or aggressive feelings. But your reaction to this brings up another set of feelings—that you might be feeling close to me, and that may make you uncomfortable and make you want to strike out for some reason. This might especially be the case if you think I'm indifferent to you. I wonder if that feeling might explain what seems like an angry response—a response that includes an attack on me, but potentially an even worse attack on you, like with the murder-suicide pact. This sequence of beginning to feel a little close to me, then feeling rejected and indirectly counterattacking could make relationships really hard.

Throughout the first months of therapy, the less obvious side of Mira's relationship with Dr. Z was her basic longing for a trusted caretaker. He saw this in her regular attendance early in treatment even when she was complaining about his "robot" nature. He referred to a pattern where subtle good interactions between them seemed to be followed by crises. He encouraged reflection on what seemed threatening during these moments of a burgeoning relation. In subsequent sessions, they explored the interaction: Mira's wish to be close to Dr. Z was interfered with by disappointment and anger that he was, in her view, indifferent. She got involved with Peter to show 1) what she considered an active engagement with someone, 2) how his indifference led to her getting into dangerous situations, and 3) that she could make him intervene to save her and to "prove his love" for her. The involvement with Peter might also have been a way to "turn the tables"—to have someone experience the humiliation that she so often felt when she felt uncared for by others.

Working together, they understood that her insistence on a "pure" relation—one with no tinge of disappointment or doubt—activated an aggressive response that then threatened the developing relation. In sum, part of her had sensed in the first months of therapy that Dr. Z's commitment to her was authentic—that was the part that motivated her to continue coming to therapy. However, insofar as it was not the ideal commitment she yearned for, part of her attacked it. She then lived in fear and anxiety that her attacks would destroy what had begun to develop, through the combination of her rage that it was not everything she longed for and her effort to keep Dr. Z involved with her by controlling him.

This line of interpretation over a period of weeks helped Mira begin to integrate the split-off parts that she had repeatedly acted out. Mira ended the relationship with Peter and continued in therapy with no further self-destructive acting out. The beginning of the process of integration seemed to free her to experience deeper levels of her internal experience and its conflicts, such as conflicts about her erotic feelings and impulses toward Dr. Z that emerged in a later stage of the therapy. In short, three principal dyads emerged during the first year of treatment, notably 1) the neglected child in relation to the neglectful "robot" parent, 2) the tortured victim in relation to the torturer/persecutor, and 3) the person longing for a caring relation in relation to the perfect provider.

A discussion and case example of how TFP addresses oedipal issues as they develop in the transference in later phases of treatment can be found elsewhere (Diamond and Yeomans 2007). As a rule, if a BPD patient responds to the structure of TFP and to the process of interpretation of the dissociated psychological structure, the therapy moves on to resemble more standard psychodynamic psychotherapy.

In summary, clarification, confrontation, and interpretation of affects and attributions in the here and now enhance reflective capacity by helping the patient consider the material he externalizes and reflect on its role within his psychological makeup. Acknowledgment of some measure of this material within the self opens the way for integration and mastery of what had previously seemed external and therefore immutable. As projections are accepted internally, they become part of a richer appreciation of self and others, which in turn increases the capacity to reflect on internal states.

Key Clinical Concepts

◆ The *object relations dyad* is an internalized representation of self and other linked by an affect. Dyads are basic elements of personality structure that influence an individual's affective and cognitive experiences.

◆ *Identity diffusion* is the lack of a coherent sense of self and others and is central to borderline personality disorder (BPD).

◆ Traditional psychodynamic techniques must be modified to work successfully with BPD patients. The treatment must be more structured to contain potential acting out, and the therapist must participate with a higher level of activity than in traditional psychodynamic psychotherapy. Transference-focused psychotherapy offers this structure in the form of a twice-weekly outpatient therapy that is guided by a clear treatment frame.

◆ The extreme internal representations of self and other that are at the root of BPD emerge in the patient's experience of the therapist.

◆ The therapist can intervene with tact to help the patient observe and reflect upon aspects of his or her experience that are split off and are acted out and/or projected. The patient's increasing grasp of these aspects of internal experience helps create a coherent self and an increasing ability to master and modulate intense affects.

Suggested Readings

Caligor E, Diamond D, Yeomans FE, et al: The interpretive process in the psychoanalytic psychotherapy of borderline personality pathology. J Am Psychoanal Assoc 57:271–301, 2009. [The most detailed discussion to date of interpretation in TFP.]

Clarkin JF, Yeomans FE, Kernberg OF: Psychotherapy for Borderline Personality: Focusing on Object Relations. Washington, DC, American Psychiatric Publishing, 2006. [The most advanced manual of TFP for the clinician.]

Clarkin JF, Levy KN, Lenzenweger MF, et al: Evaluating three treatments for borderline personality disorder: a multiwave study. Am J Psychiatry 164:922–928, 2007. [A discussion of the randomized controlled trial and symptom change.]

Diamond D, Yeomans FE: Oedipal love and conflict in the transference-countertransference matrix: its impact on attachment security and mentalization, in Attachment and Sexuality. Edited by Diamond D, Blatt S, Lichtenberg J. New York, Analytic Press, 2007, pp 201–235. [A discussion of working at more advanced phases of TFP when issues of sexual and oedipal conflicts can be addressed and resolved.]

Kernberg OF, Yeomans FE, Clarkin JF, et al: Transference focused psychotherapy: overview and update. Int J Psychoanal 89:601–620, 2008

Levy KN, Meehan KB, Kelly KM, et al: Change in attachment patterns and reflective function in a randomized control trial of transference-focused psychotherapy for borderline personality disorder. J Consult Clin Psychol 74:1027–1040, 2006. [A discussion of changes in reflective functioning and attachment status in the randomized controlled trial.]

Yeomans FE, Clarkin JC, Kernberg OF: A Primer on Transference-Focused Psychotherapy for Borderline Patients. Northvale, NJ, Jason Aronson, 2002. [The introductory-level manual for students and clinicians.]

References

Adolphs R: Cognitive neuroscience of human social behavior. Nat Rev Neurosci 4:165–178, 2003

Bateman A, Fonagy P: Psychotherapy for Borderline Personality Disorder: Mentalization-Based Treatment. New York, Oxford University Press, 2004

Bion WR: Second Thoughts: Selected Papers on Psychoanalysis. New York, Basic Books, 1967

Caligor E, Kernberg OF, Clarkin JF: Handbook of Dynamic Psychotherapy for Higher Level Personality Pathology. Washington, DC, American Psychiatric Publishing, 2007

Caligor E, Diamond D, Yeomans FE, et al: The interpretive process in the psychoanalytic psychotherapy of borderline personality pathology. J Am Psychoanal Assoc 57:271–301, 2009

Clarkin JF, Foelsch PA, Levy KN, et al: The development of a psychodynamic treatment for patients with borderline personality disorders: a preliminary study of behavioral change. J Pers Disord 15:487–495, 2001

Clarkin JF, Levy KN, Lenzenweger MF, et al: The Personality Disorders Institute/Borderline Personality Disorder Research Foundation randomized control trial for borderline personality disorder: rationale, methods, and patient characteristics. J Pers Disord 18:52–72, 2004

Clarkin JF, Yeomans FE, Kernberg OF: Psychotherapy for Borderline Personality: Focusing on Object Relations. Washington, DC, American Psychiatric Publishing, 2006

Clarkin JF, Levy KN, Lenzenweger MF, et al: Evaluating three treatments for borderline personality disorder: a multiwave study. Am J Psychiatry 164:922–928, 2007

Depue RA, Lenzenweger MF: A neurobehavioral dimensional model of personality disturbance, in Major Theories of Personality Disorder, 2nd Edition. Edited by Lenzenweger M, Clarkin JF. New York, Guilford, 2005, pp 391–453

Diamond D: Attachment to internal objects in patients with severe narcissistic disorders. Paper presented at the Confer Seminar Series on the Pain of Narcissism and Its Psychotherapeutic Treatment, Tavistock Institute, London, November 5, 2007

Diamond D, Yeomans FE: Oedipal love and conflict in the transference-countertransference matrix: its impact on attachment security and mentalization, in Attachment and Sexuality. Edited by Diamond D, Blatt S, Lichtenberg J. New York, Analytic Press, 2007, pp 201–235

Diamond D, Yeomans F: [Narcissism, its disorders and the role of TFP] (in French). Sante Ment Que 33:115–139, 2008

Diamond D, Stovall-McClough C, Clarkin JF, et al: Patient–therapist attachment in the treatment of borderline personality disorder. Bull Menninger Clin 67:224–257, 2003

Doering S, Hörz S, Rentrop M, et al; Transference-focused psychotherapy v. treatment by community psychotherapists for borderline personality disorder: randomized controlled trial. Br J Psychiatry (in press)

Donegan NH, Sanislow CA, Blumberg HP, et al: Amygdala hyperreactivity in borderline personality disorder: implications for emotional dysregulation. Biol Psychiatry 54:1284–1293, 2003

Fertuck EA, Lenzenweger MF, Clarkin JF, et al: Executive neurocognition, memory systems, and borderline personality disorder. Clin Psychol Rev 26:346–375, 2006

Fertuck EA, Grinband J, Hirsch J, et al: Convergence of psychoanalytic and social neuroscience approaches to borderline personality disorder. Paper presented at the winter meeting of the American Psychoanalytic Association, New York, 2009

Fonagy P, Bateman A: Attachment theory and mentalization-oriented model of borderline personality disorder, in The American Psychiatric Publishing Textbook of Personality Disorders. Edited by Oldham JM, Skodol AE, Bender DS. Washington, DC, American Psychiatric Publishing, 2005, pp 187–207

Fonagy P, Leigh T, Steele M, et al: The relation of attachment status, psychiatric classification and response to psychotherapy. J Consult Clin Psychol 64:22–31, 1996

Fonagy P, Gergely G, Jurist EL, et al: Affect Regulation, Mentalization, and the Development of the Self. New York, Other Press, 2002

Gabbard GO: The interface of neurobiology and psychoanalytic thinking in borderline personality disorders. Paper presented at the American Psychoanalytic Association meetings, New York, January 2009

Gabbard GO, Miller L, Martinez M: A neurobiological perspective on mentalizing and internal object relations in traumatized patients with borderline personality disorder, in Handbook of Mentalization-Based Treatment. Edited by Allen JG, Fonagy P. Chichester, UK, Wiley, 2006, pp 123–140

Grossmann KE, Grossmann K: Universality of human social attachment as an adaptive process, in Attachment and Bonding: A New Synthesis. Edited by Carter CS, Ahnert L, Grossmann KE, et al. Cambridge, MA, MIT Press, 2003, pp 199–288

Gunderson JG, Lyons-Ruth K: BPD's interpersonal hypersensitivity phenotype: a gene-environment-developmental model. J Pers Disord 22:22–41, 2008

Harman C, Rothbart MK, Posner MI: Distress and intention interactions in early infancy. Motiv Emot 21:27–43, 1997

Høglend P, Bøgwald K-P, Amlo S, et al: Transference interpretations in dynamic psychotherapy: do they really yield sustained effects? Am J Psychiatry 165:763–771, 2008

Jurist E: Mentalized affectivity. Psychoanal Psychol 22:426–444, 2005

Kernberg OF: Borderline Conditions and Pathological Narcissism. New York, Jason Aronson, 1975

Kernberg OF: Severe Personality Disorders: Psychotherapeutic Strategies. New Haven, CT, Yale University Press, 1984

Kernberg OF: Aggressivity, Narcissism, and Self-Destructiveness in the Psychotherapeutic Relationship: New Developments in the Psychopathology and Psychotherapy of Severe Personality Disorders. New Haven, CT, Yale University Press, 2004

Kernberg OF, Caligor E: A psychoanalytic theory of personality disorders, in Major Theories of Personality Disorder, 2nd Edition. Edited by Lenzenweger M, Clarkin JF. New York, Guilford, 2005, pp 114–156

Kernberg OF, Diamond D, Yeomans F, et al: Mentalization and attachment in borderline patients in transference focused psychotherapy, in Mind to Mind: Infant Research, Neuroscience, and Psychoanalysis. Edited by Jurist E, Slade A, Bergner S. New York, Other Press, 2008, pp 167–198

Koenigsberg HW: Neural correlates of emotional dysregulation in borderline personality disorder. Paper presented at the winter meeting of the American Psychoanalytic Association, New York, 2009

Krohn AJ: Borderline "empathy" and differentiation of object representations: a contribution to the psychology of object relations. Int J Psychiatry 3:142–165, 1974

Levy KN, Clarkin JF, Yeomans FE, et al: The mechanisms of change in the treatment of borderline personality disorder with transference-focused psychotherapy. J Clin Psychol 62:481–502, 2006a

Levy KN, Meehan KB, Kelly KM, et al: Change in attachment patterns and reflective function in a randomized control trial of transference-focused psychotherapy for borderline personality disorder. J Consult Clin Psychol 74:1027–1040, 2006b

Levy KN, Yeomans FE, Diamond D: Psychodynamic treatments of self-injury. J Clin Psychol 63:1105–1120, 2007

Linehan MM: Cognitive-Behavioral Treatment of Borderline Personality Disorder. New York, Guilford, 1993

Main M: Attachment theory: eighteen points with suggestions for future studies, in Handbook of Attachment: Theory, Research, and Clinical Applications. Edited by Cassidy J, Shaver P. New York, Guilford, 1999, pp 845–887

Main M, Kaplan N, Cassidy J: Security in infancy, childhood, and adulthood: a move to the level of representation. Monogr Soc Res Child Dev 209:66–104, 1985

Posner MI, Rothbart MK, Vizueta N, et al: Attentional mechanisms of borderline personality disorder. Proc Natl Acad Sci U S A 99:16366–16370, 2002

Rinne T, de Kloet ER, Wouters L, et al: Hyperresponsiveness of hypothalamic-pituitary-adrenal axis to combined dexamethasone/corticotropin-releasing hormone challenge in female borderline personality disorder subjects with a history of sustained childhood abuse. Biol Psychiatry 52:1102–1112, 2002

Rockland LH: Supportive Therapy for Borderline Patients: A Psychodynamic Approach. New York, Guilford, 1992

Sandler J, Sandler AM: The past unconscious, the present unconscious, and the vicissitudes of guilt. Int J Psychoanal 8:331–341, 1987

Silbersweig D, Clarkin J, Goldstein M, et al: Failure of frontolimbic inhibitory function in the context of negative emotion in borderline personality disorder. Am J Psychiatry 164:1832–1841, 2007

Slade A, Grienenbrener J, Bernbach E, et al: Maternal reflective functioning, attachment and the transmission gap: a preliminary study. Attach Hum Dev 7:283–298, 2005

Sroufe LA, Egeland B, Carlson E, et al: Placing early attachment experiences in developmental context: the Minnesota Longitudinal Study, in Attachment From Infancy to Adulthood: The Major Longitudinal Studies. Edited by Grossmann KE, Grossmann K, Waters E. New York, Guilford, 2005, pp 48–70

Steele H, Steele M, Croft C, et al: Infant-mother attachment at one year predicts children's understanding of mixed emotions at 6 years. Soc Dev 8:161–178, 1999

Suess G, Grossmann KE, Sroufe LA: Effects of infant attachment to mother and father on quality of adaptation to preschool: from dyadic to individual organization of self. Int J Behav Dev 15:43–65, 1992

Waters E, Merrick S, Treboux D, et al: Attachment security in infancy and early adulthood: a 20-year longitudinal study. Child Dev 71:684–689, 2001

Wupperman P, Neumann CS, Axelrod SR: Do deficits in mindfulness underlie borderline personality features and core difficulties? J Pers Disord 22:466–482, 2008

Yeomans FE, Selzer MA, Clarkin JF : Treating the Borderline Patient: A Contract-Based Approach. New York, Basic Books, 1992

Yeomans FE, Clarkin JC, Kernberg OF: A Primer on Transference-Focused Psychotherapy for Borderline Patients. Northvale, NJ, Jason Aronson, 2002

Yeomans FE, Clarkin JC, Diamond D, et al: An object relations treatment of borderline patients with reflective functioning as the mechanism of change, in Mentalization: Theoretical Considerations, Research Findings, and Clinical Implications. Edited by Busch F. New York, Analytic Press, 2008, pp 159–181

Zaki J, Ochsner KN: You, me, and my brain: self and other representation in social cognitive neuroscience, in Social Neuroscience: Toward Understanding the Underpinnings of the Social Mind. Edited by Todorov A, Fiske ST, Prentice D. New York, Oxford University Press (in press)

CHAPTER 8

Therapeutic Action in the Psychoanalytic Psychotherapy of Borderline Personality Disorder

Glen O. Gabbard, M.D.

How does psychoanalytic psychotherapy work? Let me state at the outset that the answer is clear—we don't know. Therapeutic action has been much discussed in the psychoanalytic literature, but many of the discussions are inextricably bound to particular psychoanalytic theories. Times have changed; we no longer practice in an era in which interpretation is regarded as the exclusive therapeutic arrow in the analyst's quiver (Gabbard and Westen 2003). Abend (2001) observed that "no analyst today would suggest that the acquisition of insight is all that transpires in a successful analysis, or even that it identifies the sole therapeutic influence of the analytic experience" (p. 5). As Abend implies in his distinction between psychoanalysis and "therapeutic influence," there has been an unfortunate divide between what is analytically pure and what helps the patient. In recent contributions (Gabbard 2007; Gabbard and Westen 2003), I have argued that we need to identify what strategies help patients change, rather than worrying about adherence to a particular analytic ideal. In any case, Wallerstein (1986) stressed that after reviewing the data from the monumental 30-year follow-up of the Menninger Foundation Psychotherapy Research Project patients, differentiating therapeutic change from analytic change is virtually impossible anyway.

There is no single path to therapeutic change. Single-mechanism theories of therapeutic action, no matter how complex, are unlikely to prove therapeutically useful, simply because there are a variety of targets of change and a variety of strategies for effecting change in those targets.

Although there once was a debate regarding whether insight or the therapeutic relationship was the key vehicle for change, that either/or polarization of interpretation versus the relationship with the therapist has given way to a broad consensus that both aspects of treatment contribute to change in the patient (Cooper 1989; Gabbard 2000; Gabbard and Westen 2003; Jacobs 1990; Pine 1998; Pulver 1992).

Another shift over time has been away from an archaeological approach to psychoanalytic treatment. Rather than focusing on the excavation of buried relics in the patient's past, most contemporary analytic therapists, especially those who work with borderline personality disorder (BPD), focus more on the here-and-now interaction between the therapist and the patient. The therapist's participation in enactments and projective identification allow her to identify a characteristic "dance" that the patient recreates in a variety of settings based on that patient's internal object relations. Hence by studying what transpires between therapist and patient, one has a sense of what has come before and what is going on every day outside the treatment relationship.

Attempting to study the therapeutic action of psychotherapy is a complex undertaking. If one asks patients what was helpful some time after their treatment, what one hears is often disappointing to the psychoanalytic therapist. One of my patients came back to see me several years after she had terminated a multi-year analytic process. I asked her what she had found most helpful, and she replied, "Each day when I came to your office, you were there." She evidently failed to recall any of my carefully formulated interpretations or any of the insights she had gathered in the course of her treatment with me. I realized, however, that my "being present" meant a lot to her because she had a father who was perennially absent. Hence what was important to her and what was important to me may have been entirely different. Patients may not really know what helped them.

If one investigates the issue of how therapy works by interviewing therapists, one immediately has to deal with the stark reality that they are a biased group. They are narcissistically invested in the outcomes of their patients, and they may view the patient's improvement in terms that shed favorable light on how they conceptualized and formulated the treatment. Moreover, those who are adherents to a particular theoretical school will emphasize strategies deriving from that school regardless of whether or not they were helpful to the patient.

Researchers, on the other hand, have the advantage of objectivity when studying therapeutic action. However, they also are viewing the process from a disadvantaged point of view in some respects. Psychoanalytic psychotherapy is largely about the interior spaces of the patient and the subtle interactions that occur unconsciously between two people. The therapist who is immersed in the transference-countertransference vicissitudes has an immediate sense of who the patient is and what the patient needs in the way of specific therapeutic strategies. Moreover, there are moments of meeting (Stern et al. 1998) that may be extraordinarily meaningful to both patient and therapist but are not part of a therapeutic plan. They occur spontaneously when the two parties share a joke or a deeply moving experience where tears come to the eyes of both. A psychotherapy researcher studying a transcript may entirely miss such moments.

Because all the methodologies to study therapeutic action have a set of problems associated with them, we must acknowledge that we may continue to be in the dark for some time in solving this puzzle. Greenberg (2005) has suggested that the therapeutic action of psychoanalytic treatment may ultimately be unknowable for any specific patient.

Empirical Research on Transference Interpretation

Despite the fact that the therapeutic action of psychoanalytic psychotherapy may be unknowable, I nevertheless will embark on an overview of what is known about effective treatment for BPD, with the assumption that the research seeking to find an efficacious treatment will shed some light on therapeutic action. We know that at least five different types of therapy have now been empirically validated in randomized, controlled trials: mentalization-based treatment (MBT; Bateman and Fonagy 1999), dialectical behavior therapy (DBT; Linehan et al. 2006), transference-focused psychotherapy (TFP; Clarkin et al. 2007), schema-focused therapy (SFT; Giesen-Bloo et al. 2006), and supportive psychotherapy (SP; Clarkin et al. 2007).

Two of these empirically validated treatments are psychodynamic forms of therapy: mentalization-based treatment and transference-focused therapy. One of the central controversies in the discussion of these two treatments is the role played by transference interpretation. While there is no head-to-head comparison in the literature between MBT and TFP, there is a small body of literature that has investigated the relative role of psychoanalytic treatments that focus on transference interpretation versus those that do not.

In a landmark Norwegian study, Høglend et al. (2006) conducted a randomized, controlled trial of dynamic psychotherapy designed to determine the impact of a moderate level of transference interpretations (1–3 per session) in a once-weekly psychotherapy for a duration of 1 year. One hundred patients were randomly assigned to a group using interpretation of the transference or a group that did not use such interventions. The authors included brief vignettes from the therapy so the reader could gain some understanding of the types of interventions considered to be transference interpretations. They attempted to avoid the "allegiance effect" so common in psychotherapy research, where researchers pit their favored treatment against one that they do not really think will work. The investigators cross-trained therapists in each of the therapies used and arranged for the same therapists to conduct both treatments. The results came as something of a surprise: there were no overall differences in outcome between the two treatment cells, but the subgroup of patients with impaired object relations benefited more from the therapy using transference interpretation than from the alternative treatment.

The conventional wisdom in predicting psychotherapy outcome has long been that "the rich get richer" (Gabbard 2006). In other words, patients who have greater psychological resources and more mutually gratifying relationships tend to form a solid therapeutic alliance with the therapist and gain greater benefit from the therapy. Such patients would, according to conventional thinking, be more capable of tolerating transference interpretation than those who are more disturbed and have a shakier therapeutic alliance with the therapist. Moreover, studies of transference interpretation in brief dynamic therapy indicate that there is not a positive correlation between that particular intervention and outcome (Piper et al. 1991).

In the Høglend study, when the patients who had lower scores on the quality of object relations ($n=44$) were examined, it was discovered that 61% of those subjects were diagnosable with personality disorders on the Structured Clinical Interview for DSM-III-R Personality Disorders (SCID-II; Spitzer et al. 1990). By contrast, only 20% of those measured as having had high-quality object relations ($n=55$) had personality disorders. Hence there appeared to be a correlation between presence of personality disorders and improvement with transference interpretation.

The study design had shortcomings that must be taken into account. Axis I disorders were not rigorously diagnosed using standard research interviews. For example, the effects of depression on outcome could not be evaluated with precision. It is also possible that some experienced therapists secretly felt that the patients deprived of transference work were getting less than optimal treatment. Similarly, while investigators attempted to "blind" the raters who were listening to the audiotapes, the content of these tapes might well indicate to which group the patient belonged (Gabbard 2006). Nevertheless, a subsequent report from Høglend et al. (2008) showed that the beneficial effect of transference interpretation for this subgroup of patients with lower-quality object relations was sustained at 3-year follow-up.

Therapeutic Action and Borderline Personality Disorder

Although the findings of the Norwegian study are of heuristic value, they are not specific for any particular personality disorder. When we focus on borderline personality disorder in particular, we have at least one randomized, controlled trial that emphasizes transference interpretation (Clarkin et al. 2007). In a head-to-head comparison of transference-focused psychotherapy, dialectical behavior therapy, and supportive therapy at Cornell-Westchester, 90 patients with BPD were randomly assigned to one of these three treatment groups. Over a 12-month period, six domains of outcome measures were assessed at 4-month intervals by raters blind to the treatment group. When results were analyzed using individual growth-curve analysis, all three treatments appeared to have brought about positive change in multiple domains to a roughly equivalent extent. However, in some areas, TFP seemed to do better than the alternative treatments. In fact, TFP was associated with significant improvements in 10 out of the 12 variables across the six symptom domains, compared with improvement of six variables with SP, and five with DBT. Only TFP brought about significant changes in impulsivity, irritability, verbal assault, and direct assault. Both TFP and DBT—therapies that specifically target suicidal behaviors—did better than supportive therapy in reducing suicidality.

In a report from the same study on a different dimension of these findings, Levy et al. (2006) demonstrated that TFP produced additional improvements that were not found with either DBT or SP. The study subjects who received TFP were more likely to move from an insecure attachment classification to a secure one. In addition, they showed significantly greater changes in mentalizing capacity (measured by reflective functioning) and in narrative coherence, compared with those in other groups. Problems in mentalization (that is, in the capacity to attribute independent mental states to the self and others in order to explain and predict behavior) have been identified as a specific area of psychopathology in BPD, and another empirically validated treatment, MBT, has been designed to address it. This randomized, controlled trial (Levy et al. 2006) of the three therapies at Cornell-Westchester provided suggestive evidence that other therapeutic approaches may also have beneficial effects on the capacity to mentalize.

Although this particular study suggests that TFP is superior to either DBT or SP, it is also important to note that supportive psychotherapy did almost as well as TFP but was provided once weekly instead of twice weekly like the TFP. To be sure, SP in this study was a psychoanalytically sophisticated treatment that shared much in common with TFP, though it proscribed transference interpretations. It was not simply a control condition involving giving praise and advice. The study also raises a provocative question that goes unanswered with the data: Would reflective functioning and the other symptom domains have improved to the same degree as with TFP if the supportive therapy had been offered twice weekly?

Giesen-Bloo et al. (2006) did a direct comparison between transference-focused psychotherapy and schema-focused therapy that lasted 3 years. In this randomized, controlled trial, SFT seemed to produce better outcomes than TFP. However, Yeomans (2007), a consultant to the project, clarified that the therapists doing TFP in the study were actually not well trained in that approach so that the comparison was not valid. In his view, they were using a more generic form of dynamic therapy rather than the specific transference-focused psychotherapy developed by Kernberg, Clarkin, and the other members of the research team.

MBT Versus TFP

As noted earlier, two different psychodynamic psychotherapies, mentalization-based treatment and transference-focused psychotherapy, have both been shown to be efficacious for BPD patients in randomized, controlled trials. Moreover, TFP, a treatment not specifically designed to improve mentalizing, nevertheless showed greater gains in that area than either of the control treatments.

In view of the differences between MBT and TFP, one has difficulty attributing the therapeutic action to the transference interpretation component. The two modalities approach transference interpretation quite differently.

MBT explicitly de-emphasizes the provision of insight through transference interpretation. The rationale is that transference interpretation, especially of anger, is likely to destabilize borderline patients (Gunderson et al. 2007). Instead, MBT focuses on the current mental state and mental functioning of the patient. This strategy is designed to help patients become introspective and develop more of a sense of self-agency. In other words, the patient begins to find a sense of interiority and subjectivity through interaction with a therapist who is curious about the mental functioning of both patient and therapist and through their alternative perspectives on shared experiences. An MBT therapist would not be likely to interpret that a particular feeling the patient is having has its origins in childhood experiences with a parent.

By contrast, TFP sees unintegrated anger as a core problem. Therapists trained in this modality address the splitting off of anger and its associated self and object representations. Through the use of interpreting transference developments, they attempt to integrate anger and the object- and self-representations associated with it into whole-object rather than split-off part-object relations (Gunderson et al. 2007). Given these differences, how do we understand that both MBT and TFP are effective in promoting mentalizing and improving the symptoms of BPD?

There are several possible answers:

1. All therapeutic approaches provide a systematic conceptual framework that organizes the internal chaos of the borderline patient. Patients with BPD characteristically are in a health care system that is chaotic. Because of the splitting mechanism typical of borderline patients, they often receive highly disparate advice from different treaters and diverse treatment agencies. They may feel pulled from all directions by their health care system or may even be thrown out of the system because they are thought to be "manipulators" or "splitters." Any therapeutic strategy based on an overarching theoretical premise makes them feel there is a coherent treatment plan that offers hope.

2. Different borderline patients may respond to different elements of the therapeutic action. BPD has a diverse etiology that involves such elements as childhood abuse, childhood neglect, highly confusing and problematic family interactions that do not involve overt abuse, genetic vulnerability, neuropsychological difficulties, and the influence of Axis I disorders that are more than often present (Gabbard 2005). Although we lack sufficient data to determine which patients

with BPD are likely to respond to which components of therapeutic action, the work of Blatt and Ford (1994) suggests that this form of research is possible. They have delineated two broad subgroups of character pathology that require different therapeutic strategies. The *anaclitic* subtype is concerned mainly about relationships with others, and individuals with this type of pathology have longings to be nurtured, protected, and loved. They appear to respond more to the relational aspect of psychotherapy than to insight delivered through interpretation. On the other hand, the *introjective* subtype is primarily focused on self-development, and individuals with this pathology struggle with feelings of unworthiness, failure, and inferiority. They are highly self-critical, perfectionistic, and competitive, and they appear to do better with a predominantly interpretive approach.

3. The therapeutic action may largely be attributed to secondary strategies that are not emphasized by the therapist. Gabbard and Westen (2003) have identified a number of such strategies that may receive less attention than transference interpretation and the therapeutic relationship. Various forms of confrontation carry implicit or explicit suggestions for change. For example, therapists frequently confront dysfunctional beliefs in the same way they confront problematic behaviors in the borderline patient. Whereas cognitive therapy emphasizes confrontation, dynamic therapy does not, but few therapists would deny that it is involved in the psychoanalytic psychotherapy of BPD. Therapists also engage in directive interventions that are designed to address the patient's conscious problem-solving or decision-making processes. This effort to help patients solve problems may assist them in making more adaptive life choices or also help them master strong affect states by using more explicit reasoning. Exposure, one of the central mechanisms of change in behavioral treatments, is almost always present in dynamic psychotherapy of BPD, even though few dynamic therapists write about it. In brief, exposure involves presenting the patient with a situation that provokes anxiety and assisting the patient in confronting the situation until it no longer creates anxiety because the patient has habituated to it. The diminution of transference anxieties over time is in part related to exposure, as the patient recognizes that the original fears of being criticized or attacked by the therapist are unrealistic. At the same time, the therapist encourages the patient to confront feared situations outside the therapy. Judicious self-disclosure is yet another mode of action. The therapist may share a particular feeling with the patient to promote mentalizing. The careful use of self-disclosure may help the patient see that

her own perception of the therapist is simply a representation rather than an absolute truth. Finally, affirmation may be critically important for patients who have experienced severe trauma (Killingmo 1989). Such patients may have had parents who invalidated their experiences, and the therapist's affirmative validation of the patient's experience can be highly beneficial.

4. The other possibility is that the nature of the therapeutic alliance is responsible for improvement in the patient. Norcross (2000) notes that psychotherapy research indicates that the therapeutic relationship accounts for most of the outcome variance; technique generally accounts for only 12%–15% of the variance across different kinds of therapy. The therapeutic alliance, often defined as the degree to which the patient feels helped by the therapist and is able to collaborate with the therapist in pursuit of common therapeutic goals (Gabbard 2004), has been shown in research to be the most potent predictor of outcome in psychotherapy (Horvath and Symonds 1991; Martin et al. 2000).

Role of the Therapeutic Alliance

Considerations of the therapeutic alliance provide a context for considering the role that transference interpretation plays. It is possible that the emphasis on the frequency or centrality of transference interpretation may be misplaced. Timing may be of much greater importance. Gabbard et al. (1994) studied psychotherapy process involving audiotapes of long-term dynamic psychotherapy with three BPD patients. One group of investigators in the project looked at the impact of the therapist's interventions on the therapeutic alliance. A second group collaborated on identifying the interventions used to effect the therapeutic alliance. These investigators found that transference interpretation had greater impact on the therapeutic alliance—both positive and negative—than other interventions. They concluded that transference interpretation is a high-risk, high-gain intervention in the psychotherapy of BPD patients.

When the researchers looked at the interventions made by the therapist leading up to the transference interpretation, they found that the most effective interpretations of transference, those that had a positive impact on the therapeutic alliance, had something in common. Namely, the way had been paved for the interpretation by a series of empathic, validating, and even supportive interventions that created, in Winnicott's sense, a holding environment. The patient felt understood and validated. A surgeon needs anesthesia to operate, and the psychotherapist of a borderline patient needs a solid therapeutic alliance to interpret transference. Hence the therapeutic alliance and transference interpretation may work synergistically. In this regard, Høglend et al.'s study (2006) could be understood as demonstrating that interpretive work in the therapeutic relationship strengthens the therapeutic alliance. Patients with poor object relations may be able to see the therapist as a trusting, helpful figure when the distortions in the relationship are clarified and understood (Gabbard 2006).

The therapeutic alliance, though, can work independently of transference interpretation, and the therapeutic action does not necessarily depend on their linkage. The relationship between therapist and patient can be strengthened through experiential means without resorting to interpretation or clarification within the transference. The therapist's role as a *witness* of the patient's internal experience may itself be therapeutic (Poland 2000). By the therapist's listening nonjudgmentally to the patient's narrative, the patient is provided with an experience of someone who is "present" with him and able to bear the affect states that he finds unbearable. Wallerstein (1986) studied the original Menninger Foundation psychotherapy research project patients in a 30-year follow-up. Although these patients were not rigorously diagnosed at the time, most would now be diagnosed with BPD. Wallerstein found that supportive treatments appear to be as effective and as durable as expressive treatments in patients with poor object relations.

Among the mechanisms of therapeutic action Wallerstein identified in these patients who had successful supportive treatments, he noted that many "transferred their transference" to someone else. In other words, these patients may have found a supportive romantic partner who could contain their affect states and love them nonjudgmentally in such a way that the relationship itself was healing, independent of the transference to the therapist. He also noted that some patients improved through "transference cure"—that is, they improved to gain the therapist's approval and unconditional positive regard. Others became "therapeutic lifers," patients who never really terminated therapy but continued to see their therapist at intervals varying from months to years. As long as these patients knew that no definitive termination was planned, they functioned well, but faced with the possibility of terminating, they would experience a recurrence of symptoms.

Neurobiological Factors

In looking at the research in recent years on the neurobiological correlates of BPD, we may discover some clues as to the types of psychotherapeutic interventions that are helpful. Examining neurobiological correlates is not an exercise in reductionism. Rather, it is an attempt to expand or understand psychodynamic therapy interventions by investigating how they work on the brain. For example, patients with BPD who have histories of childhood trauma have been shown to have hyperreactive amygdala responses (Herpertz et al. 2001). The amygdala is part of the limbic system and serves to increase vigilance and to evaluate the potential for a novel or dangerous situation. This hyperreactivity extends to faces. Two different studies (Donegan et al. 2003; Wagner and Linehan 1999) found that patients with BPD, compared with control subjects, show significantly greater left amygdalar activation to varied facial expressions. Of even greater importance, however, was the tendency for patients with BPD to attribute negative qualities to neutral faces. Standardized pictures of neutral faces were regarded as threatening, untrustworthy, and possibly nefarious by BPD subjects but not by control subjects. Hence a hyperreactive amygdala may be involved in the predisposition to be hypervigilant and overreactive to relatively benign emotional expressions. This misreading of neutral facial expressions is probably related to the transference misreadings that occur in psychotherapy of patients with BPD. These patients tend to develop "bad object" transferences even when the therapist is behaving professionally and empathically.

Another factor that influences the development of the negative transference in BPD is a hyperreactive hypothalamic-pituitary-adrenal (HPA) axis. Rinne et al. (2002) studied 39 female BPD patients who were given combined dexamethasone/corticotropin-releasing hormone (CRH) tests, using 11 healthy subjects as controls. In the patient group, 24 women had histories of sustained childhood abuse and 15 had no histories of childhood abuse. When the authors examined the results, the chronically abused BPD patients had significantly enhanced adrenocorticotropic hormone (ACTH) and cortisol responses to the dexamethasone/CRH challenge compared with nonabused subjects. They concluded that a history of sustained childhood abuse is associated with hyperresponsiveness of ACTH release.

Along with the misinterpretation of faces associated with a hyperreactive amygdala, we can infer that this hypervigilance related to the overly active HPA axis contributes to a specific form of object relatedness. This paradigm is illustrated in Figure 8–1. An affect state of hypervigilant anxiety links a perception of others as persecuting to perception of the self as victimized. One of the implications for psychotherapy is that the patient's quasi-delusional conviction that the therapist is up to

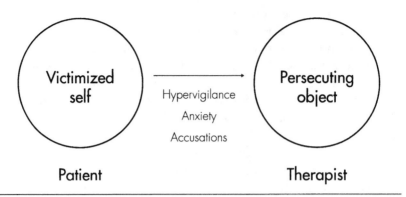

FIGURE 8–1.   An affect state of hypervigilant anxiety links a perception of others as persecuting to perception of the self as victimized.

something malevolent must tactfully be challenged. Consider the following vignette.

> Ms. A, a 27-year-old patient with BPD, was ending a session with me after doing some good work on understanding her affective storms. As she took her coat off the coat hanger on the back of my office door, she got her left arm stuck trying to slip it into the sleeve. I moved over to assist her by holding up the collar of her coat so she could more easily get her arm through the sleeve. She erupted in rage and shouted, "I can do it myself!" I backed off and told her it was fine if she preferred to do it on her own. She then left the session without making further comment.
>
> When she returned the following week, she made no mention of the incident. I brought up what had happened, and she said that it no longer applied to her since she didn't feel that way today; hence there was no reason to discuss it. She said, "Besides, that's not me. I'm not like that." I explained to her that in fact, there was a part of her that was like that. She reluctantly reflected on the last session. She said that her perception was that I was treating her like a small child who didn't know how to put on her coat. I asked, "Is there any other possible perspective on this situation besides that one?" She said that she was sure that was how I had viewed her. I persisted in exploring other options with her. Ultimately, she conceded, now that she was no longer affectively distressed, that it was possible that the therapist had other intentions. She went on to say that she hated the way her mother had infantilized her and didn't want that to be repeated with me. I also offered an interpretive understanding after several minutes of exploring it with her: "It could be that if you acknowledge that the "not me" part of you is here now, you're concerned that that's all I'll see. What would worry you is that all the loving, posi-

tive parts of you would be destroyed by that rage, and I would be driven away." The patient contemplated the possibility and said she would have to think about it.

In this vignette, I challenged the patient's emotional certainty—namely, that she was viewing me in the only way possible: as an infantilizing mother. I helped her explore other possibilities to enhance her mentalizing capacity about her own subjective state and that of others. After paving the way, I also offered an interpretive understanding of her fears in the transference—namely, that if she integrated the "bad" part of her with the more positive, loving part of her, the hate would destroy the love and I would be driven away. Hence a major effort was made to help the patient reflect on what had transpired and see other possible perspectives.

Both TFP and MBT encourage reflection by the patient on the perceptions and conclusions that the therapist draws from interactions. Ochsner et al. (2002) have shown that actively rethinking or reappraising feelings activates the prefrontal area of the brain that modulates amygdala-based negative feelings such as fear. Hence one possibility in terms of therapeutic action is that the reflection and contemplation of affective states and their meaning may increase the prefrontal control of the amygdalar hyperreactivity.

At least one study not involving borderline personality disorder suggests that conscious effort to think may increase the prefrontal volume. Peterson et al. (1998) found that in Tourette's patients, some were able to consciously suppress the motor tics when they had a premonitory urge that they were coming. Others were not good at consciously suppressing them. Those who made a stronger effort to consciously suppress the tics actually increased the volume of their frontal cortex compared to those who were not able to consciously suppress the motor tics, according to functional magnetic resonance imaging scans. Whether a similar change in prefrontal volume is part of the therapeutic action with BPD remains to be studied.

Further research suggests there may actually be a frontolimbic network that is central to the emotional dysregulations in BPD (Schmahl and Bremner 2006). This network consists of the anterior cingulate cortex (ACC), orbitofrontal cortex (OFC), dorsolateral prefrontal cortex, hippocampus, and amygdala. The ACC may be regarded as the brain area involved in mediating emotional control, and studies show that it is deactivated in response to stressful stimuli in BPD. Hence ACC dysfunction is probably a key component in the emotional dysregulation seen in BPD.

Silbersweig et al. (2007) designed an ingenious study to examine the mechanisms involved in frontolimbic dysfunction. BPD patients were asked to push a button for words in standard font but not for those in italicized font. BPD patients, as expected, were more impulsive than non-BPD control subjects, particularly when the italicized words were negative. In contrast to controls, BPD patients showed increased amygdalar reaction and decreased activity in the subgenual cingulate and the medial OFC. Also in response to negative words, the BPD subjects showed increased activity in the dorsal ACC. Hence even though they were not able to exercise impulse control, this finding suggests that they were aware they needed to devote other resources to monitoring it.

We can conclude, then, that neuroimaging data implicates the prefrontal cortex and the ACC as target areas for psychotherapeutic intervention to help decrease emotional dysregulation in BPD patients.

Another contribution to understanding neurobiological correlates of the therapeutic action involves timetables for change in the neurobiology of learning. Wiltgen et al. (2004) stressed that insight and repeated experience have quite separate and different effects on changing what has been learned in the past. Insight based on hippocampal learning provides quick new ways of looking at new information and adapting to new situations. Other neuronal connections, however, are based on implicit, nonhippocampal learning and have never been conscious, nor do they have the capacity to be easily retrieved by shifting one's attention. These types of neuronal associations, developed through intense repeated experiences early in life, are likely to remain strong despite interpretation and insight. Hence explicit and declarative memory systems may change with insight, while implicit and procedural memories may require multiple exposures over an extended period of time for change to be achieved (Folensbee 2007).

Structural change is often regarded as a strengthening of the ego or modification of the superego. However, with our growing knowledge of neural networks, we also know that changes can be understood in terms of what happens in the brain. Through repeated experiences, certain representations of object and self, connected by an affect state, are embedded in neural networks. Those that occur on a regular basis, such as a father who repeatedly hits his son when angry, will become activated automatically when there is a threat. Over time, a psychotherapist offers a new model of relationship for internalization. In this way, the neural network associated with the old object- and self-representations gradually weakens while new associative linkages are occurring that are strengthened through repeated exposure to the psychotherapist, who is a benign and caring figure instead of an abusive one. The capacity for conscious self-reflection allows the patient to override unconscious dynamics once they are recognized and to begin resetting some of the relevant connections. Hence the old neural networks do not disappear but are relatively weakened while the new neural networks, containing the new object relationship of the therapy, are strengthened.

Key Clinical Concepts

- ◆ Summarizing what we know about therapeutic action, we can conclude that there is no single path to therapeutic change.
- ◆ Diverse models of psychotherapy appear to be effective with patients who have borderline personality disorder.
- ◆ Some principles of change and some techniques for eliciting change are likely to be useful for all patients, whereas others may be useful only for some.
- ◆ Patients with impaired object relations may respond well to interpretive techniques, so it is not accurate to assume that strictly supportive techniques are necessary for all patients with borderline psychopathology.
- ◆ Both transference-focused psychotherapy and mentalization-based therapy may improve mentalizing capacity.
- ◆ A solid therapeutic alliance may be essential in all forms of psychotherapy.
- ◆ Transference interpretation is a high-risk, high-gain strategy in the dynamic therapy of borderline personality disorder.
- ◆ Structural change involves weakening old networks while strengthening new ones formed in the therapy and other positive relationships.
- ◆ Neurobiological research suggests that insight may be helpful for phenomena involving hippocampal learning, but repetition of new experience over time may be more mutative for problems stemming from nonhippocampal learning, such as early trauma.

Suggested Readings

Bateman A, Fonagy P: Mentalization-Based Treatment for Borderline Personality Disorder: A Practical Guide. Oxford, UK, Oxford University Press, 2006

Clarkin JF, Yeomans FE, Kernberg OF: Psychotherapy for Borderline Personality Disorder. New York, Wiley, 1999

Gabbard GO: Gabbard's Treatments of Psychiatric Disorders, 4th Edition. Washington, DC, American Psychiatric Publishing, 2007

Gunderson JG, Links PS: Borderline Personality Disorder: A Clinical Guide, 2nd Edition. Washington, DC, American Psychiatric Publishing, 2008

Horwitz L, Gabbard GO, Allen J, et al: Borderline Personality Disorder: Tailoring the Psychotherapy to the Patient. Washington, DC, American Psychiatric Press, 1996

References

Abend SM: Expanding psychological possibilities. Psychoanal Q 70:3–14, 2001

Bateman A, Fonagy P: Effectiveness of partial hospitalization in the treatment of borderline personality disorder: a randomized controlled trial. Am J Psychiatry 156:1563–1569, 1999

Blatt SJ, Ford TQ: Therapeutic Change: An Object Relations Perspective. New York, Springer, 1994

Clarkin JR, Levy KN, Lenzenweger MF, et al: Evaluating three treatments for borderline personality disorder: a multiwave study. Am J Psychiatry 164:922–928, 2007

Cooper AM: Concepts of therapeutic effectiveness in psychoanalysis: a historical review. Psychoanalytic Inquiry 9:4–25, 1989

Donegan NH, Sanislow CA, Blumberg HP, et al: Amygdala hyperreactivity in borderline personality disorder: implications for emotional dysregulation. Biol Psychiatry 54:1284–1293, 2003

Folensbee RW: The Neuroscience of Psychological Therapies. Cambridge, UK, Cambridge University Press, 2007

Gabbard GO: Psychodynamic Psychiatry in Clinical Practice, 4th Edition. Washington, DC, American Psychiatric Press, 2005

Gabbard GO: Long-Term Psychodynamic Psychotherapy: A Basic Text. Washington, DC, American Psychiatric Publishing, 2004

Gabbard GO: When is transference work useful in dynamic psychotherapy? Am J Psychiatry 163:1667–1669, 2006

Gabbard GO: Do all roads lead to Rome? New findings on borderline personality disorder. Am J Psychiatry 164:853–855, 2007

Gabbard GO, Westen D: Rethinking therapeutic action. Int J Psychoanal 84:823–841, 2003

Gabbard GO, Horwitz L, Allen JG, et al: Transference interpretation in the psychotherapy of borderline patients: a high-risk, high-gain phenomenon. Harv Rev Psychiatry 2:59–69, 1994

Giesen-Bloo J, van Dyck R, Spinhoven P, et al: Outpatient psychotherapy for borderline personality disorder: randomized trial of schema-focused therapy vs. transference-focused therapy. Arch Gen Psychiatry 63:649–658, 2006

Greenberg J: Theories of therapeutic action and their technical consequences, in The American Psychiatric Publishing Textbook of Psychoanalysis. Edited by Person ES, Cooper AM, Gabbard GO. Washington, DC, American Psychiatric Publishing, 2005, pp 217–228

Gunderson JG, Bateman A, Kernberg O: Alternative perspectives in psychodynamic psychotherapy of borderline personality disorder: the case of "Ellen." Am J Psychiatry 164:1333–1339, 2007

Herpertz SC, Dietrich TM, Wenning B, et al: Evidence of abnormal amygdala functioning in borderline personality disorder: a functional MRI study. Biol Psychiatry 50:292–298, 2001

Høglend P, Amlo S, Marble A, et al: Analysis of the patient-therapist relationship in dynamic psychotherapy: an experimental study of transference interpretations. Am J Psychiatry 163:1739–1746, 2006

Høglend P, Bøgwald K-P, Amlo S, et al: Transference interpretations in dynamic psychotherapy: do they really yield sustained effects? Am J Psychiatry 165:763–771, 2008

Horvath AD, Symonds BD: Relation between working alliance and outcome in psychotherapy: a meta-analysis. J Couns Psychol 38:139–149, 1991

Jacobs TJ: The corrective emotional experience—its place in current technique. Psychoanalytic Inquiry 10:433–454, 1990

Killingmo B: Conflict and deficits: implications for technique. Int J Psychoanal 70:65–79, 1989

Levy KN, Meehan KB, Clarkin JF, et al: Change in attachment patterns and reflective function in a randomized controlled trial of transference-focused psychotherapy for borderline personality disorder. J Consult Clin Psychol 74:1027–1074, 2006

Linehan MM, Comtois KA, Murray AM, et al: Two-year randomized controlled trial and follow-up of dialectical behavior therapy vs therapy by experts for suicidal behaviors and borderline personality disorder. Arch Gen Psychiatry 63:757–766, 2006

Martin DJ, Garske JP, Davis MK: Relation of the therapeutic alliance with outcome and other variables: a meta-analytic review. J Consult Clin Psychol 68:438–450, 2000

Norcross JC: Toward the delineation of empirically based principles in psychotherapy: commentary on Beutler. Prevention and Treatment 3:1–5, 2000

Ochsner KN, Bunge SA, Gross JJ, et al: Rethinking feelings: an fMRI study of the cognitive regulation of emotion. J Cogn Neurosci 14:1215–1229, 2002

Peterson BS, Skudlarski P, Anderson AW, et al: A functional magnetic resonance imaging study of tic suppression in Tourette syndrome. Arch Gen Psychiatry 55:326–333, 1998

Pine F: Diversity and Direction in Psychoanalytic Technique. New Haven, CT, Yale University Press, 1998

Piper WE, Azim HF, Joyce AS, et al: Transference interpretations, therapeutic alliance, and outcome in short-term individual psychotherapy. Arch Gen Psychiatry 48:946–953, 1991

Poland WS: The analyst's witnessing and otherness. J Am Psychoanal Assoc 48:16–35, 2000

Pulver SE: Psychic change: insight or relationship? Int J Psychoanal 73:199–208, 1992

Rinne T, de Kloet ER, Wouters L, et al: Hyperresponsiveness of hypothalamic-pituitary-adrenal axis to combined dexamethasone/corticotropin-releasing hormone challenge in female borderline personality disorder subjects with a history of sustained childhood abuse. Biol Psychiatry 52:1102–1112, 2002

Schmahl C, Bremner JD: Neuroimaging in borderline personality disorder. J Psychiatr Res 40:419–427, 2006

Silbersweig D, Clarkin JF, Goldstein M, et al: Failure of frontolimbic inhibitory function in the context of negative emotion in borderline personality disorder. Am J Psychiatry 164:1832–1841, 2007

Spitzer RL, Williams JBW, Gibbon N, et al: Structured Clinical Interview for DSM-III-R Personality Disorders (SCID-II). Washington, DC, American Psychiatric Press, 1990

Stern DN, Sander LW, Nahum JP, et al: Non-interpretive mechanisms in psychoanalytic therapy: the "something more" than interpretation. Int J Psychoanal 79:903–921, 1998

Wagner AW, Linehan MM: Facial expression recognition ability among women with borderline personality disorder: implications for emotion regulation? J Pers Disord 13:329–344, 1999

Wallerstein R: Forty-Two Lives in Treatment. New York, Guilford, 1986

Wiltgen BJ, Brown RA, Talton LE, et al: New circuits for old memories: the role of the neocortex in consolidation. Neuron 44:101–108, 2004

Yeomans F: Questions concerning the randomized trial of schema-focused therapy vs transference-focused psychotherapy (letter). Arch Gen Psychiatry 64:609–610, 2007

CHAPTER 9

Narcissistic Personality Disorder

Otto F. Kernberg, M.D.

Definition and Classification

Traditional psychoanalytic metapsychology defines *narcissism* as the libidinal investment of the self. *Narcissistic libido* is libido invested in the self. Although the traditional view of libido as one of the two basic drives (aggression is the other) is currently being questioned in psychoanalysis, as opposed to affectively positive or rewarding investments, the self is here conceived as a substructure of the ego as a system, a substructure reflecting the integration of self representations that develop as the result of experiences with other human beings—objects. Narcissistic libido, in my currently proposed reformulation, is the sum total of positive affective investments in the self as a substructure of the system ego, a sum total equivalent to the "drive" libido. *Object libido,* the sum total of positive affective investment in objects and their psychic representations, is in a dynamic relation with narcissistic libido.

Narcissism defined at the clinical level is the normal or pathological regulation of self-esteem or self-regard. Self-esteem or self-regard normally fluctuates according to the gratifying or frustrating experiences one has in relations to others, and according to how one evaluates the distance between goals and aspirations, on the one hand, and one's achievements and success, on the other. Clinical experience, however, tells us that the relations between self-esteem, moods, the extent to which various self representations are integrated or dissociated, and the vicissitudes of internalized object relations are extremely complicated.

The regulation of self-esteem depends, among other factors, on the pressures exerted by the superego on the ego. A harsh superego—because of its unconscious demands for perfection and its infantile prohibitions—can diminish self-esteem. The regulation of self-esteem may also be affected by the absence of gratification of both libidinal and aggressive instinctual needs. Furthermore, self-esteem regulation depends on internalizing libidinally invested objects. Libidinally invested object representations provide the self with reinforcement of the images of those the person loves and by whom the person feels loved. Should excessive conflicts around aggression weaken the libidinal investment of others and affect the corresponding object representations, the libidinal investment of the self and self-love also suffer.

I find it useful to classify narcissism as normal adult, normal infantile, and pathological narcissism. *Normal adult narcissism* is characterized by normal self-esteem regulation. Here we find a normal self structure, "total" or well-integrated internalized object representations, a mature superego, and gratification of instinctual needs occurring within the context of stable object relations and value systems.

Because fixation at or regression to normal infantile narcissistic goals (infantile mechanisms of self-esteem regulation) is an important characteristic of all character pathology, normal infantile narcissism is important. *Normal infantile narcissism* consists in the regulation of self-esteem by age-appropriate gratifications, including or implying normal infantile "value systems," demands, and/or prohibitions. The mildest type of narcissistic pathology can be understood as fixation at or regression to a functioning at the level of normal infantile narcissism. In this type of pathology the regulation of self-esteem seems to be overly dependent on expressing or defending against childish gratifications that, later on, are normally abandoned. This frequent and relatively mild disturbance need not concern us further at the present time.

A second, relatively infrequent but more severe type of narcissism, *pathological narcissism*, was first described by Freud (1914/1957) to illustrate "narcissistic object choice." Here the patient's self is identified with an object and the representation of the patient's infantile self is simultaneously projected onto that very object. This creates a libidinal relation in which the functions of self and object have been interchanged, a condition often found among male and female homosexuals: they love another in the way they would have wished to be loved.

The most severe type of pathological narcissism is the narcissistic personality disorder proper. This syndrome is one of the most challenging met within clinical psychiatry. The narcissistic personality disorder constitutes the focus of the rest of this chapter. It is a specific type of character pathology that centers around the presence of a pathological grandiose self, to be described below.

The Clinical Syndrome

Individuals with narcissistic personality disorder present, clinically, at three levels of severity. In the mildest cases, the individuals appear "neurotic" and usually present indications for psychoanalysis. They typically seek treatment only because of a significant symptom that seems so linked to their character pathology that anything but the treatment of their personality disorder would seem inadequate. In contrast, other narcissistic patients at that level present with symptoms that may be treated without an effort to modify or resolve their narcissistic personality structure. All these patients seem to be functioning very well, in general, except for typically presenting with significant problems in long-term intimate relationships and in long-term professional or work interactions. The second level of severity of illness of narcissistic personalities reflects the typical syndrome with all the various clinical manifestations to be described below. Patients at this level of severity definitely need treatment for their personality disorder, and here the alternative between standard psychoanalytic treatment and psychoanalytic psychotherapy depends on individualized indications and contraindications. At the third level of severity of narcissistic personality disorder, patients function on an overt borderline level: in addition to all the typical manifestations of narcissistic personality disorder, these patients present with a general lack of anxiety tolerance and of impulse control and a severe reduction in sublimatory functions (i.e., in their capacity for productivity or creativity beyond gratification of survival needs). They usually show severe and chronic failure in their work and profession, and chronic failure in their efforts to establish or maintain intimate love relations. At this same level of severity, another group of patients may not show overt borderline features, but present with significant antisocial activity, which, prognostically, places them in the same category as those who function on a borderline level.

All these low-level, severely narcissistic patients may respond to a psychoanalytic, transference-focused psychotherapy, unless, for individualized reasons, this approach would seem contraindicated, in which case a more supportive approach or cognitive-behavioral approach might be the treatment of choice (O.F. Kernberg 2004; Levy et al. 2005). Patients whose antisocial behavior is predominantly passive and parasitic present less of a threat to themselves and to the therapist than do those others who present with severe suicidal and parasuicidal behavior or violent attacks against others. Aggression against others or self is typical for antisocial behavior of the aggressive type, particularly when the criteria for the syndrome of malignant narcissism are fulfilled. The syndrome of malignant narcissism includes, in addition to narcissistic personality disorder, severe antisocial behavior, significant paranoid trends, and ego-syntonic, self-directed, or other-directed aggression.

Now, let us review briefly the dominant features of narcissistic personality disorder as typically represented, particularly at the second, or intermediate, level of severity described (O.F. Kernberg 1997).

1. *Pathology of the self.* Patients show excessive self-centeredness, overdependency on admiration from others, prominence of fantasies of success and grandiosity, avoidance of realities that are contrary to their inflated image of themselves, and bouts of insecurity disrupting their sense of grandiosity or specialness.
2. *Pathology of the relationship with others.* Patients suffer from inordinate envy, both conscious and unconscious. They show greediness and exploitativeness of others, entitlement, and devaluation of others and an incapacity to really depend on them (in contrast to ongoing need for admiration from others). They show a remarkable lack of empathy with others, shallowness in their emotional life, and a lack of capacity for commitment to relationships with others or for working toward shared goals or at joint purposes.
3. *Pathology of the superego (conscious and unconscious internalized value systems).* At a relatively milder level, patients evince a deficit in their capacity for sadness and mourning. Their self-esteem is regulated by severe mood swings rather than by limited, focused self-criticism; they appear to be determined by a "shame" culture rather than by a "guilt" culture, and their values have a childlike quality. More severe superego pathology, in addition to defective mourning, entails chronic antisocial behavior and significant irresponsibility in all their relationships. In their lack of consideration of others, there is no capacity for guilt or remorse for such devaluing behavior. A particular syndrome—mentioned before, reflecting severe superego pathology, characterized by the combination of narcissistic

personality disorder, antisocial behavior, ego-syntonic aggression (directed against self and/or others), and marked paranoid trends— is the syndrome of malignant narcissism.

4. *Chronic sense of emptiness and boredom.* A basic self state of these patients is a chronic sense of emptiness and boredom, resulting in stimulus hunger and the wish for artificial stimulation of affective response by means of drugs or alcohol that predisposes to substance abuse and dependency.

Patients with narcissistic personality disorder may present with typical complications of this disorder, including sexual promiscuity or sexual inhibition, drug dependence and alcoholism, social parasitism, severe (narcissistic type) suicidality and parasuicidality, and, under conditions of severe stress and regression, the possibility of significant paranoid developments and brief psychotic episodes.

Narcissistic Personality Disorder and Antisocial Personality Disorder

Antisocial personality disorder is the most severe form of narcissistic character pathology; it may be defined as a narcissistic personality disorder with extreme absence of superego functions. Clinically, the antisocial personality proper may be divided into an aggressive type and a passive-parasitic type (Henderson 1939; Henderson and Gillespie 1969).

Careful exploration of nearly all antisocial personality disorders shows that symptoms of this disorder were already present in early childhood. The tendency in the DSM-IV nomenclature (American Psychiatric Association 1994) to separate "conduct disorders" in childhood from the antisocial personality disorder in adulthood, with an artificial limit set at age 18 before the diagnosis of an antisocial personality may be established, ignores this continuity (Hare 1970; Hare and Shalling 1978; P.F. Kernberg 1989). The distinction between conduct disorder and antisocial personality disorder seems absurd from a psychopathological and clinical viewpoint. Given the grave implications of an antisocial personality disorder at any age, it is important that the clinician examining an adolescent with significant antisocial behavior be prepared to diagnose this disorder. I have explored the differential diagnosis between antisocial personality disorder, the syndrome of malignant narcissism, and narcissistic personality disorder in earlier work (O.F. Kernberg 1989), and shall summarize briefly the main characteristics of the antisocial personality disorder proper that enable the clinician to distinguish it from the syndrome of malignant narcissism and the less severe narcissistic personality disorder, both of which may present antisocial behaviors.

It is important to keep in mind that the passive-parasitic type of antisocial personality usually goes unnoticed during early childhood, particularly if antisocial features of the patient's family and social background absorb the patient's antisocial behavior into culturally tolerated patterns. Thus, for example, early cheating in school, stealing, and habitual lying may not be taken seriously in an ambiance of social disorganization and severe family pathology, whereas such behavior would stand out in a relatively stable and healthy social and family environment. Antisocial tendencies or severe narcissistic pathology of the parents may provide convenient "cover-ups" for a child's passive-parasitic antisocial behavior, characterized by manipulativeness, exploitativeness, lying, stealing, and cheating at school.

The predominantly aggressive type of antisocial personality disorder is usually more readily recognized because of the impact of this pathology on the immediate social environment of the child. As Paulina Kernberg (1989) has pointed out, the aggressive type of antisocial personality disorder in children is characterized by extreme aggression from early childhood on, to the extent that violent and destructive behavior may be expressed toward siblings, animals, and property; the parents are usually afraid of these children. The children show an "affectless" expression of aggression, chronic manipulativeness and paranoid tendencies, and a marked inability to keep friends, and sometimes effect a true reign of terror at home or in their immediate social circle at school. Often the parents are unable to convince mental health professionals of the gravity of the situation. In early adolescence, this aggression extends beyond the family circle and may include criminal behavior.

From a diagnostic viewpoint, the essential characteristics of the antisocial personality proper are, first, the presence of a narcissistic personality disorder as described before and, second, in the case of the antisocial personality of a predominantly aggressive type, the symptoms of malignant narcissism. In the case of the predominantly passive-parasitic type, there is no violence, only passive-exploitative behavior, such as lying, cheating, stealing, and exploitation of others. Third, careful evaluation of the past history reveals the presence of antisocial behavior beginning in early childhood.

Fourth, and fundamentally, these patients prove incapable of experiencing feelings of guilt and remorse for their harmful actions. They may express remorse when these are discovered, but not so long as they believe their prohibited behavior is unknown to anybody else. It is also striking that they are unable to identify with the moral dimension in the mind of the diagnostician, to the extent that, while they may be very skilled in assessing other people's motivations and behavior, the possibility of an ethical motivation is so foreign to them that the exploration of this issue—for example, in wondering how they believe the therapist may be reacting to their antisocial behavior—often reveals their striking incapacity to imagine the sense of sadness, concern, or moral shock evoked by acts of cruelty or exploitation.

Fifth, these patients are incapable of nonexploitative investment in others; they display an indifference and callousness that extends also to pets, which they may mistreat or abandon without any feelings. Sixth, their lack of concern for others is matched by lack of concern for themselves; they lack a sense of time, of future, and of planning. While they may carry out concrete antisocial acts with excellent short-term planning, the long-term effects of cumulative antisocial behavior are emotionally insignificant to these patients and hence totally ignored. A sense of future is a superego function, in addition to an ego function, and glaringly absent in these cases.

Seventh, the lack of an affective investment in significant others is matched by a lack of normal love for the self, expressed in defiant, fearless, potentially self-destructive behavior and a proneness to impulsive acts of suicide when they experience themselves driven into a corner; and of course, under the impact of intense rage, they present the risk of severely aggressive and homicidal behavior toward others.

Eighth, these patients show remarkable stunting of the capacity for depressive mourning and grief, and marked limitation of anxiety tolerance. The latter shows up in the prompt development of new symptoms or antisocial behavior when they feel threatened or controlled by external structure.

Ninth, these patients show a remarkable inability to learn from experience, or to absorb the information or moral support provided by the therapist: behind this imperviousness is a radical devaluation of all value systems, a sense that life is an ongoing struggle either among wolves or between wolves and sheep, with many wolves disguised as sheep.

Finally, these patients are incapable of falling in love. They cannot experience the integration of tenderness and sexuality, and their sexual involvements have a mechanical quality that renders them eternally unsatisfactory. When antisocial personalities develop a sadistic perversion, they can become extremely dangerous to others. The combination of severe aggression, the absence of any capacity for compassion, and the lack of superego development is the basis for the psychopathology of mass murder as well as murder in the context of sexual involvements.

In the diagnostic interviews with these patients, their manipulativeness, pathological lying, and shifting rationalizations create what Paulina Kernberg has called "holographic man": they are able to evoke flimsy, rapidly changing, completely contradictory images of themselves and of their lives and interactions. The diagnostic evaluation of these cases requires taking a complete history from these patients so as to identify shifts in the versions of their past presented on different occasions, to observe their interactions with the therapists as well as with significant others, and to obtain a very full social history in order to compare external observations and information with the patient's communication.

The exploration of these patients' history should include tactful questions of why they did not engage in what would seem, under some specific circumstances, expectable antisocial behaviors in their case; this often reveals the lack of the capacity to identify with ethical systems even while the patients are trying to portray a picture of themselves as honest and reliable individuals. Naturally, patients who lie to the diagnostician should be confronted with that in nonpunitive ways, mostly so that the therapist can assess the extent to which the capacity for guilt, remorse, or shame is still available. Patients with narcissistic personality disorder with passive-parasitic tendencies will show the same general characteristics mentioned for patients with the aggressive type, except for direct aggressive attacks on others, on property, on animals, and on the self. Patients with the syndrome of malignant narcissism, but without an antisocial personality proper, will present with the capacity for guilt, concern for self, some nonexploitative relations, some remnants of authentic superego functions, and some capacity for dependency; their prognosis is significantly better.

Antisocial behavior is not in itself a diagnosis. It may appear in patients with borderline personality organization and other personality disorders, as well as some patients with neurotic personality organization and good ego identity integration. Antisocial behavior may, at times, reflect a neurosis with strong rebellious features in an adolescent, and even a normal adaptation to a pathological social subgroup (the "dissocial" reaction). In all these cases, the antisocial behavior has an excellent prognosis with the psychotherapeutic treatment of the underlying character pathology or neurotic syndrome. Therefore, in all adolescent patients with antisocial behavior, it is essential to rule out the syndrome of identity diffusion, the presence of a narcissistic personality disorder, the syndrome of malignant narcissism, and the presence of an antisocial personality proper.

Therapeutic Approaches

GENERAL CONSIDERATIONS

As mentioned earlier in this chapter, the indications for psychoanalytic and other modalities of treatment of narcissistic personality disorder vary with the severity of the illness and the individual combination of particular symptoms and character pathology. The general techniques of standard psychoanalysis and psychoanalytic psychotherapy have to be modified or enriched by specific approaches to deal with the narcissistic transference/countertransference binds (Koenigsberg et al. 2000). Without further exploring here the general differences between these modalities of treatment and their respective indications, I shall spell out particular issues that typically emerge in the treatment of narcissistic patients and that become especially dominant in treatment encounters with the "almost untreatable narcissistic patients" that we shall explore, and that, within the entire spectrum of psychoanalytically derived treatments, require certain specific technical approaches.

A core issue for narcissistic patients is their incapacity to depend on the therapist, because such dependency is experienced as humiliating. Such fear of dependency, often unconscious, is defended against with attempts to omnipotently control the treatment (O. F. Kernberg 1984; Rosenfeld 1987). Clinically, this takes the form of the patient's efforts at "self-analysis" as opposed to a collaboration with the therapist leading to integration and reflection. These patients treat the therapist as if he were a "vending machine" of interpretations, which they then appropriate as their own, at the same time being chronically disappointed for not receiving enough or not the right kind of interpretations, unconsciously dismissing everything they might learn from him. For this reason, treatment often maintains a "first session" quality over an extended period of time. Narcissistic patients show themselves as intensely competitive with the therapist and are suspicious of what they consider his indifferent or exploitative attitude toward them. They cannot conceive the therapist as spontaneously interested and honestly concerned about them, and as a result of this belief, they evince significant devaluation and contempt of the therapist.

Conversely, narcissistic patients may also show a defensive idealization of the therapist, considering him as "the greatest," but such idealization is frail and can rapidly be shattered by devaluation and contempt. It also may be part of omnipotent control, in that these patients unconsciously attempt to force the therapist to be always convincing and brilliant, as befitting their grandiosity, but not superior to them, as that would generate envy. The patient needs the therapist to remain "brilliant," and thus protected against the patient's tendency to devalue him, because devaluing the therapist would leave the patient feeling totally lost and abandoned in the treatment.

A major feature involved in all these manifestations is the patient's conscious and unconscious envy of the therapist—the patient's consistent sense that there can only be one great person in the room, who necessarily will depreciate the other, inferior one, which motivates the patient to try to stay on top, with the risk of feeling abandoned because of the loss of the devalued therapist. Envy of the therapist, at the same time, is an unending source of resentment of what the therapist has to give, and it may take many forms. The most important one is the envy of the creativity of the therapist, of the fact that he can creatively understand the patient rather than providing him with pat, cliché answers that can be memorized by the patient. Also, the very capacity of the therapist to invest in a relationship, which the patient is aware he does not have himself, is envied. The most important consequence of conflicts around envy comprises negative therapeutic reactions: typically, the patient feels worse following a situation in which he clearly acknowledged having been helped by the therapist. Acting out of the envious resentment of the therapist may take many forms, such as playing one therapist against another; an aggressive pseudo-identification with the therapist by playing the therapist's role in a destructive interaction with third parties; and, quite frequently, the patient's constructing a view that it is he himself alone who is the cause of his progress.

The analysis of the constituent, idealized self and idealized object representations that jointly consolidate into the pathological grandiose self of these patients gradually tends to reduce the grandiosity in the transference and the pseudo-integration of that pathological grandiose self, and brings about the emergence of more primitive internalized object relations in the transference and more primitive affective investments related to them. This development shows clinically in the breakthrough of aggressive reactions as part of such primitive object relations, including suicidal and parasuicidal behavior in unconscious identification with powerful yet hostile objects: the "victory" of these primitive object representations over the therapist may be symbolized by the destruction of the body of the patient.

Chronic suicidal tendencies of narcissistic patients have a premeditated, calculated, coldly sadistic quality that differs from the impulsive, "momentarily decided upon" suicidality of ordinary borderline patients (O. F. Kernberg 2001). The projection of persecutory object representations onto the therapist in the form of severe paranoid transferences also may become predominant, as may a form of narcissistic rage that expresses the patient's sense of entitlement as well as his envious resentment. "Stealing" from the therapist may take the form of learning the therapist's language in order to apply it to others rather than to the patient himself, as well as the syndrome of perversity, reflected in taking what was received from the therapist as an expression of the therapist's concern and commitment, and using it as a way of expressing aggression against others. In other words, perversity is a malignant transformation of what the patient received from the therapist. The corruption of superego values may be acted out as antisocial behavior that the patient, unconsciously, perceives as caused by the irresponsibility of the therapist and not by himself.

Narcissistic entitlement and greedy incorporation of what the patient feels is denied to him may take the form of apparently erotic transferences, demands to be loved by the therapist, or even efforts to seduce the therapist as part of a general effort to destroy his role. These are severe complications, very different from the erotic transferences of higher-level, neurotic patients.

When improvement occurs, typically, the severe envy diminishes, and the capacity for gratitude gradually emerges both in the transference and in extra-transferential relations, particularly in the relationship with intimate sexual partners. Envy of the other gender is a dominant unconscious conflict of narcissistic personalities, and the decrease of the envy of the other sex permits a decrease of unconscious devaluing attitudes toward intimate partners, and the capacity for maintained love relations improves. Narcissistic patients may become more tolerant of their own feelings of envy without having to act them out, and, with increased awareness, tendencies toward defensive devaluation gradually decrease in this process. The development of more mature feelings of guilt and concern over their aggressive and exploitative attitudes indicates the consolidation of the superego, as well as the deepening of their object relations. At times, however, that integration may imply such a severity of the now integrated but sadistic superego that these patients may experience severe depression at a point where improvement in their character pathology is evident.

Under optimal conditions, patients who had experienced dominant psychopathic transferences (their conviction of the therapist's dishonesty, or the direct expression of conscious dishonesty and deceptiveness on these patients' part) over an extended period of time may shift into paranoid transferences, against which the psychopathic transferences, typically, had been a defense. And, later on, such paranoid transferences (related to the projection of persecutory object representations and superego precursors onto the therapist) may shift into depressive transferences, as the patient becomes able to tolerate ambivalent feelings and to recognize his experiencing both intense positive and negative feelings toward the same object (O.F. Kernberg 1992).

Perhaps the transference development most difficult to manage is that of patients with an extreme intensity of aggression, which may present itself in the form of almost uncontrollable suicidal and parasuicidal behavior outside the sessions and in chronic sadomasochistic transferences in the sessions. In the latter case, the patient sadistically attacks the therapist over an extended period of time, clearly attempting to provoke him to respond, in his countertransference, in the same way, only to then accuse the therapist of being aggressive and destructive. In all of this, the patient experiences himself as the therapist's helpless victim. This development of a secondary masochistic relation to the therapist may be followed, in turn, by self-directed aggression in which the patient accuses himself exaggeratedly of his "badness," only, eventually, to revert again to an extremely sadistic behavior toward the therapist, thus reinitiating the cycle. Here the technical approach involves pointing out to the patient these patterns of experiencing self and other as either the aggressor or his victim in the transference, with frequent role reversals.

Another manifestation of severe aggression in the transference is the syndrome of arrogance, quite frequently present in patients with narcissistic personalities functioning on an overt borderline level: the combination of intense arrogant behavior, an extreme curiosity about the therapist and his life but little curiosity about himself, and "pseudo-stupidity" (Bion 1967). The last-mentioned symptom consists in a lack of capacity to accept any logical, rational argument: the main defensive purpose of this entire syndrome, on the patient's part, is to protect himself against the very awareness of the intense aggression that controls him. Aggressive affect is expressed in behavior rather than in an affectively marked representational process.

While these transference developments may evolve in any treatment modality, the advantage of psychodynamic psychotherapies and psychoanalysis, where indicated, is that they may permit resolution of these transference manifestations by means of the interpretive focus. In contrast, supportive and cognitive-behavioral treatments may control and reduce the most severe effects of these transference developments on the relationship with the therapist, but their continued unconscious control of the patient's life continues to be a major problem. Supportive and cognitive-behavioral approaches may reduce, by educational means combined with a general supportive attitude, the inappropriate nature of the patient's interactions at work or in a profession. However, in my experience, work at this level is not sufficient to modify the incapacity of these patients to establish significant love relations in depth and to maintain gratifying intimate relations in general. And, not infrequently, the difficult transference developments described earlier may undermine supportive or cognitive-behavioral approaches. Therefore, when it seems reasonable to conclude that the patient may tolerate an analytic approach, regardless of the severity of the symptoms, that indication usually is a prognostically positive feature. But, as we shall see in the next section, such an analytic approach has definite limits.

There are references in the psychoanalytic literature, particularly within the Kleinian approach, that indicate successful treatment with nonmodified analytic approaches of some severely ill narcissistic patients (Bion 1967; Spillius 1988; Spillius and Feldman 1989; Steiner 1993). The work of Steiner (1993), particularly, clearly refers to the analysis of narcissistic patients, whom he designates as presenting a "pathological organization," and Hinshelwood (1994) points to the use of this term, within Kleinian literature, for "inaccessible personalities." One problem, however, is that the overall description of such patients in that literature usually lacks sufficiently detailed information about their general symptomatology and personality characteristics, so that it is difficult to compare them with the patients referred to in our work at Cornell. In addition, the subtle and convincing descriptions in the Kleinian literature of particular interpretations of the transference of these patients convey a sense of effectiveness of these interventions that leaves open, however, the overall questions of the long-range effectiveness of the treatment and of indications and contraindications.

ALTERNATIVE VIEWS

All three contemporary psychoanalytic approaches to the treatment of narcissistic personalities (Kohut's self psychology, Rosenfeld's Kleinian approach, and Kernberg's ego psychology object relations views) agree that psychoanalysis is the treatment of choice for these patients. It needs to be pointed out, however, that Kohut has limited himself to discussing the treatment of analyzable patients with this disorder, whereas Rosenfeld and Kernberg have broadened the spectrum of their investigations to include narcissistic personalities with overtly borderline features. Rosenfeld still maintains that this latter group should also be treated by psychoanalysis, but O.F. Kernberg (1984) proposes that narcissistic patients with overtly borderline functioning usually have serious contraindications for psychoanalysis proper and should be treated by exploratory or expressive psychotherapy. If psychoanalytic psychotherapy is contraindicated, Kernberg proposes supportive psychotherapy as the treatment of choice.

Rosenfeld's psychoanalytic technique pretty much coincides with the general technical approach of the Kleinian school of psychoanalysis. It is modified for narcissistic personality disorders only insofar as the specific primitive defenses and object relations of these patients should be explored systematically in the transference. Rosenfeld stresses the importance of interpreting both positive and negative transferences and only modifies his techniques with narcissistic patients functioning at the overtly borderline level by exploring very carefully the reality situation that triggers paranoid psychotic transference regressions, in order to contain and reduce such regressions (Rosenfeld 1978).

Kohut (1971) stresses the need to permit the development of the patient's narcissistic idealization of the analyst, avoiding premature interpretation or reality considerations. This approach permits the gradual unfolding of mirror transferences. The patient relives the earlier traumatic experiences with a more mature psyche and acquires new psychic structures, with the help of the analyst as self-object, by the process of transmuting internalization. The psychoanalyst must be basically empathic, focusing on understanding the patient's narcissistic needs and frustrations rather than on the drive derivatives and conflicts that emerge at times of narcissistic frustration in the analytic situation. In each of these conditions of narcissistic frustration, the psychoanalyst explores with the patient where and how the analyst has failed in being appropriately empathic and how this relates to past failures of the significant object of the patient's childhood. Kohut insists that this does not require establishing parameters of technique, that it represents a modification of the standard psychoanalytic technique for non-narcissistic patients only in that it stresses the analyst's empathy in contrast to "objective neutrality" and focuses on the vicissitudes of the self rather than on drives and (not yet existent) interstructural conflicts.

In this author's view, the most important aspect of the psychoanalytic treatment of narcissistic personalities is the systematic analysis of the pathological grandiose self as presented in the transference. The activation of the grandiose self can be detected in the psychoanalytic situation by the patient's emotional unavailability, a subtle but persistent absence of the normal or "real" aspects of the relationship between the patient and analyst in which the patient treats the analyst as a specific individual. In contrast, the activation of the patient's pathological self-idealization, alternating with the projection of such self-idealization onto the analyst, conveys the impression that there is only one (ideal, grandiose) person and an admiring yet shadowy complement to it in the room. Frequent role reversals between patient and analyst illustrate this basically stable transference pattern. In this author's view, the analyst has to interpret this transference pattern and the primitive defense mechanisms recruited in its service. This includes the interpretation of the expression of omnipotent control in the transference, of the defensive use of rage reactions, of sudden devaluation of the analyst and his comments, and of negative therapeutic reactions following times when the patient experiences the analyst as helpful. Generally speaking, the primitive defensive operations of omnipotent control, projective identification, primitive idealization, and devaluation are prevalent in the transference of narcissistic patients throughout their treatment and require systematic working through.

Behind the apparently simple activation of narcissistic rage lies the activation of specific primitive unconscious internalized object relations of the past, typically of split-off self and object representations reflecting condensed oedipal-preoedipal conflicts. These conflicts may gradually emerge as the pathological grandiose self is analytically resolved, with a breakthrough of primitive transferences expressing paranoid distrust, direct aggression in the transference, and, eventually, differentiated enactments of internalized object relations in a repetitive alternation or interchange with the analyst of representations of the patient's real and ideal self, ideal objects, and real objects. In the final stage of resolution of the grandiose self, the treatment situation usually resembles that of the psychoanalysis of neurotic patients in that the patient can now establish a real dependence on the analyst, can explore both his oedipal and preoedipal conflicts in a differentiated fashion, and can simultaneously normalize his pathological object relations and his narcissistic regulatory mechanisms.

The detailed aspects of psychoanalytic technique within any of these competing formulations are beyond the limitations of the present summary. So far, there are no controlled empirical studies available comparing these competing treatment approaches. The discussions regarding their respective merits and problems are based exclusively upon the clinical experience of psychoanalysts specializing in this area.

Prognostic Considerations and Complications

Usually, negative prognostic features become evident during the initial evaluation of patients, but we are all familiar with cases in which, despite careful history taking and assessment, important data emerge only after treatment has begun, altering our initial diagnostic and prognostic impressions. There are, however, typical manifestations of what may eventually prove almost insurmountable obstacles to the treatment that may be identified in the initial evaluation. The following cases reflect such frequent danger signals.

CHRONIC WORK FAILURE IN CONTRAST TO HIGH EDUCATIONAL BACKGROUND AND CAPACITY

Some patients have worked for many years below their level of training or capacity and often drift into a "disabled" status so that they must be cared for by their families (if they are wealthy) or the public social support system. Such a chronic dependency on the family or on a social support system represents a major secondary gain of illness, one of the principal causes of treatment failure. In the United States, at least, these patients are high consumers of therapeutic and social services; however, were they to get well, they would no longer qualify for the supports that maintain their existence. These patients come to treatment, consciously or unconsciously, not because they are interested in improvement but to demonstrate to the social system their incapacity to improve and, therefore, their need for ongoing social support. Because they are usually required to be in some kind of treatment in order to get, for example, supportive housing, Supplemental Security Insurance, or Social Security Disability, they go from program to program and therapist to therapist. Michael Stone, a senior member of our Personality Disorders Institute at Cornell, has concluded that, for practical purposes, if a patient is potentially able to earn by working at least 1.5 times the amount of money he is receiving from social support systems, there may be a chance that eventually he will be motivated to work again. Otherwise, the secondary gain of illness may carry the day (Stone 1990).

This condition of work failure may merge with grandiose fantasies of capacities and success that remain unchallenged as long as the patient does not become part of the workforce; the rationalization of this pattern of social parasitism may include a fantasized profession or talent the patient has and that nobody has recognized as yet: the unknown painter, the inhibited author, the revolutionary musician.... Often such a patient is perfectly willing to enter treatment as long as somebody else pays for the treatment, and will abandon it the day when this payment is no longer available, even if there existed the possibility of continuing the treatment if the patient were willing and able to take on some remunerated employment.

The therapeutic approach in such cases needs to include the reduction or elimination of the secondary gain of illness. Clinically, I would point out to the patient that an active involvement in work and its related interactional experiences and/or acceptance of conceptual responsibility for financing the treatment are essential for the treatment to help the patient, and that such an engagement is a precondition for the possibility of carrying out a psychoanalytic psychotherapy. Depending on the situation, I might give the patient a period of time, say 3–6 months, to achieve this goal, with a clear understanding that should it not be possible to achieve it, treatment would be interrupted at that point. This condition constitutes a limit setting that will become part of the treatment frame and, therefore, require interpretation as part of its transference implications from the beginning of the treatment. Practically speaking, these interpretations may focus on the unconscious motivation for the refusal of work, the importance of the gratification of secondary gain, the resentment the patient may experience toward the therapist's threat to the patient's equilibrium, and the self-defeating aspects of the patient implied in his denying himself the possibility of well-being, success, self-respect, and enrichment of life linked to a potentially successful and creative engagement in a work or a profession.

PERVASIVE ARROGANCE

The symptom of pervasive arrogance may dominate in patients who, while recognizing that they have significant difficulties or symptoms, obtain unconscious secondary gain of illness by demonstrating the incompetence and incapacity of the mental health professions to alleviate such symptoms. They become super-experts in the field of their suffering, diligently research the Internet, check out therapists for their background and orientation, compare their merits and shortcomings, present themselves for treatment "to give the therapist a chance," but consistently obtain an unconscious degree of satisfaction in defeating the helping profession. They may have symptoms such as chronic marital conflicts, bouts of intense depression when threatened with failures at work or in their profession, anxiety and somatizations, and even significant chronic depression. Such severe, chronic depressions respond only "partially" to whatever psychopharmacological treatment they receive (and even to the electroconvulsive treatment that sometimes is questionably recommended for patients with chronic and severe characterological depression). Not infrequently, the combination of a psychotherapeutic treatment with psychopharmacological treatment temporarily leads to a surprising improvement, which, in these patients' view, is due to "the medication alone"; the psychotherapeutic treatment is "not helpful" and becomes "unnecessary" (although later, the medication, too, "does not work anymore").

The sudden shift from frail idealization to complete devaluation of the therapist mentioned before may occur at any point, and, sometimes, a treatment of many months' duration that seemed to be progressing satisfactorily is unexpectedly disrupted because of an intense onslaught of envy of the therapist that triggers a radical devaluation of him. The initial evaluation of these patients usually reveals an ego-syntonic arrogance that, in some cases, may evolve into grossly inappropriate behavior and rudeness or, in others, be thinly masked by a surface facade of appropriate tactfulness. This characterological arrogance has to be differentiated from the syndrome of arrogance referred to earlier, described by Bion (1967), that coincides with intense affect storms in the transference and that, in the context of a psychoanalytic psychotherapy in which the patient's relationship with the therapist is firmly established, has a better prognosis.

The technical approach to these patients must include a very tactful confrontation and systematic analysis of the defensive functions of arrogance in the transference, pointing out to the patient in the process, from the very start, that, given that patient's emotional disposition, there is a risk that the treatment will end prematurely because of the devaluation of the therapist. Typically, the patient fears, by projective identification, that the therapist has a similar depreciatory disposition toward him, and therefore, if the patient's superiority is challenged or destroyed, he will be subject to a humiliating devaluation by the therapist. Whenever possible, it is very helpful, from early on, to interpret the unconscious identification of the patient with a grandiose parental object that often is at the bottom of this characterological disposition (and an important component of the pathological grandiose self). The identification with such a grandiose and sadistic object, on the surface, seems to bolster the patient's self-esteem by protecting the patient's sense of superiority and grandiosity; at the bottom, in this identification, the patient is submitting to an internalized object that stands against any real involvement in a relationship with somebody else that might be helpful, and is profoundly hostile to the dependent and true relational needs of the patient.

DESTRUCTIVENESS OF THE THERAPEUTIC PROCESS AND EXPRESSION OF A DOMINANT UNCONSCIOUS SELF-DESTRUCTIVENESS AS A MAJOR MOTIVATIONAL SYSTEM

Cases in which destructiveness of the therapeutic process and a dominant unconscious self-destructiveness represent a major motivational system include what, usually from the very beginning of their evaluation, impresses the experienced clinician as extremely grave conditions. These are patients with severe, repetitive suicidal attempts of an almost lethal nature, suicidal attempts that happened "out of the clear sky," though often carefully prepared over a period of time, and even glee-fully engineered under the eyes of concerned therapists. Chronic self-destructiveness may also manifest itself, in addition to such suicidal at-tempts, by self-destructive behavior in what potentially might become gratifying love relations, a promising work situation, the opportunity for professional advancement—in short, success in crucial areas of any aspects of life. Sometimes these individuals are seen in relatively early years of adolescence or young adulthood, when many opportunities lie still ahead of them in life. In other cases, these individuals come to the therapist's attention much later, after many failed treatments and a gradual deterioration of the patient's life situation, in an apparent search for treatment as a "last resort"; this may induce a sense of hope-fulness, or an illusion, in the therapist, who believes the patient's life may still change. At times, the patient may very openly state that he or she is committed to death by suicide, defiantly challenging the therapist to see whether he can do anything about it. Sometimes this defiant chal-lenge comes to a head early, at the time of setting up of the treatment contract, with the patient refusing to commit himself to such contractual arrangements. Usually the family background of these patients evinces severe and chronic traumatizations, including severe sexual or physical abuse, an unusual degree of family chaos, or a practically symbiotic re-lationship with an extremely aggressive parental figure.

If antisocial features complicate the picture, the patient may be de-ceptive about suicidal tendencies, and the chronic lack of honesty and a psychopathic type of transference may preclude any possibility to build up a helpful human relationship with a therapist. For example, one of our patients would ingest rat poison for suicidal and parasuicidal pur-poses. She was able to smuggle rat poison into the hospital, and she developed internal hemorrhages. While she steadfastly denied the on-going consumption of rat poison to the therapist, her blood tests showed a continuous increase in the prothrombin time. Eventually, this psychotherapeutic treatment had to be interrupted because of her obvi-ous unwillingness or incapacity to adhere to the treatment contract that committed her to stop ingesting rat poison as a precondition for ongo-ing psychotherapy. André Green (1993) has described, in connection with the syndrome of the "dead mother," the unconscious identification with a psychologically dead parental object. The unconsciously fanta-sized union with this object justifies and rationalizes the patient's com-plete dismantling of all relationships with psychologically important objects. In fact, the onset of this patient's ingestion of rat poison was co-incident with a visit to her mother's gravesite.

Unconsciously, the patient may deny the existence of both others and the self as meaningful entities, and this radical dismantling of all object relations may constitute, at times, an insurmountable obstacle to treatment. In other cases, the self-destructiveness is more limited, being expressed not in suicidal behavior proper, but in severe self-mutilation that repetitively punctures the psychotherapeutic treatment and signals the unconscious triumph of the forces in the patient that promote self-destructiveness as a major life goal. Such self-mutilation may lead to the loss of limbs or severely crippling fractures but stop short of the risk of immediate death.

This disposition may emerge in a patient's relentless effort to pro-voke the therapist into an aggressive disposition or action against the patient, to transform the relationship into a sadomasochistic one. At the same time, this reaction usually is accompanied by desperate efforts to transform the assumedly "bad" therapist into a "good" one—to trans-form the persecutory object into an ideal one—an effort that fails be-cause of the relentless need to reenact this sadomasochistic transference by repetition compulsion. In contrast to patients whose main motiva-tion is a total dismantling of the object relationship, here there is an im-plicit recognition that the therapist has attempted to be helpful: in fact, this experience is what triggers this particular negative therapeutic re-action. If the therapist is not provoked to an extent that may, indeed, lead to a disruption of the treatment, the consistent interpretation of this fantasy and unconscious provocativeness may resolve the impasse. One might also say that, as part of the effort to deal interpretively with this whole area of severe dominance of self-destructiveness, efforts to disen-tangle this kind of relationship from the more extreme ones mentioned before are part of the therapeutic task.

The technical approach to this entire group of patients implies, first, taking very seriously the danger that the patient could end up destroy-ing himself physically. The patient's self-destructiveness is an ongoing threat to the treatment, making this danger a selected theme of the in-terpretive work from the very beginning of treatment. The therapeutic contract that is negotiated with the patient is intended to establish the minimal preconditions that will ensure that the treatment will not be used as a "cover story" for providing the patient with further freedom or incentives for self-destructive action. This may not be an easy task, as the therapist has to make it very clear that the treatment will not proceed if these minimal conditions for ensuring the patient's survival are not met. Such conditions may include, for example, the patient's commitment to immediate hospitalization if suicidal impulses are so strong that the patient believes he will not be able to control them; or the absolute commitment to stop behaviors that threaten the continuation of treatment and/or the patient's survival.

PREDOMINANCE OF ANTISOCIAL FEATURES

Here we are dealing with the aggressive infiltration of the pathological grandiose self, both in cases where this is expressed mostly in a passive/ parasitic tendency, and in cases where it takes an aggressive/paranoid form (in the syndrome of malignant narcissism). All cases of narcissistic personality disorder with significant antisocial features have a relatively reserved prognosis. Patients with the syndrome of malignant narcissism are at the very limit of what we can reach with psychoanalytic approaches within the field of pathological narcissism. The next degree of severity of antisocial pathology, the antisocial personality proper, has practically zero prognosis for any psychotherapeutic treatment.

Paradoxically, the very severity of the aggressive-paranoid behavior of patients with the syndrome of malignant narcissism, its function to confirm the power and grandiosity of the patient, facilitates the interpretation of this behavior in the transference. Suicidal behavior (i.e., self-directed aggression), for example, clearly represents a triumphant aggression toward the family or the therapist, or a triumphant "dismissal" of a world that does not conform to the patient's expectations; parasuicidal, self-mutilating behavior may indicate the patient's triumph over all those others who are afraid of pain, lesions, or bodily destruction.

These are also patients who, in the treatment situation, may show the syndrome of arrogance in a restricted sense, and the interpretation of this may effectively resolve it. This interpretive work includes pointing out to the patient his intolerance of his own intense, envious aggression, which is expressed in behavior or somatization as a way to avoid acquiring full consciousness of it. The pseudo-stupidity seen in this syndrome, through the defensive dismantling of ordinary reasoning and cognitive communication, defends against the humiliating possibility of the therapist's interpretive work reaching the patient in meaningful ways. The inordinate curiosity about the therapist's life that is also a feature of this syndrome is a way to control the therapist and also to control any new sources of envious resentment.

The consistent interpretation of the syndrome of arrogance may, in fact, be a key feature in the transformation of the transference from a psychopathic one into a paranoid one—a transformation that marks the beginning of the patient's capacity for self-exploration of his primitive aggression rather than having to act it out. Helping the patient to become aware of the intensely pleasurable nature of his sadistic behavior against the therapist and others is an important aspect of this interpretive work. This requires that the therapist feel comfortable in an emotional empathy with such sadistic pleasure: the therapist's fear of his own sadism may interfere with his fully exploring this issue with the patient.

Therapeutic Management of Complications

We may summarize briefly the major negative prognostic features that emerge in this overall category of "almost untreatable" narcissistic patients as including the following: secondary gain of illness, including social parasitism; severe antisocial behavior; severity of primitive self-directed aggression; drug and alcohol abuse as chronic treatment problems; pervasive arrogance; general intolerance of a dependent object relation, and the most severe type of negative therapeutic reaction. The evaluation of these prognostic features is facilitated by a careful and detailed initial evaluation of the patient.

For example, regarding the nature of antisocial behavior, it is important to elucidate the extent to which it corresponds to simple, isolated antisocial behavior in a narcissistic personality disorder without other major negative prognostic implications; or the extent to which it corresponds to severe, chronic, passive parasitic behavior that augments the secondary gain of illness; or whether what is present is a syndrome of malignant narcissism; or, finally and most importantly, whether we are facing an antisocial personality proper, either of the passive parasitic type or of the aggressive type.

At times, antisocial behavior may be strictly limited to intimate relationships, where it expresses aggression and revengefulness, particularly when accompanied by significant paranoid features. This may be important when, in the transference, antisocial behavior is directed at the therapist, because at times the behavior may create such a high risk for the therapist that treatment under such circumstances might not be wise to attempt. In some patients, aggressive, revengeful acting out takes the form of litigious behavior against therapists, with the patient initiating a lawsuit against a first therapist while idealizing a second one who is "recruited" into a treatment for the damage done by the first one, only to be involved in turn with a lawsuit initiated by the patient as he transfers to a third therapist for help, and so on. It may be wise not to accept a patient of this kind for intensive psychotherapeutic treatment

while legal procedures related to the involvement with another therapeutic situation are still going on. Some patients with a hypochondria-
cal syndrome who are prone to accuse previous therapists of not having
recognized the severity of some somatic symptom or illness may be related to this group.

In the case of patients with chronic suicidal attempts, it is extremely
important to differentiate suicidal behavior that corresponds to the authentic severity of a depression from suicidal behavior "as a way of life,"
not linked to depression, and typical for borderline personality disorder
as well as for narcissistic personality disorder (O. F. Kernberg 2001).
Here, the differential nature of the suicidal attempts referred to before
may be extremely helpful in diagnosing the patient's case.

The elimination or reduction of secondary gain of illness is one of the
most important and often difficult aspects of the treatment, particularly
in setting up the initial treatment contract and a viable treatment frame.
The parameters of the treatment contract provide the assurance that the
agreed-upon treatment frame will protect both parties (and the therapist's belongings and life situation) from the patient's acting out that
may evolve in the course of the treatment. In the course of the psychoanalytic psychotherapy of all patients with borderline personality organization—and this includes the patients explored in this chapter—the
emergence of severe regression in the transference is practically un-
avoidable and frequently takes the form of efforts to challenge and
break the therapeutic frame. In any such challenge, the therapist's physical, psychological, professional, and legal safety takes precedence over
the safety of the patient. That means that, while the therapist has to ensure the safety of the patient by means of the setting up of the contract
and a treatment frame that protects both of them, the therapist's own
safety is an indispensable precondition for his being able to help the patient, even for setting up conditions that assure the patient's safety. This
point would seem obvious or trivial, if it were not that so often therapists are seduced into a treatment situation in which their safety is at
risk. Concrete conditions, relevant to each individual case, which
clearly would indicate discontinuation of the treatment if not fulfilled,
must be spelled out and, if necessary, reiterated as part of the treatment
arrangements, and then, as mentioned before, immediately interpreted
regarding their transference implications.

Summarizing the indications for differential treatment approaches
mentioned so far: For the mildest cases of narcissistic psychopathology,
a focused psychoanalytic psychotherapeutic approach or even a focal
supportive psychotherapy may be the treatment of choice, and standard
psychoanalysis is chosen only if the severity of the corresponding char-

acter pathology warrants it. Standard psychoanalysis would be the treatment approach for the second, or intermediate, level of severity described earlier, and possibly, in some cases, for the severe spectrum of narcissistic functioning on an overt borderline level, when, for individual reasons, such a treatment is possible. For most cases of narcissistic pathology functioning on an overt borderline level or with severe antisocial pathology, the specialized psychoanalytic psychotherapy that we have developed at the Weill Cornell Medical College—namely, transference-focused psychotherapy—is recommended as the treatment of choice (Levy et al. 2005). When individualized preconditions for treatment cannot be met in the initial contract setting (Clarkin et al. 1989), a cognitive-behavioral or a supportive psychotherapeutic approach may be the treatment of choice.

In general, a supportive psychotherapeutic modality based on psychoanalytic principles is indicated for cases in which the patient's need for "self-curing" is so intense that any dependency is precluded, and obtaining active counseling and advice in a supportive relationship may be much more acceptable to the patient (Rockland 1992). When severe secondary gain cannot be overcome, and the patient's prognosis, therefore, would be severely limited with an analytic approach, a supportive psychotherapy focused on the amelioration of predominant symptoms and behavioral manifestations may be helpful. In cases with severe antisocial features that require ongoing information from outside sources and social control, technical neutrality may be too affected to carry out an analytic approach, and a supportive one would appear preferable. For patients who, as a consequence of their long-standing illness, already have suffered severe regression into social incompetence, all their "bridges burned" behind them, making a realistic adaptation to life much more difficult, a supportive psychotherapeutic approach may be preferable to a psychoanalytic modality of treatment. In the latter approach, the patient would have to come to terms with the extremely painful recognition of having destroyed much of their lives: here the subtle and empathic judgment of the therapist regarding what the patient may be able to tolerate becomes very important.

It needs to be kept in mind that before psychoanalytic knowledge advanced in the understanding of the psychopathology of pathological narcissism and helped us to develop specific techniques to deal with these patients analytically, the prognosis was much more limited for a much larger number of cases than is true today. New developments in the psychoanalytic psychotherapy for those cases of narcissistic personality disorder where standard psychoanalysis would seem contraindicated have significantly improved our therapeutic armamentarium.

Continuous efforts to explore the cases at the limits of our present psychoanalytic understanding and capacity to help should expand this field further in the future. Given the high prevalence of this kind of pathology and its severe social repercussions in many cases, this is an important task for the psychoanalytic researcher and clinician at this time.

Recent Developments and Empirical Research

Psychoanalytic psychotherapy and psychoanalysis have originated new knowledge regarding the psychopathology of narcissistic patients that is increasing our understanding of their dynamics, as well as broadening the spectrum of those reachable by psychotherapeutic methods. An important contribution to our understanding of narcissism has been the observation of the paradoxical presence of masochistic characteristics embedded in the narcissistic structure, as frequently observed in the clinical material of these patients (Cooper 1989). In such cases, as described by Cooper (1989), we see a tendency toward victimization, an unconscious search for or provocation of circumstances of humiliation and failure, a tendency to relate preferentially to frustrating or damaging objects, and a systematic undermining or rejection of potential help, all of which reflect the patient's unconscious fantasy that he is the "greatest sufferer," the "greatest victim." All the while, the patient persists in self-defeating behavior while simultaneously expressing the entitlement and rights to "specialness" derived from this victim status. In other cases, narcissistic personality disorder covers deeper underlying masochistic dynamics that may be uncovered in the course of psychoanalytic treatment, revealing primitive, severely masochistic internalized object relations.

An additional development in our understanding of the psychopathology of narcissistic personality disorder has been the increasing attention paid to the two main negative prognostic indicators—namely, antisocial features and secondary gain of illness. In fact, the extent to which antisocial features not only dominate the clinical condition but are accompanied by ego-syntonic aggression against self or others, together with paranoid trends—that is, the syndrome of malignant narcissism—has gained more attention because of the prognostic severity of the syndrome and yet the possibility of a positive response to psychotherapeutic methods. Also, this syndrome, as well as the most severe spectrum of narcissistic personality disorder in general, is frequently confused, in hospital practice, with borderline personality disorder (O.F. Kernberg and Yeomans, in press). Of utmost importance is the differentiation between the syndrome of malignant narcissism, which is amenable to treatment, and the antisocial personality disorder proper, which, from a psychopathological point of view, may be considered the most extremely severe level of pathological narcissism and, to this point, is not reachable with a psychotherapeutic approach.

Contributions from the Kleinian school have pointed to different subtypes of narcissistic personalities. Rosenfeld (1987) differentiated "thin-skinned" and "thick-skinned" narcissistic patients. The latter are characterized by marked self-assurance, grandiosity, and callousness in spite of superficially engaging behavior, while the former are extremely sensitive to any sort of criticism or threat to their self-esteem. This grouping has been confirmed by other clinicians and by empirical research. Russ et al. (2008) has described three subtypes of narcissistic patients: grandiose-malignant, fragile, and high-functioning/exhibitionistic. The last-mentioned group, while grandiose, competitive, and attention seeking, shows much better adaptive functioning and represents the highest level of narcissism mentioned earlier. John Steiner (1993) has described a series of patients with narcissistic personality disorders undergoing psychoanalytic treatment, referring to them as having "pathological organizations," and described in detail the characteristic defensive emotional distancing of these patients under the heading "psychic retreats."

Regarding the etiology of narcissistic personality disorder, psychoanalytic investigation of these patients has pointed to the consistent finding of severely traumatic experiences in early childhood, most frequently abandoning, aggressive, and/or rejecting maternal images, and chaotic combinations of frustration and overstimulation. The psychoanalytic formulations relating such developmental features to the structural characteristics of these patients vary, but most take as their starting point the theories of Herbert Rosenfeld, Kohut, and Kernberg. Regardless of theoretical adherence, there is little disagreement in the description of the clinical characteristics of the disorder, dominated by the presence of a grandiose self, although its origin and structural characteristics are understood differently.

From the point of view of self psychology, this psychic structure corresponds to an archaic, primitive, normal self that was stunted in its early development because of the empathic failure of the caregiver, leading to a specific defect in the capacity for forming mature "self-object" ties. These patients' transferences are dominated by infantile unconscious idealizing and mirroring tendencies related to primitive grandiosity and exhibitionism of the immature self-structure, resulting in a reduced capacity for empathy and object relatedness. Psychoanalytic treatment, from a self psychological viewpoint, relates to the capacity of the analyst to immerse himself empathically in a patient's inner world, with gratification of the patient's early narcissistic needs, and the patient's consequent capacity to construct the missing self-structures that would permit resumption of normal growth.

In contrast, Rosenfeld (1987) and Kernberg (1975) view pathological narcissism as not simply a fixation at a primitive normal narcissism, but rather a defensive construction of a pathological grandiose self derived from the integration of one-sided, positive aspects of self and object representations and ego ideal, constituting a secondary defense against an underlying dominance of primitive splitting mechanisms and of intense negative internalized object relations related to the aggressive consequences of early childhood deprivation. Here, psychoanalytic treatment focuses on the activation and gradual resolution of the pathological grandiose self in the transference, with consequent development of a normal capacity for dependency, maturation of the normal self-concept, and the capacity for establishment of normal object relations.

More recently, our expanding knowledge regarding the structural consequences of insecure attachment (Fonagy et al. 2003) has pointed to the relationship between the avoidant type of insecure attachment and the development of narcissistic personality features. Insofar as normal, as well as insecure, attachment reflects the behavioral manifestations of normal or disturbed internalization of object relations ("internal working models" within attachment theory), these behavioral manifestations may constitute important developmental markers of early internalized object relations derivative structures. They also may pinpoint the predominance of pathological internalized object relations under the predominance of noncontextualized, intense negative affect states. Undoubtedly, later developments in the dynamics of intrapsychic structural developments, under the influence of family dynamics, also play an important role in the consolidation of narcissistic personality disorder. Paulina Kernberg (1989) first described narcissistic personality disorder in childhood and pointed to the general importance of exploring the development of personality disorders, at least the most severe ones, in childhood, while expanding our knowledge regarding narcissistic personality disorders in adolescence.

To this point, there has been no systematic empirical research reported on the effects of psychoanalysis and psychoanalytic psychotherapy with patients presenting with narcissistic personality disorder (Levy et al. 2009). Such outcome studies as have been reported do not seem to have been carried out with specific technical psychoanalytic approaches geared to the analysis of narcissistic transferences; at least, there has been no specific reference to such specialized therapeutic approaches, in contrast to the application of more general psychodynamic and cognitive-behavioral approaches. Clinical cases with significant resolution of narcissistic psychopathology following psychoanalytic treatment and psychoanalytic psychotherapy have been reported (O. F. Kernberg 2004), but this field still requires a systematic exploration of the effects of treatments specifically structured to deal with the particular challenges of narcissistic personality disorder.

Key Clinical Concepts

- ◆ Narcissism defined at the clinical level as normal or pathological regulation of self-esteem may be classified as normal adult narcissism, normal infantile narcissism, or pathological narcissism. The narcissistic personality disorder represents the most severe type of pathological narcissism.

- ◆ Narcissistic personality disorder centers around the presence of a pathological grandiose self. Its main features are excessive self-centeredness, overdependency on admiration, grandiose fantasies, and bouts of insecurity.

- ◆ Patients with narcissistic personality disorder present pathological relations with others: excessive envy, exploitativeness, entitlement, devaluation, and lack of empathy.

- ◆ Narcissistic patients may present significant superego pathology reflected in antisocial behavior, and a differential diagnosis from the antisocial personality disorder proper is required. This differential diagnosis carries essential prognostic implications because of the poor prognosis of antisocial personality disorder.

- ◆ Psychoanalysis may be the treatment of choice for the better-functioning patients, and modified psychoanalytic psychotherapy, particularly transference-focused psychotherapy, may be best for patients with severe cases.

- ◆ In psychodynamically oriented treatments, the analytic exploration of the manifestations of the pathological grandiose self is essential. The transferences of these patients are characterized by incapacity to depend on the therapist, frail idealization and devaluations, and acting out of envy and primitive forms of aggression.

- ◆ The prognosis depends strongly on the secondary gain from symptoms, the patient's degree of arrogance, self-destructiveness as a major motivation, and the presence of antisocial tendencies.

◆ For patients with contraindications for a psychodynamic approach, and for those with overwhelming negative prognostic indicators, a supportive or cognitive-behavioral approach may be indicated.

Suggested Readings

Kernberg O (ed): Narcissistic Personality Disorder. Psychiatr Clin North Am 12:505–776, 1989

Kernberg O: Aggressivity, Narcissism, and Self-Destructiveness in the Psychotherapeutic Relationship: New Developments in the Psychopathology and Psychotherapy of Severe Personality Disorders. New Haven, CT, Yale University Press, 2004

Kernberg O (ed): Narcissistic personality disorder. Psychiatr Ann 39 (part 1): 1–171, 2009

Kernberg O (ed): Narcissistic personality disorder. Psychiatr Ann 39 (part 2): 172–235, 2009

Kohut H: The Analysis of the Self. New York, International Universities Press, 1971

Kohut H: The Restoration of the Self. New York, International Universities Press, 1977

Rosenfeld H: Impasse and Interpretation. London, Tavistock, 1987

References

American Psychiatric Association: Diagnostic and Statistical Manual of Mental Disorders, 4th Edition. Washington, DC, American Psychiatric Association, 1994

Bion WR: Second Thoughts: Selected Papers on Psychoanalysis. New York, Basic Books, 1967

Clarkin J, Yeomans F, Kernberg OF: Psychotherapy for Borderline Personality. New York, Wiley, 1989

Cooper AM: Narcissism and masochism: the narcissistic masochistic character. Psychiatr Clin North Am 12:541–552, 1989

Fonagy P, Gergeley G, Jurist EL, et al: Affect Regulation, Mentalization, and the Development of the Self. New York, Other Press, 2003

Freud S: On narcissism: an introduction (1914), in The Standard Edition of the Complete Psychological Works of Sigmund Freud, Vol 14. Translated and edited by Strachey J. London, Hogarth Press, 1957, pp 67–102

Green A: On Private Madness. Madison, CT, International Universities Press, 1993

Hare RD: Psychopathy: Theory and Research. New York, Wiley, 1970

Hare RD, Shalling D: Psychopathic Behavior: Approaches to Research. New York, Wiley, 1978

Henderson DK: Psychopathic States. London, Chapman & Hall, 1939

Henderson DK, Gillespie R: Textbook of Psychiatry: For Students and Practitioners, 10th Edition. Revised by Batchelor IRC. London, Oxford University Press, 1969

Hinshelwood RD: Clinical Klein. London, Free Association Books, 1994

Kernberg OF: Borderline Conditions and Pathological Narcissism. New York, Jason Aronson, 1975, pp 230–238

Kernberg OF: Technical aspects in the psychoanalytic treatment of narcissistic personalities, in Severe Personality Disorders: Psychotherapeutic Strategies. New Haven, CT, Yale University Press, 1984, pp 197–209

Kernberg O (ed): Narcissistic Personality Disorder. Psychiatr Clin North Am 12:505–776, 1989

Kernberg OF: Psychopathic, paranoid, and depressive transferences. Int J Psychoanal 73:13–28, 1992

Kernberg OF: Pathological narcissism and narcissistic personality disorders: theoretical background and diagnostic classification, in Disorders of Narcissism: Diagnostic, Clinical, and Empirical Implications. Edited by Ronningstam EF. Washington, DC, American Psychiatric Press, 1997, pp 29–51

Kernberg OF: The suicidal risk in severe personality disorders: differential diagnosis and treatment. J Pers Disord 15:195–208, 2001

Kernberg OF: Aggressivity, Narcissism, and Self-Destructiveness in the Psychotherapeutic Relationship. New Haven, CT, Yale University Press, 2004

Kernberg OF, Yeomans FE: [The differential diagnosis of borderline personality disorder], in Handbuch der Borderline Störungen, 2nd Edition. Edited by Dulz B, Herpertz S, Kernberg OF, et al. Stuttgart, Germany, Schattauer (in press)

Kernberg PF: Narcissistic personality disorder in childhood. Psychiatr Clin North Am 12:671–694, 1989

Koenigsberg HW, Kernberg OF, Stone MH, et al: Borderline Patients: Extending the Limits of Treatability. New York, Basic Books, 2000

Kohut H: The Analysis of the Self. New York, International Universities Press, 1971

Levy KN, Meehan KB, Weber M, et al: Attachment patterns in borderline personality disorder: implications for psychotherapy. Psychopathology 38:64–74, 2005

Levy KN, Chauhan P, Clarkin JF, et al: Narcissistic pathology: empirical approaches. Psychiatr Ann 39:203–213, 2009

Rockland LH: Supportive Therapy for Borderline Patients: A Psychodynamic Approach. New York, Guilford, 1992

Rosenfeld H: Notes on the psychopathology and psychoanalytic treatment of some borderline patients. Int J Psychoanal 59:215–221, 1978

Rosenfeld H: Impasse and Interpretation: Therapeutic and Anti-therapeutic Factors in the Psychoanalytic Treatment of Psychotic, Borderline and Neurotic Patients. London, Tavistock, 1987

Russ E, Shedler J, Bradley R, et al: Redefining the construct of narcissistic personality disorder: diagnostic criteria and subtypes. Am J Psychiatry 165:1473–1481, 2008

Spillius EB (ed): Melanie Klein Today: Developments in Theory and Practice, Vols 1 and 2. London, Routledge, 1988

Spillius EB, Feldman M (eds): Psychic Equilibrium and Psychic Change: Selected Papers of Betty Joseph. London, Tavistock/Routledge, 1989

Steiner J: Psychic Retreats. London, Routledge, 1993

Stone MH: The Fate of Borderline Patients. New York, Guilford, 1990

CHAPTER 10

Treatment of Histrionic Personality Disorder

Mardi J. Horowitz, M.D.
Uma Lerner, M.D.

The word *histrionic,* from the Latin word for actor, refers to a style of dramatic self-presentation. When this style is excessive, symptomatic, and maladaptive, it contributes to a diagnosis of histrionic personality disorder (Horowitz 1977). Emotional displays to obtain attention from others are so demanding that they are socially inappropriate. The pattern is maladaptive because it is repeated despite the fact that sometimes it has disastrous personal consequences. The DSM-IV-TR (American Psychiatric Association 2000) diagnostic criteria for histrionic personality disorder are shown in Table 10–1.

Following similar criteria in the earlier DSM-III (American Psychiatric Association 1980) nosology, Samuels et al. (1994) found that 2.1% of an epidemiologically selected sample of 762 Baltimore, Maryland, residents assessed in 1988 warranted this diagnosis. An additional 1.5% of subjects were assessed with a provisional diagnosis of histrionic personality disorder, making a total of 3.6% of these categorizations of mental disorder in an urban population. On the other hand, Blagov and Westen (2008) found significant overlap among histrionic, borderline, dependent, and antisocial personality disorders and diversity within the histrionic diag-

---

TABLE **10–1.**   DSM-IV-TR diagnostic criteria for histrionic personality disorder

---

A pervasive pattern of excessive emotionality and attention seeking, beginning by early adulthood and present in a variety of contexts, as indicated by five (or more) of the following:

(1) is uncomfortable in situations in which he or she is not the center of attention

(2) interaction with others is often characterized by inappropriate sexually seductive or provocative behavior

(3) displays rapidly shifting and shallow expression of emotions

(4) consistently uses physical appearance to draw attention to self

(5) has a style of speech that is excessively impressionistic and lacking in detail

(6) shows self-dramatization, theatricality, and exaggerated expression of emotion

(7) is suggestible, i.e., easily influenced by others or circumstances

(8) considers relationships to be more intimate than they actually are

---

Source.   Reprinted from the *Diagnostic and Statistical Manual of Mental Disorders,* 4th Edition, Text Revision. Washington, DC, American Psychiatric Association, 2000. Copyright 2000, American Psychiatric Association. Used with permission.

nosis that could warrant subtyping. Although personality disorders are typically thought of as being persistent and enduring, histrionic and other Cluster B personality disorders have been shown to become significantly less pronounced over time (Seivewright et al. 2002).

Formulation is crucial to treatment design (Wallerstein 1986). We begin with discussion of a sample approach to systematic case formulation and then discuss prototypical phases of treatment. The first phase emphasizes therapist interventions to increase state stability and reduce current crises. The second phase of treatment emphasizes work to increase connection with others and deal with obstacles to personality growth. The third phase focuses on increasing self-coherence and improving intimacy with integrity. This is a didactic approach, and actual treatments combine all phases.

Formulation

The terms *state, defensive control processes,* and *person schema* pertain to categories of a systematic approach to case formulation that is called *configurational analysis* (Horowitz 2005). By analyzing states of mind, the clinician takes a dynamic rather than a static approach to pathological phenomena, recognizing that symptoms and behavior problems vary in different states of mind. Special attention is paid to the emotionality, relationality, and apparent self-regulation in each of the patient's significant states. A feature usually important in histrionic personality disorders is the explosive entry into undermodulated states of intense negative emotionality and impulsive relationship behaviors. That is why during the first phase of treatment, focusing on state control is emphasized.

The second phase of therapy emphasizes ways to clarify verbal communication and modify defensive control processes. In histrionic personality disorders, a cloudy communicative style often results from inhibition of thoughts. The obscurity makes it hard to select topics for a focus of attention during psychotherapy sessions. Once relative safety has been achieved, the emphasis in phase two of psychotherapy is on modification of excessive defenses, especially distortions and inhibitions. The goal is to increase skills of self-reflection and self-governance as well as attitudes of responsibility for self.

In the third phase of treatment, change in irrational and conflicted belief structures becomes a therapeutic focus. Formulation of the patient's role relationship configurations is revised and deepened in this phase of therapy. This usually means deeper levels of exploration of wishes and fears.

Histrionic personality disorder patients often have segregated, dissociated, distorted, and contradictory role relationship models. A systematic approach is helpful to the clinician as self–other views are gradually clarified. Benjamin (2003) devised a system for operationalizing descriptions of these interpersonal patterns and their effect on the self-concept (structural analysis of social behavior). In addition, the Core Conflictual Relationship Theme pattern of Luborsky and Crits-Christoph (1990) is a system for such formulation. Horowitz (1991a, 1991b, 1997, 2005) amplified such precursors in developing a configurational analysis system. Different models of self and others are formulated in configurational analysis as enduring unconscious belief structures. Different role relationship models organize different, more conscious states of mind (Horowitz 2005). Patients explosively shift in state when a change occurs in the role relationship model that is dominant in organizing the unconscious mental processing that leads to conscious ideas, emotions, and actions. Triggers to activation of repetitive but inappropriate views of self and other can be gradually identified and counteracted.

The first step in the systematic procedure called configurational analysis involves stipulating a list of *problems* and strengths or resources.

The second step involves defining the patient's various *states of mind* in which these symptoms, signs, and problems may or may not occur; and the third step identifies the key *topics of concern and defensive obstacles to clarity* about these themes of concern. These first three steps deal with conscious attitudes that can be raised into self-reflective consciousness for appraisal and reappraisal. These first three layers of formulation set the stage for identifying how and why specific dysfunctional concepts about self and relationships function in unconscious conflicts involving wishes and fears. These wish-wish dilemmas are related to unconscious fantasies, which are irrational expectations about life.

PHENOMENA: SYMPTOMS AND REPETITIVE MALADAPTIVE BEHAVIORS

Patients seeking treatment for a histrionic personality disorder commonly show configurations of out-of-control impulses, emotions, perceptions, and actions. Many complain of feeling inundated by floods of intense negative affect. Feelings emerge involuntarily, and storms of emotion are hard to understand or dispel. Thoughts are jumbled but seldom grossly irrational or delusional.

Mood variation, impulsive shifts in goals, social friction, intolerance for frustration, insistence on immediate gratification, and rage on frustration are usually associated with interpersonal relationships, which are unsatisfactory and end explosively. New relationships are entered precipitously, out of a sense of desperation. The ability to wait for new attachments to develop gradually is low. The patient's values may fluctuate according to the interests of current companions rather than the self. Self-esteem decreases and relationship traumas mount—leading to mixtures of fear, bitterness, depression, and self-disgust. Alcohol or other self-prescribed drugs may be used impulsively to stop negative feelings. A variety of secondary effects from addiction and impaired mind-brain functioning can complicate the presenting picture (Horowitz 1977, 1991b, 1995; Kernberg 1975, 1992).

STATES OF MIND

Patients with a histrionic personality disorder commonly show an animated, attention-seeking state of mind in the wrong setting. For example, the person dresses too seductively for a business meeting or presents needs for sympathy when there are other pressing issues. A transition into a sullen or hurt pouting state may occur when the attention sought is not given. Although the dramatic state may have maladaptive consequences, it is, nonetheless, preferred by the patient because the excitement reduces apathy, pining, and a sense of being weak. With minor triggers, the person may go rapidly from excited gaiety to tears.

Shy, inhibited states of mind also may occur; these may help the individual avoid the danger of excessive self-display. The person wants to gain attention rather than give in to feelings of despair, but he or she fears that when the desired attention is attained, it will be too exciting and lead to a loss of self-control.

TOPICS OF CONCERN AND DEFENSIVE STYLES

The most frequent conflicted topics involve experiencing inadequate or "wrong" attention from others, with an emphasis on flip-flopping from too much (being sexually exploited, for example) to too little (and then being abandoned) attention. The relevant goals are learning how to get the right amount of attention on the basis of reciprocal intimacy, balanced self-esteem, and authenticity. Making such plans involves habitual obstacles.

Many persons with this form of personality disorder inhibit conscious information processing to blunt strong emotions that could catapult them into dreaded states of mind or self-disgust (Shapiro 1965). They deploy attention globally and diffusely. They also focus on whether another person is paying attention to them. This appraisal of others remains on the surface; the deeper intentions of the other person are not contemplated. Attention to planning the future may be excessively brief and magically wishful rather than rationally organized and long sustained.

Because of their vivacious emotionality, such persons may be quite interesting. However, the clinician, who pays closer attention, may note that they relate stories about maladaptive interpersonal actions in such a way that it is difficult to know what happened and in what sequence. Who really instigated which course of action? The patient may seek to avoid self-blame by remembering only passive roles and disavowing active gambits or provocations.

Attention may shift rapidly. One concept is not well linked to another. Images, bodily gestures, and postures are used as signals and invitations but are poorly translated into conscious words for thoughtful self-contemplation. Nonverbal modes of expression may even contain meanings that contradict concepts expressed verbally. Instead of staying with problems to consider alternative solutions, individuals with this personality style characteristically short-circuit to quick, inadequate solutions.

Saying "I don't know" may function unconsciously as if it means "I must not know." The more that defensive control processes are used (externalization, projection, and projective identification), the deeper the level of pathology in character structure.

PERSON SCHEMAS: IDENTITY CONCEPTS AND ROLE RELATIONSHIP MODELS

Theatrical self-presentations are used to attract the attention of others. The displayed aspects of self may be dissociated from authentic inner experiences or an enduring sense of identity. Sexual body parts may be exhibited even though erotic arousal is low; real symptoms of illness or handicaps may be exaggerated to get attention. A person with this pattern is at risk of being seen as manipulative or malingering.

As Lilienfeld et al. (1986) found, histrionic and antisocial personality disorders as well as histrionic personality and somatization disorder may be significantly associated in some individuals. However, the person with a histrionic personality usually is not consciously aiming to deceive and may be unaware of feigning or fabrication; fear of such accusations may even prevent the patient from getting optimum medical or psychiatric treatment in the case of real illness (Slavney and McHugh 1984).

During the theatrical state of mind, the functioning role relationship model may guide the individual to try to experience the present self as a sexy movie star, a wounded hero, or a worthy invalid. Displaying these role attributes, the self expects to gain interest from a desired other. Roles of the other are complementary ones, such as interested suitor, devoted rescuer, or responsible caregiver. The self, having gained interest, then feels restored, grateful, and loving. The person has a deep desire for such attachments but, with stress, may believe security is forthcoming when, in fact, exploitation and abandonment may be experienced.

In a dreaded role relationship model, once the self gains interest, the self is then misused and finally abandoned by the other. The self becomes angry about the misuse and despairs over the rejection. The result can become a smoldering sense of grievance and desire for revenge.

These scripts may be a state cycle from excitation to dismay, with intervals of rage and/or suicidal despair. The state cycle may begin again with the individual soliciting interest to relieve despair.

A variety of scenarios in which victim, aggressor, and rescuer roles are enacted becomes a series of repeated life stories. These vague scripts in which the person is frequently exploited and abandoned emphasize a passive self that drifts through life. The reason is that awareness of the intentions and feelings of others is shallow and is influenced by "cardboard" stereotypes rather than sagacious estimates of intentions of the other person (Standage et al. 1984).

These dramatic repetitions of victim-aggressor-rescuer state cycles may be enacted without cause-and-effect reasoning about what may be realistically expected. The person "wakes up" to threats. The self is then perceived as an innocent, passive, injured victim. However, there may also be self-critical, self-punitive, and despairing suicidal impulses.

A victim role may be used to evoke the interest of a potential rescuer. The rescue may lead to transient euphoric states, but dysphoria ensues. The once-praised rescuer may be criticized as an exploitative aggressor or an inadequate helper; the cycle repeats. With aging, the person may feel that he or she has led a wasted life because the maladaptive pattern has not led to any sustained and deepened sense of true intimacy (Pfohl et al. 1984; Pilkonis and Frank 1988).

Sadomasochistic themes are common. The person with a histrionic style may take the submissive role and make a masochistic prepayment on the often erroneous assumption that after a sadistic aggressor has caused hurt, the perpetrator will feel remorse and provide compensatory attention. Alternatively, in other patterns, there may be chronic dependency on a person who likes to feel strong in relation to a fragile, grateful companion. These patients come to therapy with transferences that can evoke countertransference reactions. On first meetings, the people with histrionic personality disorder, with their dramatic stories and eager appeals for interest, may activate a sense in the clinician that he or she can give dramatic help. A rescue fantasy, in both the patient and the clinician, may result, and a period of mutual enthusiasm follows. This is likely to be brief and to end in turmoil.

On becoming aware of therapeutic boundaries, the patient may react with anger or hostility. The clinician then may respond with hostile, rejecting impulses. The patient may feel abandoned just when most in need of help, and may then seek help elsewhere, presenting the former therapist to a new clinician as an exploitative seducer, a cold fish, or an incompetent doctor. A special-rescuer fantasy may be evoked in the new professional and the cycle repeated.

People with a narcissistic level of character and the interpersonal style of a histrionic personality disorder may use other persons as selfobjects (Kohut 1971, 1977). They seem self-centered to the point of lacking concern for the needs and sensitivities of others, which may evoke negative countertransferences. Demands for praise from mirroring selfobjects, obsequious sidling up to idealized figures, or inappropriate twinning with complementary others may characterize their patterns.

Irrational grandiosity may occur as a restitutive effort to avoid deflation of self-esteem.

The person with borderline levels of histrionic personality disorder may dissociate views of self and others into all-good and all-bad variants (Gunderson 1996; Gunderson and Singer 1975; Kernberg 1975). If a critical comment comes from a desired person, the view of self may change from worthwhile to worthless, and the view of the other's role may shift from well-intentioned to malevolent. Short-term psychotic states may occur.

The less patients are able to integrate ambivalences and contradictions in identity within a supraordinate, umbrella-like structure, the more difficult it will be for clinicians to attain initial treatment goals such as state stabilization. Such behaviors necessitate combining psychotherapy with brief hospitalization and/or psychiatric medications for some disrupted patients. Some concepts that aid in such formulation of level of self-organization may be found in Table 10–2.

Suggested Phases of Treatment

PHASE ONE: STATE STABILIZATION

In addition to intense negative emotions such as rage, fear, shame, and disgust, patients may report moods colored by a sense of being out of control. In discourse, the clinician may find them in states during which they are unable to rationally plan their next activities. Some patients are so deeply depressed that they cannot provide a clear or accurate psychiatric history. Others are so highly anxious that hypervigilance and confusion lead to an incoherent or at least rambling and disjointed communicative style. That is why initial treatment stages may need to focus on stabilizing mental states. The first goal is to help the patient avoid substance abuse, other addictions, sexual promiscuity, dangerous thrills, and desperate engagements in self-destructive actions.

In some patients, clinical judgment may indicate comorbid major depressive disorder. In such instances, appropriate psychiatric medications may be indicated as a way to improve state control. As noted by Davis et al. (1995), it is important with such patients to point out repeatedly that drugs are not a panacea and to address unrealistic expectations as soon as possible. Because habitual clinging to medications, progressively increasing dosages, or impulsive overdosing may occur, use of medication should be limited to cases in which it is essential. Clear instructions probably should be written down for repeated review. Clinicians should be aware that such patients who are taking medication often complain intensely of negative effects, even after an initial period of elation, over positive effects. A patient might even use any side effects of the drugs to provoke a sense of guilty helplessness in the therapist.

Because of the vulnerability of patients to impulsive decisions, they may use alcohol or street drugs, which can interact with prescribed medications. Psychopharmacological agents should be selected with an eye to avoiding intended or subintended self-destructive effects, including suicide.

Even after relative state control has been achieved in the first phase of treatment, subsequent and episodic regressions are likely to occur. Stressor events and emergent memories and fantasies can trigger increases in undermodulated and impulse-ridden states. Transference reactions can also threaten the patient. Patients of this type often fear that their intrusive thoughts, unbidden images, and out-of-control impulses signify that they are going crazy. They dread and fearfully expect abandonment or exploitation by helpers. Anticipation of dreaded states can be confronted directly, and that may help stabilize a mood of preparedness. The patient plans and rehearses a sequence of steps on how to handle incipient, feared out-of-control states. Some of these phase one techniques are summarized in Table 10–3.

PHASE TWO: MODIFICATION OF COMMUNICATIVE STYLE AND DEFENSIVE CONTROL PROCESSES

After supportive techniques stabilize states, the therapist can begin to teach the patient how to think and talk about conflict. The patient usually will need to learn how to reflect on his or her intentions and motives as well as those of others.

This second phase begins with a reexamination of the reasons for treatment. A step-by-step reinventory of problems already presented usually helps the patient establish a new focus. This approach may include asking about roles, emotions, phenomena, and actions that are desired but seldom experienced. Some questions to consider at this point include the following:

- What does the patient want?
- What is the patient afraid of?
- How does the patient plan to cope with past stress or present and future situations?
- Are better ways available for defending against excessive emotional excitement or entry into dreaded, undermodulated mood states?

TABLE 10–2.	Level of character psychopathology defined by organization of self and other schematization

Level	Description
Normal	Such persons have a well-developed supraordinate self (a large schema connecting and so containing several self schemas). They function from a relatively unitary position of self as agent and maintain consistent values and commitments over time. They have conflicts and negative moods and own these as "of the self." Conflicts are between various realistic pros and cons or limitations of real relationships. Conflicts tend to be handled well through the appropriate use of rational choices, restraints, renunciations, sublimations, wisdom, humor, or even resignation. The person is able to relate intimately and intuitively and knows that another person is separate and has his or her own intentions and expectations. (A person at this level might have a theatrical style but would not have a histrionic personality disorder.)
Neurotic	Such persons have long-standing unresolved themes of conflict. These themes contain antitheses of intention, expectation, and values. Defensive styles ward off emotional flooding but prevent the connection of meanings into supraordinate schemas that might reduce or integrate contradictions in identity and relationships. Discrepancies between views of self as agent of action and self as critic of actions are not resolved in a reasonable time by rational choices. For example, they may see themselves as both expressing sexual interest in another person and opposing such expression on moral grounds. Rigid inhibitions, indecisive, repetitive ruminations, and doing and undoing become habitual. Enactments of conflict lead to repetitive maladaptive relationship cycles in spheres of work, intimacy, and caregiving. (A person at this level could have a neurotic histrionic personality disorder.)

TABLE 10–2. Level of character psychopathology defined by organization of self and other schematization *(continued)*

Level	Description
Narcissistically vulnerable	Such persons have relatively dissociated ideal, real, and deflated self schemas. Even without high connectivity of meanings into a supraordinate self schema, they are often able to maintain a state organized by a cohesive and relatively realistic self schema, but they also have states when they are vulnerable to feeling extremely self-impoverished or grandiose. With further stress, they may either lose a sense of self-cohesion or use irrational distortions to inflate illusions of perfection in spheres of creativity, power, or sexuality. Such people usually also view some others irrationally as if they were extensions of self (selfobjects). (A person at this level would have problems of demandingness, irrational illusions, and expectations of the therapist becoming a selfobject, in addition to having the problems of a neurotic histrionic personality disorder.)
Borderline	Such persons have various self schemas, each of which is only part of the actual self, and various schemas of others that include only part of the actual behavior of others. Composites of person schemas that are all good may be dissociated from composites that are all bad. Under stress, to prove the validity of such segregations of meaning, negative emotions such as rage may be projected and provoked in others. (Borderline-level histrionic personality disorders give rise to even more vulnerability than do narcissistic ones to states of delusional thinking and impulsive self-attack when rage, perhaps activated by expected abandonment or abuse, cannot be externalized.)

Note. Histrionic personality disorder is usually conceptualized as neurotic, but comorbidity with narcissistic and borderline personality disorders may occur.

TABLE 10–3.   Phase one: focus on state control

1. Encourage restraint from actions that will provide immediate relief but that risk harm.

2. Do not rush excessively to prescribe medications or engineer social living solutions in response to imperative demands to end problems quickly, *yet* do not become or appear indifferent to suffering.

3. Listen empathically without regarding intense expressions of emotion as "theatrical."

4. Describe states with specific words.

5. Ask a series of questions to establish cause-and-effect sequences of events.

6. Encourage attention to mental and external incidents while establishing a temporal order of what has happened and is likely to happen next.

7. Help the patient use dose-by-dose reflections on conflictual topics to avoid emotional flooding.

8. Help the patient anticipate future dilemmas and pitfalls.

9. Rehearse "thinking before acting" by planning how to relieve dreaded states of feeling in advance.

The answers to these questions seldom will be clear, but new ways of thinking may begin to develop. The therapist may help the patient to consider how feelings vary between different states of mind. Dreaded or problematic states of mind are likely to be presented first. If so, after first showing empathic receptivity, the therapist may begin to ask questions that focus attention beyond complaints. These questions ask about beliefs and behavior patterns that cause problems. The therapist also may explore questions related to positive functioning. During what states of mind are the symptoms and problems less present? Are there desired states of mind that the patient tries to enter and finds difficult to achieve? Are there rational routes into desired states? Can these become alternative future possibilities?

Some histrionic patients engage in a dangerous search for partners to provide succor. Seeking contact, they may feign erotic interest. Such patients are likely to connect only with exploitative or obtuse partners. Establishing an understanding of this pattern and learning to recognize red flags to prevent sequences of abuse and abandonment are important aspects of this phase of treatment.

During this phase, it is usually helpful to convey back to the patient, through clear verbal communication, an empathic awareness of the intensity of the patient's emotions. The therapist's responses should

TABLE 10–4. Phase two: clarify communications

1. Model contemplation by speaking clearly and calmly while talking about topics that have been unspeakable.

2. Do not respond to behavioral provocations to shift social roles. Avoid flirtation, inappropriate humor, and criticism.

3. Interpret shifts into pretended emotions. Compassionately label feelings that are like those feigned and that can be felt authentically.

4. Encourage verbal expression as a way to get attention.

5. Show the patient how to use words to translate somatic enactions and emergent images into verbal meanings. Do not use hypnosis, somatic movement, or guided imagery as a fast route to intense emotional expression; these techniques are likely to result in undermodulated states without insight.

remain balanced and appropriate, neither too close nor too remote. Techniques that may clarify communication in this second phase of psychotherapy are summarized in Table 10–4.

Patients with histrionic personality disorder use a variety of defensive control processes to ward off emotionally dangerous ideas. Defenses may inhibit memories and fantasies, intentions, and expectations. Patients may feel emotions but not be aware of their associations to particular thoughts or events. Modification of defensive inhibitions and avoidances (Table 10–5) may lead to further clarification of communication. As the patient learns to tolerate feeling sad, angry, and fearful without excessive shame and guilt, the habitual defensive control processes will become less necessary. Internal connections of meaning gradually can be made.

TABLE 10–5. Phase two: modify defensive control processes

1. Counteract the tendency to quickly drop a topic that contains conflicts (often manifested by saying "I don't know" or "I will just do this").

2. Counteract the tendency to leave concepts within a cloudy matrix of loose associations; do this by repeating key chains of concepts.

3. Show the patient how to infer intentions rationally rather than making habitual irrational assumptions about other people.

4. Teach the patient to reappraise and revise decisions.

5. Discourage efforts to rationalize impulsive decisions and disavow personal responsibility for actions.

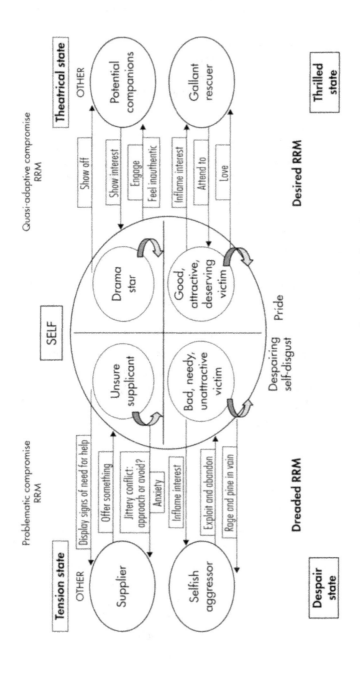

FIGURE 10–1.   Sample configuration of role relationship models (RRMs) from a patient with histrionic personality disorder.

WISH-FEAR DILEMMA: Seeking love leads to despair

The adaptive value of planning is emphasized to the patient. This requires the patient to slow down his or her train of thought or discourse. Such change reduces the chance of emotional flooding. The therapist facilitates slowing down mental activities by repeating what the patient has said and by helping the patient organize the sequence of expressions. Emotions and cause-and-effect sequences can be connected by using this technique.

The therapist may help the patient learn to think about emotions and ideas by putting nonverbal messages, which are a part of the patient's paralinguistic or physical discourse, into verbal expressions. The patient's monitoring of nonverbal messages may gradually increase. This may reduce some maladaptive interpersonal patterns outside of therapy.

A vital technique is to help patients stay with an unresolved topic longer than they ordinarily would. Patients typically will declare an unresolved topic over or impossible to solve, or they may just trail off with the hallmark statement "I don't know." The therapist can clarify the dysfunctional, irrational, or conflictual concepts. Exploring how and why a style of not-knowing was learned in the past also may help modify the avoidant habitual style. Is the style an emulation of other people important to the patient, perhaps those she or he knew in childhood or adolescence? Not-knowing may have been encouraged in the context in which the patient grew up, but now knowing is encouraged.

One aspect of teaching how to use thought to plan action and forestall threats is to help the patient learn to focus on different frameworks of time. Patients with histrionic personality disorder often skip around in conceptualizing past, present, and future. Memory and imagination that are really time-, place-, and person-differentiated may become jumbled or falsely combined in their minds. With some encouragement and repetition, patients can learn to keep appropriate segregations of meanings in person, place, and time, as well as forge new and more appropriate connections. A periodic effort to focus on the very near, short-range future of alternative possibilities may be especially useful.

PHASE THREE: MODIFICATION AND INTEGRATION OF INTERPERSONAL PATTERNS AND PERSON SCHEMAS

A problematic or dreaded state of mind can be clarified by inferring what concepts of self and others occur prominently in that state. Reduction in defensive control processes will make this more possible. Use of role relationship models as summary statements can lead to a configuration of desired, dreaded, and compromise models, as illustrated in Figure 10–1.

A role relationship model for a theatrical state shows off appealing traits of self that are intended to inflame the interest of another person. Without this display, the expectation is that the other person will not be interested. Even victim roles may be used to attract attention, especially from a health professional. That is, the role of abused victim may be exaggerated and shown to provoke rescue from a gallant figure.

Unfortunately, the role in the patient's mind, namely as someone who is found to be of interest and worthy of being saved by a gallant rescuer, does not correspond to what usually happens. Instead, in outside life, these individuals attract someone who will exploit and abandon them. Thus, it is not surprising that instead of thrills, the patient experiences being degraded, desperate, and alone. This maladaptive but repetitive interpersonal pattern, once specified in therapy, becomes a focal target for change. The cognitive analytic therapy model actually diagrams on paper the patient's self states and how the person gets in and out of these states (Kellett 2007). Creating and reflecting on these images during therapy assists the patient in intervening in maladaptive patterns of behavior and interaction.

Transference patterns may clarify the concepts that are often misapplied to the current self and to current others. The role of rescuer initially may be projected onto the therapist. The patient may feel grateful, but as therapy becomes more difficult and more work is expected, the patient may shift views and then feel more like a bad, needy, unattractive victim. The therapist seems to demand self-observation, self-control, and effort to change the future. The patient may even assume that the therapist is about to abandon the patient because he or she cannot comply with these demands. The patient may complain of the therapist to others. It is helpful to predict and prepare for this shift with the patient.

Interpretations made within a context of frank disclosure and expert help can be used to compare the actual immediate properties of the therapy relationship with the patient's transference expectations and strivings. The interpersonal treatment model evaluates positive therapy interventions as facilitating collaboration, facilitating pattern recognition, blocking maladaptive patterns, strengthening will to give up maladaptive patterns, and facilitating new learning (Benjamin 2003). Discussing the progress made in therapy and the reality of the therapy relationship may foster a therapeutic alliance. As already mentioned, with patients who are narcissistically vulnerable or borderline in organizational level of character psychopathology, these interpretations need to be early, short, tactfully worded, and frequently repeated in a sympathetic manner.

Wishes for attention (lower right quadrant of Figure 10–1, p. 302) are often linked to fears of attention. The patient may expect despair to be a consequence of love even while desperately seeking love. Acting to get close to someone is expected to lead to exploitation (lower left quadrant of Figure 10–1). This wish-fear dilemma leads to the jittery shifts noted in the Tension State and the Problematic Compromise RRM (role relationship model) shown in the upper left quadrant of Figure 10–1.

Rejection is anticipated as likely because the self is unworthy of attention unless some personal quality is exaggerated. The self is cast into a "worthy" role only by inflated presentations of some attribute, such as sexual attractiveness or physical infirmity. As shown in the upper right quadrant, Quasi-Adaptive Compromise RRM, of Figure 10–1, the person has to stand out—be the "star"—in some way. The problem is that identity feels inauthentic when in these roles of presenting self as remarkably special through a bodily attribute or a talent. Beck et al. (2007) assert that lasting change in a person with histrionic personality disorder is made through repeatedly stimulating thought about his or her concept of identity, decatastrophizing beliefs about relationship loss and rejection, and, ultimately, challenging the most basic assumption that "I am inadequate and have to rely on others to survive."

The parents of the patient may have been unstable in state and inconsistent in care. They may have disavowed negative behaviors in their own past when in positive caregiving states. This may have led to the patient having a variety of dysfunctional beliefs about why care was inconsistent. In addition, the patient may have a variety of contradictory and unintegrated memories and fantasies of past life. Developing an image of the self as bad may have been an aspect of magical explanations as to why bad things happened in childhood. Reconstructions of life stories may be valuable in the therapist's efforts to help the patient review memories and fantasies of the past. However, it is important to take an equidistant and "don't be too sure" stance on what elements in a reappraisal are real events and what elements are fantasies.

In addition to clarifying dysfunctional beliefs in self-concepts, it may be useful to facilitate recognition of personal skills and real accomplishments. Some of these techniques of the third phase of therapy are summarized in Table 10–6.

PHASE FOUR: TERMINATION OF TREATMENT

Phase four of treatment focuses on separation. The therapeutic relationship may have become one of the most significantly authentic experiences in the patient's adult life. The quality of this experience may have

TABLE **10–6.**   Phase three: help the patient modify interpersonal behaviors and integrate concepts of identity and relationships

1. Identify fears of being abandoned and the dysfunctional belief that the self is incapable of managing basic life tasks.

2. Define excessive dependence on and idealization of unreliable others. Discourage premature confiding, unwitting seductions, and going along with exploitations.

3. Clarify and challenge irrational beliefs identifying the self as devalued, degraded, unworthy, dirty, bad, or weak.

4. Bolster realistic, positive, and competent self-concepts in opportunity-appropriate role relationship models. Encourage authentic ways of getting attention, affiliation, and commitments.

5. Identify and discourage patterns of masochistic prepayment for fantasized and hoped-for satisfactions.

6. Develop conscious recognition and anticipation of script sequences that otherwise tend to run automatically. Identify role reversal (from active to passive, adult to child, tempter to victim, aggressor to rescuer, lover to hater, triumphant rival to abandoned loser).

7. Help the patient consciously plan to get increments of what is desired rather than demand it all at once.

8. Compare transference and therapeutic alliance views of the here and now. Interpret the reasons for the transference attitudes, and do so without criticism.

9. Indicate that current emotional reactions are based on dysfunctional beliefs and inappropriate roles learned in the past, and show how these can be changed in the future by rehearsing and repeating new concepts and actions.

been due, in part, to development of an alliance for change that did not exploit the patient. The support and reality orientation of the therapist will have provided a sense of constancy. There may have been identification by the patient with the way the therapist calmly discussed emotionally difficult issues and reacted to turbulent provocations. The patient may doubt that he or she can maintain improved levels of functioning and contemplation of problems without the therapist. Also, he or she may anticipate pining and feelings of emptiness (Kellett 2007).

Because the therapist's attunement, containment, and commitment to the patient's long-range welfare are likely not to be duplicated in the near future, termination will be a real loss to the patient. Unrealistic but powerful unconscious fantasies about separation and loss are also activated. For these reasons, termination should not be abrupt. Many themes of work already accomplished may need to be repeated in this new context.

Termination will involve mutual agreement on a future time of cessation followed by regular meetings for months. Several sessions may be needed to reach a clear future time point for defining "the end." The sessions of a termination phase can both repeat themes of the middle phase and facilitate an anticipatory mourning process for loss of the therapy situation itself.

Conclusion

Every real case will deviate in some way from this prototype, and every real therapist will devise a different plan. The configurational analysis approach can help the clinician in individualized formulation and planning. States of mind can be labeled with highly personal descriptors. Then specific defensive maneuvers can be clearly defined, and distinctive role relationship models can be gradually sketched and revised. The guidelines are not precise maps; they are not as detailed, deep, and complex as the real individuality of each of our patients.

Key Clinical Concepts

- ◆ Clarity in communications is first learned by identifying with the therapist's exemplifications of lucidity and reasoning of cause-and-effect sequences and differentiators of reality from fantasy.
- ◆ Histrionic personality disorder is a maladaptive set of *interpersonal* patterns.
- ◆ At an *intrapsychic* level, these patterns depend on person schemas such as role relationship models. These self and other schematizations may vary in organizational level in persons at a neurotic, narcissistically vulnerable, and borderline level of having or not having supraordinate configurations.
- ◆ Technique may vary with persons at different organizational levels. State stabilization will take longer and be more frequently necessary during regressions with such patients who are at the borderline level.

Suggested Readings

Beck AT, Freeman A, Davis DD: Cognitive Therapy of Personality Disorders. New York, Guilford, 2007

Benjamin LS: Interpersonal Diagnosis and Treatment of Personality Disorders, 2nd Edition. New York, Guilford, 2003

Horowitz MJ (ed): Hysterical Personality Style and the Histrionic Personality Disorder. Northvale, NJ, Jason Aronson, 1991

References

American Psychiatric Association: Diagnostic and Statistical Manual of Mental Disorders, 3rd Edition. Washington, DC, American Psychiatric Association, 1980

American Psychiatric Association: Diagnostic and Statistical Manual of Mental Disorders, 4th Edition, Text Revision. Washington, DC, American Psychiatric Association, 2000

Beck AT, Freeman A, Davis DD: Cognitive Therapy of Personality Disorders. New York, Guilford, 2007

Benjamin LS: Interpersonal Diagnosis and Treatment of Personality Disorders, 2nd Edition. New York, Guilford, 2003

Blagov PS, Westen D: Questioning the coherence of histrionic personality disorder: borderline and hysterical personality subtypes in adults and adolescents. J Nerv Ment Dis 196:785–797, 2008

Davis JM, Janicak PG, Ayd FJ: Psychopharmacotherapy of the personality-disordered patient. Psychiatr Ann 25:614–620, 1995

Gunderson JG: The borderline patient's intolerance of aloneness: insecure attachments and therapist availability. Am J Psychiatry 153:752–758, 1996

Gunderson JG, Singer MT: Defining borderline patients: an overview. Am J Psychiatry 132:1–10, 1975

Horowitz MJ (ed): Hysterical Personality. Northvale, NJ, Jason Aronson, 1977

Horowitz MJ (ed): Hysterical Personality Style and the Histrionic Personality Disorder. Northvale, NJ, Jason Aronson, 1991a

Horowitz MJ: Person Schemas and Maladaptive Interpersonal Patterns. Chicago, IL, University of Chicago Press, 1991b

Horowitz MJ: Histrionic personality disorder, in Treatment of Psychiatric Disorders, 2nd Edition. Edited by Gabbard GO. Washington, DC, American Psychiatric Press, 1995, pp 2311–2326

Horowitz MJ: Formulation as a Basis for Planning Psychotherapy Treatment. Washington, DC, American Psychiatric Press, 1997

Horowitz MJ: Understanding Psychotherapy Change: A Practical Guide to Configurational Analysis. Washington, DC, American Psychological Association, 2005

Kellett S: A time series evaluation of the treatment of histrionic personality disorder with cognitive analytic therapy. Psychol Psychother 80:389–405, 2007

Kernberg OF: Borderline Conditions and Pathological Narcissism. Northvale, NJ, Jason Aronson, 1975

Kernberg OF: Aggression in Personality Disorders and Perversions. New Haven, CT, Yale University Press, 1992

Kohut H: The Analysis of the Self. New York, International Universities Press, 1971

Kohut H: Restoration of the Self. New York, International Universities Press, 1977

Lilienfeld BA, Van Valkenburg C, Larntz K, et al: The relationship of histrionic personality disorder to antisocial personality and somatization disorders. Am J Psychiatry 143:718–722, 1986

Luborsky L, Crits-Christoph P: Understanding Transference: The Core Conflictual Relationship Theme Method. New York, Basic Books, 1990

Pfohl B, Stangl D, Zimmerman M: The implications of DSM-III personality disorders for patients with major depression. J Affect Disord 7:309–318, 1984

Pilkonis PA, Frank E: Personality pathology in recurrent depression: nature, prevalence, and relationship to treatment response. Am J Psychiatry 145:435–441, 1988

Samuels JF, Nestadt G, Anthony JC, et al: The detection of mental disorders in the community using a 20-item interview version of the General Health Questionnaire. Acta Psychiatr Scand 89:14–20, 1994

Seivewright H, Tyrer P, Johnson T: Change in personality status in neurotic disorders. Lancet 359:2253–2254, 2002

Shapiro D: Neurotic Styles. New York, Basic Books, 1965

Slavney PR, McHugh PR: Life stories and meaningful connections: reflections on a clinical method in psychiatry and medicine. Perspect Biol Med 27:279–288, 1984

Standage K, Bilsbury C, Jain S, et al: An investigation of role-taking in histrionic personalities. Can J Psychiatry 29:407–411, 1984

Wallerstein RS: Forty-Two Lives in Treatment: A Study of Psychoanalysis and Psychotherapy. New York, Guilford, 1986

CHAPTER 11

Psychodynamic Treatment of Antisocial Personality Disorder

J. Reid Meloy, Ph.D., A.B.P.P.
Jessica Yakeley, M.B. B.Chir., M.R.C.Psych.

Many psychoanalytic clinicians and researchers experienced in working with severe personality disorders have concluded that patients with a diagnosis of antisocial personality disorder are not treatable with psychodynamic psychotherapy (Gabbard 2005; Kernberg 1984; Kernberg et al. 2008). This pessimism is based on the seeming impossibility of engaging with patients whose pervasive deception and emotional detachment forecloses any possibility of entering into a viable therapeutic relationship, while the focus of therapy is constantly being diverted from exploration of the patient's mind into managing his risky antisocial behaviors. Although there is a lack of systematic controlled empirical evidence to indicate that psychodynamic treatments are effective in these individuals, recent research into the psychopathic patient's abnormal cognitive deficits and emotional responses (Patrick 2006) and awareness that antisocial personality disorder is a disorder of attachment (Meloy 2002) are stimulating a renewed interest in psychodynamic approaches.

Treatment Studies

The early literature on individual psychoanalysis (Cleckley 1941; Freud 1916/1957) and group psychotherapy (Foulkes 1948/1983) for antisocial patients was based on individual case reports, and the most disturbed individuals were most likely not offered treatment (McGauley et al. 2007). Because of the high levels of dangerous acting out, such as violence, self-harm, substance abuse, and violations of the law, attempts to treat these patients with conventional outpatient psychotherapy have rarely been successful (Meloy 1995). These difficulties led to the development of specialized institutional settings for the treatment of antisocial and psychopathic patients and offenders that could provide sufficient containment of their risks, and the environmental setting itself became an essential therapeutic tool of the therapy. The longest established residential approach to the treatment of antisocial personality disorder is the therapeutic community (Jones 1952), a democratic structure in which all the patients take responsibility for both the care and the containment of each other. The main modality of treatment is group, both small and large, in which the patients examine and challenge each other's behavior.

Although a review of treatments for antisocial personality disorder and psychopathic disorder (Dolan and Coid 1993) suggested that therapeutic community approaches showed the most promise among forms of treatment for psychopathic disorder, this cautious optimism was seriously dented by a series of studies in the 1990s. Group interventions in therapeutic community settings for individuals with psychopathy not only led to a poorer treatment response and greater dropout rate than for nonpsychopaths (Ogloff et al. 1990), but actually increased violent recidivism in the psychopathic samples studied (Harris et al. 1991, 1994). Many clinicians concluded that psychopathic and antisocial personality-disordered patients were untreatable. Subsequent research challenged this abject pessimism (Salekin 2002; Skeem et al. 2002), but also found that lengthier and more intensive treatments were necessary.

In recent years cognitive-behavioral treatments targeting the antisocial personality-disordered patient's behaviors and associated symptoms, such as aggression, self-harm, and substance abuse, have been promoted over therapies aimed at altering the underlying abnormal personality structure. Cognitive-behavioral techniques have been adapted to create specific treatment programs that show some success with personality-disordered offenders. These include relapse prevention programs (Andrews et al. 1990); programs combining cognitive skills with social skills and problem solving (Friendship et al. 2002); anger and violence management programs (Saunders 1996; Wong and

Gordon 2000); sex offender treatment programs (Beech et al. 1999, 2001); and treatments for psychopathic individuals (Wong and Hare 2005). Much of the recent interest in the past two decades in the treatment of antisocial personality disorder has been fueled by increasing political concern about public protection from mentally ill offenders, often magnified by high-profile homicides widely reported by the media. Canada has responded with treatment programs for offenders (Wong and Gordon 2004). More recently, specialized intensive units for patients with so-called dangerous and severe personality disorder have been established in the United Kingdom (Department of Health and Home Office 1999). Although cognitive-behavioral techniques predominate in these treatment programs, some use psychodynamic ideas to both manage staff and tailor therapeutic interventions. Such applications include using the therapeutic community model of treatment, recruiting psychoanalytically trained clinicians as consultants to the team to address staff dynamics, and using psychodynamic therapy and mentalization-based approaches in group and individual treatments.

A Psychodynamic Approach to Treatment

It appears that the therapeutic pendulum may have swung too far in a behavioral direction. The limitations of treatments aimed at changing surface behaviors and symptoms, if these are not linked to changes in internal mental states, have become more evident. A psychodynamic understanding of the patient with antisocial personality disorder assumes that unconscious determinants play a major role in behavior (Gabbard 2005; Meloy 1988, 2001). Overt behaviors such as violence can be thought of as symptoms that signal disturbance in, or that defend against, internal states of mind, which are complex constellations of conscious and unconscious thoughts, affects, motivations, fantasies, and wishes. Antisocial personality disorder patients with lesser degrees of psychopathy may also have some capacity to form an attachment, albeit abnormal, and it is important to recognize that their antisocial behavior may serve to defend against or control underlying emotions. They may experience their interactions with others, including professionals, as the unconscious reenactment of earlier trauma, rejection, and abuse. Moreover, antisocial and psychopathic patients' reduced capacity for empathy and related cognitive deficits can be understood as part of a developmental failure of the ability to mentalize (Bateman and Fonagy 2004), that is, the capacity to understand one's own and others' intentional mental states. The violent or antisocial act can also be understood as a communication with unconscious meaning within an attachment paradigm: the patient's mode of relating with others is characterized by action or even predation, and one of the tasks of therapy is to insert thought between impulse and action. However, one of the pitfalls in working with psychopathic individuals is that thought without caring or feeling, or mentalizing without empathizing, may lead only to better predation.

The following psychodynamic framework considers both the management and the treatment of patients with antisocial personality disorder, activities that are not entirely separate from each other. There is inherent conflict and ambiguity in conceptualizing the aims of interventions for personality-disordered offenders. Are interventions carried out solely to reduce the risk of harm to the public, or can there be some benefit in mental health to the patient? An essential component of management is the *setting* in which treatment is delivered, wherein containment, risk, boundaries, and disclosure of information are paramount. The treatment setting must be secure enough to ensure the safety of both patients and staff before treatment planning can begin. Treatment planning commences with a careful *assessment* of the patient to ascertain the severity of psychopathy, identify any treatable Axis I or III conditions, and distinguish personality traits and characteristics that may be amenable to treatment given available resources (Meloy 2007). Treatment planners then need to consider the *modality* of therapy in which the patient engages, which may be individual, group, or occasionally family therapy; how to *engage* the patient in a therapeutic process; and *specific therapeutic interventions* used in treatment, which include psychodynamic psychotherapy with certain modifications of technique. Specific new therapies that have evolved from psychoanalytic theory have been developed for patients with personality disorder, including mentalization-based treatment (MBT; Bateman and Fonagy 2004) and transference-focused psychotherapy (TFP; Kernberg et al. 2008). Finally, recognition and analysis of the powerful *countertransference* reactions that these patients provoke in those involved in their care is a central component of both management and treatment of antisocial personality disorder patients (Meloy 1988, 2001, 2007). An understanding of how these patients' unconscious communications and utilization of immature defense mechanisms can influence the dynamics of the team looking after them can be used to refine both therapeutic interventions and the assessment and management of risk (Yakeley 2007).

ASSESSMENT

It is critical that the severity of psychopathy be determined for each patient with a history of antisocial behavior. The most valid and reliable scientific instruments for this task are the Psychopathy Checklist—Revised (PCL-R) and its short form, the Psychopathy Checklist Screening Version (PCL:SV) (Hare 2003). The PCL:SV is most useful at the level of screening for psychopathy in acute settings, or in designing a program that assesses for psychopathic risk in a cost-efficient manner. The more comprehensive PCL-R is then utilized when certain scoring thresholds are passed. Both instruments are standardized observational measures that yield a unidimensional score for degree of psychopathy following a structured clinical interview and review of all available records. We recommend thinking about psychopathy as a dimensional measure rather than a categorical measure, for several reasons: psychopathy does not appear to be a taxon; degree of severity is more useful for clinical treatment purposes; and the thrust of personality research in general is toward dimensional rather than categorical measures (Livesley 2004; Patrick 2006). Data suggest that psychopathic individuals have quite different prognoses depending on their PCL-R scores: 10–19 indicates mild psychopathy, 20–29 indicates moderate psychopathy, and 30 and above indicates severe psychopathy. Clinicians should avail themselves of training with these instruments to ensure they are competently utilized.

We also recommend that assessment of the antisocial patient be further individualized through the use of other psychological and neuropsychological measures, including the Rorschach test (Gacono and Meloy 1994), the MMPI-2 (Friedman et al. 2001), and various measures of structural and functional impairments, ranging from various neuropsychological test batteries to neuroimaging techniques. Review of research involving neuroimaging studies with psychopathic, antisocial, and habitually violent patients, for example, indicates that there are often both structural and functional impairments, the latter more significant, in the prefrontal cortex, superior temporal gyrus, amygdala-hippocampal complex, and anterior cingulate cortex (Yang et al. 2008). Brain dysfunction is clearly a risk factor for antisocial behavior, but there is within-group and between-group heterogeneity.

MODALITY OF TREATMENT

Modality of treatment refers to the mode in which it is delivered, which can be viewed as a vehicle for psychic change. The therapeutic mode can be individual, group, or family therapy, or the therapeutic community itself, using its distinctive culture (Main 1983) as a therapeutic tool. Different theoretical models of therapy (e.g., cognitive-behavioral, dialectical behavioral, supportive, or psychodynamic) can be applied within each modality.

Group Therapy

Both clinical experience and research studies indicate that for many antisocial and psychopathic patients, group therapy may be more effective than individual therapy. Foulkes (1948/1983) showed early interest in the group treatment of antisocial patients and suggested that when taking part in a group, "collectively they constitute the very norm, from which, individually, they deviate" (Foulkes 1964, p. 297). This suggestion raises a striking paradox in regard to the therapeutic group for deviant or dangerous individuals: instead of violent or antisocial behavior being potentiated by meeting with other violent members of a group, as would occur in a prison or gang subculture, engaging in a therapeutic group and seeing one's own difficulties through the eyes of others may act to attenuate such behavior and bring about therapeutic change (Schlapobersky 1996). In the United Kingdom, psychoanalytically oriented group therapy was started in Broadmoor High Secure Hospital in 1970 (Cox 1976), and since then there have been comprehensive group programs, including some psychodynamic groups, running in high secure psychiatric hospitals and many medium secure psychiatric units. Such programs have been more recently introduced into the prison and probation systems.

Many patients with antisocial personality disorder have deficits in their capacity to reflect on feelings and thoughts and find it difficult to tolerate internal anxiety. For these patients, whose capacity for mentalization is rudimentary, group therapy may be more effective than individual work. The group acts as a container of the patient's projections and as a collective auxiliary ego that can think and reflect on behalf of the patient, very gradually promoting more healthy ego functioning. Specific mentalization techniques can be used in a group setting for offender patients. Bateman and Fonagy (2004) suggest that for patients with poor affect control, group work is optimal because it is less arousing than individual therapy and also offers more opportunities to understand other people's minds. Other group processes are also important, such as modeling of more appropriate behavior and interpersonal interactions that may be internalized by the patient.

Antisocial patients whose reality testing is impaired risk forming intensely erotic or even psychotic transference relationships with the therapist in individual work. These patients may do better in group therapy, where the transference relationships are multiple and the intensity of feeling is diluted and distributed among the different members of the group. This is one of the reasons why violence may be better contained and understood within a group setting (Welldon 1996). For patients who are frightened of their own aggressive impulses, the multiple transferences that a group provides offer the patient more than one target for aggression, and this may be reassuring. Group rather than individual psychotherapy is also the treatment of choice for psychopathic patients whose activities involve secretiveness and deception, including perpetration of sexual abuse. The psychopathic individual will find it more difficult to con others in a group of similar patients who can recognize, challenge, and penetrate the pervasive patterns of deception—often not entirely conscious (Meloy 1988)—that characterize the psychopath's way of relating to himself and others.

> Mr. A was a 40-year-old man with a diagnosis of antisocial personality disorder and a history of behaving violently and conning others, including the setting up of "stings." The latter involved the deception and sexual exploitation of businessmen, whom he seduced and then robbed of their cash and expensive watches while they were asleep. While in prison he became depressed after the death of his sister, the only person he had ever felt close to, who had looked after him during their long periods in care as children when they were removed from their abusive parents.
>
> After Mr. A's release from prison he was referred by the probation service to a specialist residential unit for offenders with personality disorder, and there he started group therapy. Mr. A was an intelligent man and appeared to be an active and motivated member of the group, contributing such perceptive and insightful comments about other group patients' difficulties that the group therapist at times felt redundant. At the same time, Mr. A often dominated and frightened the group by his frequent declarations of despair and threats of suicide, which had led the worried professionals involved in his care to dedicate extra nursing staff to be with him continuously to prevent him from harming himself.
>
> Following several weeks of such behavior, another group member, Mr. B, eventually pointed out to Mr. A that he had found a way to satisfy his propensity for violence and deception in the group. Mr. B said that he was fed up with feeling terrorized by Mr. A's violent threats of self-harm, which he felt were more destructive for the group than for Mr. A himself, and that Mr. A. had successfully conned both patients and staff into thinking that he was a sick patient and needed to be the center of attention. Another patient, Mr. C, said he felt sorry for Mr. A, who appeared confused as to whether he was an omnipotent group therapist or was actually a little boy who needed to be totally looked after. The group therapist, aware of his own countertransferential sense of impotence, interpreted the group's sense of powerlessness and anger at him, the therapist, for being so asleep (like the businessmen) as not to notice that they felt Mr. A was "stealing" precious attention and care away from them-

selves. Mr. A was initially shocked and infuriated by these comments, but after much further work in the group he was able to acknowledge how he had deceived both himself and others in his adoption of the sick role.

Individual Therapy

Individual psychotherapy may complement group work. It can offer an opportunity to focus on the fine details of maladaptive behavior and psychopathology, and this can be critical to facilitating change (Livesley 2003). A short period of individual therapy may also be necessary to prepare patients for the challenges of group therapy. Although most individual psychotherapy offered for antisocial patients and offenders is cognitive-behavioral therapy based, a carefully selected minority may benefit from a more psychodynamic approach. However, the individual therapist should not work in isolation and must be constantly alert to the hazards of working with patients who are adept at leading therapists into unethical enactments and enticing them into colluding with the minimization or denial of the patient's offenses.

Family Therapy

Many studies show the effectiveness of specific child, parent, and family interventions for children with conduct disorder, who may be at risk of developing antisocial personality disorder when adults (Kazdin 1995; National Institute for Health and Clinical Excellence 2009). Although there is no published research on family therapy involving adult patients with antisocial personality disorder, Salekin's (2002) review of effective interventions for psychopathic disorders included a role for family-based interventions. Although psychopathic individuals may have no respect for the public or for cultural values in general, they may have some narcissistically based loyalty and respect for their family that may be capitalized on in therapy (Dowsett and Craissati 2008). Family therapy is not advised when a parent is severely psychopathic, because he will likely use information about other family members to sadistically hurt and control them (Meloy 2007). However, patients with antisocial personality disorder who show mild to moderate psychopathic traits may benefit, especially when their children have conduct disorder, and such interventions may ameliorate the intergenerational transmission of the disorder (Sutker et al. 1993) and reduce criminal recidivism (Gendreau and Ross 1987). Acting out on the part of the antisocial personality-disordered parent should be anticipated and the physical and emotional safety of other family members closely monitored.

ENGAGING THE PATIENT

The majority of antisocial personality disorder patients do not accept that they have mental health difficulties and do not accept a traditional sick role (Parsons 1951), let alone that of a psychotherapy patient (Norton and McGauley 1998).

One patient, when asked by his doctor if he knew his diagnosis, said, "Doc, they say I have antisocial personality disorder, but I don't believe them. I love to fuck with people!" Another patient beamed with pride when told he had scored 36 on the PCL-R. He thought the higher the score, the "better" he did.

Those patients who are available for treatment may not present voluntarily and may have been put forward by professionals concerned more about reducing risk than effecting intrapsychic change. Unlike the neurotic patient, in whom the existence of a positive working alliance with the therapist is assumed to be a prerequisite to intrapsychic work, antisocial patients will imbue the therapeutic relationship from the beginning with their transferential early object relations, which are often defined by dominance and submission, rather than reciprocal affection. The therapist will be experienced as dominant, submissive, untrustworthy, prone to deception, or easily corrupted. Motivation for therapy is often overestimated when the patient resides in a secure forensic institution or prison, and the patient often believes that signing up for a course of treatment will expedite his date of release. Most of the programs for antisocial personality disorder patients in secure settings require the person to volunteer for treatment. However, offenders who have appeared to be compliant and motivated in prison treatment programs may often revert to impulsive and risky behaviors once released into the community.

Even the minority of antisocial personality-disordered patients who may eventually benefit from psychodynamic psychotherapy may need much encouragement and preparation for such work. Dowsett and Craissati (2008) warn that the community treatment provider should anticipate that such patients will be late or miss sessions altogether, fail to complete therapeutic tasks, become verbally aggressive and socially disruptive in the treatment setting, misuse substances, and create frequent crises. To minimize attrition and noncompliance with treatment, these authors recommend that therapists prepare patients carefully for treatment; such preparation may include giving practical advice, providing psychoeducation about the personality disorder, allowing the patient to rehearse acceptable behavior with the therapist prior to group work, and in general fostering a collaborative relationship with the therapist. The therapist should be proactive in follow-up of patients to ensure attendance—for example, calling the patient to remind him of appointments and positively reinforcing the patient's engagement in therapeutic tasks. Strategies should be in place to modulate known factors likely to reduce compliance, such as substance misuse, self-harm, or a chaotic lifestyle.

Psychodynamic Psychotherapy for Antisocial Personality Disorder

Despite the many therapeutic pitfalls and hazards inevitably encountered, dedicated and experienced psychodynamic clinicians continue to embark on psychodynamic psychotherapy with antisocial personality-disordered patients. They also strive to research and develop therapeutic technique with these patients, for whom a classical psychoanalytic approach is untenable. Therapeutic enthusiasm for this population has historically been more apparent in the United Kingdom and Europe, where forensic psychiatric practice has always emphasized treatment (Gunn 2004), than in the United States, where forensic psychiatry consists mainly of medicolegal practice rather than therapeutics. In the United Kingdom, there has been a long tradition of psychoanalysts working in the high secure psychiatric hospitals, and this more recently has been formally developed into the psychiatric subspecialty of forensic psychotherapy (Cordess and Cox 1996). Currently, on both sides of the Atlantic, therapies designed for the treatment of borderline personality disorder are being applied to the treatment of antisocial patients, but the term *forensic psychotherapy* is virtually unknown in the United States. Forensic psychotherapy is, however, widely practiced by mental health clinicians, primarily in publicly funded forensic facilities.

The patient must be carefully assessed by an experienced psychodynamic clinician before psychodynamic therapy is attempted. Those with antisocial personality disorder will show serious deficits in key areas of psychic functioning such as psychological mindedness, ego strength, mature defenses, and a developed superego. The normal threshold for offering psychodynamic therapy may be lowered if sufficient expertise and support for the treatment is available. The goal is to ascertain whether the patient's potential for curiosity about his internal world and ownership of his difficulties can be nurtured and developed. Favorable selection criteria include low to moderate levels of psychopathy, presence of anxiety and/or depressive affect, a history of some capacity to form attachments with other people, the presence of higher-level or neurotic defenses, and some evidence of superego functioning. Meloy (1988) states that therapy should not be offered to, and will not benefit, psychopathic patients who manifest any of the following features: sadistic aggressive behavior resulting in serious injury, complete absence of remorse or justification for such behavior, very superior intelligence or mild mental retardation, a historical absence of capacity to form emotional attachments, and unexpected atavistic fear felt by the experienced clinician in the patient's presence (Meloy and Meloy 2002). An easily remembered acronym for clinically evaluating the usefulness of psychodynamic psychotherapy for any antisocial patient is the presence of **ABC:** anxiety, bonding, and conscience.

> Mr. P was introduced to crime at an early age by his violent and abusive father and spent his youth working as an assassin for a feared and powerful organized drug gang in an American city. He lived a glamorous life of exhilaration and triumph, fueled by cocaine and large amounts of money, which stopped only when the prominent leaders of the crime syndicate were finally arrested and convicted. Mr. P managed to escape conviction, but now deprived of the supportive structure of his criminal family of associates, he started to descend into increasing drug and alcohol addiction. Eventually rescued by a supportive partner, he was persuaded to give up his life of crime, violence, and drugs, but he became increasingly anxious and was tormented over several years by intrusive thoughts involving self-recrimination and "guilt" about what he had done to his previous victims. Feeling suicidal, he presented to his doctor, who referred him to a psychiatrist. During the first consultation he presented as very depressed, and he worried the clinician with his suicidal ideation. During this interview he revealed details of past violent exploits for which he had never been caught, which made the psychiatrist feel special and excited to be seeing such an interesting patient. At the following appointment 2 weeks later the psychiatrist was astonished when Mr. P announced that his depression of the past two years had vanished, he no longer felt any guilt, and he had a "free conscience" and was very grateful to the doctor for "curing" him.

Here we can see how Mr. P's grandiose self-structure was dependent on his circle of powerful criminal friends, who created a world of omnipotence and excitement that bolstered Mr. P's psychopathic ego. When this world collapsed after the incarceration of the members of the gang, Mr. P's own psychopathic defense mechanisms began to collapse, and he entered into a downward spiral of drug abuse until he was offered salvation by his girlfriend. Although he appeared to present with depressive symptoms, on closer examination it can be seen that he was not experiencing genuine feelings of guilt, loss, and concern for his victims, but had replicated the sadomasochistic criminal world in his mind, masochistically torturing himself, by means of a sadistic super-ego, with his intrusive thoughts of self-recrimination. Contact with the psychiatrist appeared to have fulfilled the function of the confessional: Mr. P had "off-loaded" his sins onto the doctor, resulting in the rapid resurrection of his defenses and previous functioning. This represents a manic solution rather than any real acknowledgment of painful feelings of guilt, loss, and rejection (Meloy 1988).

> Mr. P re-presented to the psychiatrist a few weeks later, again feeling depressed and suicidal and tempted to take cocaine again, as his girlfriend had left him. The psychiatrist this time took a more cautious approach and referred him for further assessment to a forensic psychiatric colleague experienced in the psychotherapeutic treatment of antisocial personality disorder. This colleague thought that Mr. P, while fulfilling criteria for antisocial personality disorder, showed some evidence of an ability to form attachments (to the girlfriend), had some, albeit pathological, superego function, and was presenting with depression, all of which he thought might be favorable indicators for treatment.

Psychotherapy should ideally be commenced while the patient is in an institutional setting so that he is contained within a structured environment. The temptations for him to act out will be increased as his internal world is opened up and anxieties and aggressive impulses mount. If such a setting is not available, sufficient community support should be organized so that the appropriate professionals are accessible to respond to crises. Modifications of technique should be employed from the start and will form part of the continuum of strategies necessary to engage the patient. The more anxious or paranoid patient is likely to experience silences as persecutory and also may not tolerate the full length of a session, necessitating briefer encounters. Therapeutic interventions should be carefully timed and titrated according to the patient's affective "temperature." As Minne (2007) describes, one of the tasks that the forensic psychotherapist has to negotiate is how to introduce the patient to the unconscious contents of his mind without either patient or therapist becoming overwhelmed by states of acute anxiety, aggression, or suicidal despair. Many therapists working with violent and antisocial patients advocate the avoidance of early interpretations of unconscious conflicts and fantasies, as these are not understood by patients with poor representational capacity and deficits in symbolic thinking. Instead, it is more useful to provide brief and simple descriptive comments about the patient's state of mind (Bateman 1999; Fonagy and Target 1999). These may include the therapist's putting words to the patient's concrete thoughts and feelings as well as using basic metaphors to introduce him to symbolic thinking. The therapist helps the patient to connect such internal states of mind to his behavioral actions (Gabbard 2005) and to gradually understand how acts of violence or misuse of substances may defend against the awareness of more painful thoughts and feelings.

> Mr. P, introduced above, was referred to a mental health service specializing in the treatment of personality disorder and started once-weekly outpatient psychotherapy with an experienced forensic psychotherapist. Mr. P was also assigned a community forensic nurse who was available if he felt suicidal, as well as a social worker to help him with practical matters such as housing and work. He also started a once-weekly psychoeducational group for substance abusers. During the first few months of psychotherapy sessions, the therapist focused on encouraging Mr. P to talk about his feelings of anxiety and aggression and to recognize that in the past he had discharged the aggressive feelings through his violent activities or numbed them with alcohol and drugs. Now that these outlets were no longer available, he was turning his aggression toward himself, as evidenced by his self-tormenting and suicidal thoughts.

For patients whose original caregivers were abusive or neglectful, being thought about by another person will be a novel, but also threatening, experience. One of the tasks of therapy is to gradually open up a space within the patient's mind where difference can be tolerated rather than feared. This is achieved by the gradual internalization of the therapist as a reliable figure who is consistent and boundaried, empathic and nonjudgmental, but able to consider different points of view. Many antisocial personality-disordered patients have experienced profound early difficulties in separation and individuation, their bodies and minds being intruded upon and treated as narcissistic extensions of their parents. Psychotherapy aims to introduce them to transitional spaces in their minds, as originally described by Winnicott (1951/1991), where playfulness and experimentation in relating can occur.

However, many of these patients will not tolerate a free-associative process, and therapeutic work may need to be more directive than in classical psychoanalytic psychotherapy. Interpretations should be focused on the here and now rather than reconstructions of the past, and the patient's denials and minimization of antisocial behavior should be repeatedly confronted (Gabbard 2005). Gabbard also advises that the patient's denigration of the therapist and contemptuous devaluation of the therapeutic process be repeatedly challenged. However, for patients with a precarious sense of self who experience the world as menacing and punitive, premature interpretations of the negative transference should be avoided, as these will be perceived by the patient as critical and retaliatory and will confirm that the world consists of only bad objects, the therapist included. This dilemma has led several authors (e.g., Bateman 1999; Cartwright 2002; Davies 1999) to recommend the use of analyst-centered interpretations (Steiner 1994) with violent and antisocial patients. An analyst-centered interpretation is one in which the therapist attempts to clarify the patient's perception of what is going on in the therapist's mind, such as by saying "You are afraid that I am angry with you," rather than offering a patient-centered interpretation about the patient's own conflicts. An analyst-centered interpretation conveys a sense of being understood by the therapist and is more containing for anxious patients than patient-centered interpretations, which can make the patient feel blamed. The invitation to observe what might be going on in the therapist's mind, when the patient's expectation of the therapist's hostile reaction is talked about but not fulfilled, reveals a cognitive dissonance between expectation and experience that can lead to a change in the patient's perception.

> After a few months, the drug and alcohol group that Mr. P had been attending stopped, and Mr. P became more erratic in his attendance at psychotherapy sessions, arriving late or missing sessions altogether. Instead of interpreting this to Mr. P as him attacking the therapy, the therapist formulated an analyst-centered interpretation, saying that she wondered whether Mr. P was feeling unsettled now that his drug and alcohol group had ended, and if perhaps he was worried that she might think he was ready to finish therapy here, too. This facilitated Mr. P's admitting that he did miss the companionship of the other patients in the group; and while he could not at this stage consciously acknowledge his dependence on his therapist, he started coming to the sessions more regularly again.

Although the therapist always keeps the transference in mind, interpretation of the transference to the patient—in the classical sense of exploring how the patient's experience of the therapist is influenced by early object relationships—may need to wait until a late stage of the therapy. The communications of patients with antisocial personality disorder are often concrete and one-dimensional; they find it difficult or impossible to experience the "as if" quality of the transference, and they tend to identify with the concrete content of interpretations rather than their symbolic meaning. Rigorous and continual monitoring of the therapist's countertransference, however, is essential both to gain insight into the internal world of the patient, and to prevent enactments on the part of the therapist.

The therapist must be prepared for the long and arduous nature of any therapeutic work with antisocial personality-disordered patients. The therapist may oscillate between therapeutic nihilism and therapeutic zeal, but with patients who are so seriously psychically abnormal or damaged, therapeutic aims should be realistically limited to effecting small shifts in their internal world. The painful paradox that a patient has to confront in therapy is that becoming more knowledgeable about his internal world brings with it, at least temporarily, more psychic distress and anguish. If the process of self-awareness is too rapid, the patient will regress to previous pathological but familiar and safer states of mind to avoid becoming overwhelmed by intolerable feelings. In practice, during the course of therapy, patient and therapist will need to endure many cycles in which apparent progress and insight are followed by negative therapeutic reactions and regression to withdrawn, depressive states or more manic, impulsive behavior, both of which serve to obliterate self-knowledge and reflection. The empathy and insight achieved in one session will be subverted and attacked in the next. Such cycles can be understood as oscillation by the patient between paranoid-schizoid and depressive states of mind (Bion 1962/1984; Klein 1946). The former characterizes the patient's familiar pathological configuration in which primitive defense mechanisms operate to keep objects split and bad parts of the self projected. If therapy is successful, the patient will gradually move toward occupying a more depressive position—in which conflicted feelings can become more integrated and directed toward the same object, ambivalence can become more tolerable, loss can be acknowledged, and concern and guilt begin to predominate over grievance. Such progress also diminishes envy in the patient, an insidious emotion in the transference that unconsciously motivates the patient to destroy any goodness being born in the treatment.

> After a year of treatment, Mr. P joined a psychodynamically oriented group for men with antisocial personality disorder, as well as continuing with his individual psychotherapy. Declaring himself less depressed and more self-confident in general, he started skipping some of his individual sessions again; when he did attend, he would make disparaging comments about his therapist, saying that she was "too nice" to him compared to the male group therapist, who "really knows how to confront us about our behavior." At this stage in the therapy, the therapist felt Mr. P could tolerate more direct transference interpretations. She said that Mr. P appeared to have found an ideal, strong father figure in

the group leader, someone whom he hoped would show him how to behave in a way his father had not, while Mr. P was experiencing her as a
weak woman, someone perhaps rather like his mother, who saw Mr. P
being pushed around by his father but did not intervene. She said that
Mr. P appeared to have located his hope and progress in the group. It
was more difficult for him to think about painful feelings evoked by his
mother's or his girlfriend's rejections—or even hers, the therapist's, for
encouraging him to join the group, which he might think meant that she
wanted to get rid of him. To avoid such thoughts and feel more in control, Mr. P was trying to get rid of her by not coming to therapy.

Several authors warn against the therapist being taken in by the apparent progress of the more psychopathic patient, who consciously or
unconsciously may learn to imitate more mature emotional states that
he observes the therapist wants him to feel (Meloy 1988). Cartwright
(2002) describes "pseudo-digestive" capacities, demonstrated by the
patient's talking about the index offense for a couple of sessions, in
which apparent remorse is verbalized, but then not referring to it again.
Glasser (1996) highlights the problems with deception in these patients,
describing the defensive process of simulation that develops in some individuals; that is, the person appears to comply with the demands others place on him, but this compliance is false, albeit unconsciously so.
Such a process, caused by severe early abnormalities in identifications,
has become part of his lifelong defensive makeup and characterizes his
way of relating to others in general. This is akin to Winnicott's (1960/
1990) notion of the "false self" personality and Gaddini's (1992) description of imitation as a defense. Meloy (1988) coined the term *malignant
pseudoidentification* for the process whereby the psychopathic individual
consciously imitates or unconsciously simulates certain behaviors of the
victim to foster the victim's identification with him, thus increasing the
victim's vulnerability to exploitation. Glasser (1996) cautioned that such
simulative processes may be very subtle and often are only detected via
an intuitive sense that something about the offender, who appears to be
making behavioral progress, does not ring quite true.

Countertransference

A central feature of successful work with antisocial personality disorder
patients is an understanding of the countertransference of the psychotherapist *while or shortly after it is experienced*. Such skill, in our opinion,
almost always requires a personal psychoanalysis or intensive psychoanalytic psychotherapy for the professional, often secured during train-

ing, but also not to be neglected as a "tune-up" throughout the professional's career. There is a developing literature on these countertransference reactions, ranging from therapeutic nihilism—the belief that no patient with any antisocial acts in his history can be treated—to excitement and fascination, often imbued with erotic feelings, especially if the therapeutic relationship involves opposite-sex participants (Meloy 1988, 2001, 2007).

By far the most common countertransference reaction, especially with the severely psychopathic patient, is an atavistic fear of being prey to an intraspecies predator. This is viscerally experienced by the therapist as autonomic arousal, most commonly affecting somatosensory neurons. Clinicians report, "He made the hair stand up on my neck," "He gave me the willies," "He gave me goose bumps," or "The way he looked at me sent chills down my spine." Survey research of mental health clinicians indicates that the vast majority—77%, to be exact—will experience some form of autonomic arousal in the presence of a severely psychopathic individual, even in the absence of any overtly threatening behavior (Meloy and Meloy 2002). We urge those who work with antisocial patients of any stripe to closely monitor their reactions, whether these emerge as spontaneous fantasies, disturbing emotions, or visceral responses, and use them as a basis for further objective exploration of the patient's psychopathology.

A forensic clinician was tasked with the evaluation of a notorious sexual murderer of a child. He spent 16 hours with this individual over the course of 4 days, the goals being to understand the personality and psychopathology of the subject and communicate his findings to the subject's defense attorneys. The evaluation went well, and all evidence pointed toward a severely psychopathic individual who had enjoyed sexually assaulting and then killing his 12-year-old victim, kidnapped from her home and previously unknown to him.

What was most troubling, however, was the clinician's countertransference reactions. He had a spontaneous detailed fantasy after the evaluation—which continued intermittently for days—of pulling a .45-caliber handgun out of his briefcase during the evaluation and shooting the defendant in the head and the chest. In the fantasy, when the smoke cleared he surrendered to the correctional guards and was jailed and prosecuted, but the jury found him not guilty of any crime. The second reaction, much less edifying, was experiencing symptoms of posttraumatic stress: he would alternately feel numb, and then intensely furious; he had intrusive recollections of the subject's laughing with pleasure as he recounted the killing to the evaluator; and he would be acutely anxious at times. These feelings subsided after several weeks.

He came to realize that he both identified with the homicidality of the subject and also condemned himself and the subject for a horrendous crime, desiring to murder as the subject had murdered—the primitive rule of *lex talionis*—and avenge the death of the young girl.

New Therapies for Personality Disorder

Specific therapies have been developed and empirically supported for the treatment of severe personality disorders, mostly in the treatment of patients with borderline personality disorder. Although based on very different theoretical models, such therapies show some overlap in technique, and in recent years they have been applied to the treatment of antisocial offenders. The most widely used therapies from a cognitive-behavioral model are dialectical behavior therapy (Linehan 1993) and schema-focused therapy (Young et al. 2003), whereas the two most prominent therapies to emerge from the psychoanalytic school are mentalization-based treatment (MBT) and transference-focused psychotherapy (TFP). The latter two will be briefly described here in relation to the treatment of the antisocial personality disordered patient, and the reader is referred to a fuller account of these therapies elsewhere in this book (see especially Chapter 6, "Mentalization-Based Treatment and Borderline Personality Disorder," and Chapter 7, "Transference-Focused Psychotherapy and Borderline Personality Disorder").

MENTALIZATION-BASED TREATMENT

MBT has been developed in the United Kingdom by Bateman and Fonagy (2004) for patients with borderline personality disorder. Bateman and Fonagy believe that these patients have an unstable or reduced capacity to mentalize. Mentalizing is an essential human capacity underpinning interpersonal relations that develops in the first few years of life in the context of safe and secure child-caregiver relationships. The infant finds its mind as represented in the mind of the other and therefore develops a sense of self as a social agent, learns to differentiate and represent affect states, and regulates its impulse control—prerequisites for discovering the minds of others. Such mental structure, from an object relations perspective, defines a normal or neurotic personality organization (Tyson 1996). This developmental process is severely disrupted in environmental conditions of neglect, emotional abuse, or physical or sexual maltreatment during childhood. Inadequate mirroring and disorganized attachment undermine the capacity to mentalize, so that internal states remain confusing, unsymbolized, and difficult to regulate.

Such development can also be impeded by deficits and defects as well as by conflict (Pine 1994): the nexus of psychodynamics, psychobiology, and the parental environment. Allen et al. (2008) offer five helpful and handy definitions of mentalizing: holding mind in mind, attending to the mental states of self and others, understanding misunderstandings, seeing yourself from the outside and others from the inside, and giving a mental quality to or cultivating mentally (p. 3).

MBT involves the therapist facilitating the patient's finding of his own mind through representations in the mind of the other in the context of a securely attached therapeutic relation. Therapists attempt to construct an image of the patient's mind by naming affects and cognitions and by spelling out implicit beliefs. MBT can be applied in individual, group, or family settings and involves a spectrum of interventions, from supportive and empathic, through clarification and elaboration, to basic mentalizing, interpretive mentalizing, and mentalizing the transference (Allen et al. 2008).

Clinicians have recently started to apply mentalization techniques in the treatment of antisocial personality disorder patients. It is too early, however, for the effectiveness of the techniques to be evaluated in this population. Bateman and Fonagy (2006) postulate that antisocial patients show some enhanced areas of mentalization; for example, their ability to deceive and exploit others necessitates an ability to understand the mind of the other to predict what he will and will not believe. However, they caution that this apparently highly tuned capacity to mentalize is actually very restricted and rarely generalizable to complex interpersonal situations, and that psychopathy exemplifies a partial but fundamental impairment of mentalizing, what Baron-Cohen (2005) called "mindreading without empathizing." Neurobiological differences in the severely psychopathic patient may preclude the use of mentalizing techniques, which may increase risk toward others due to greater behavioral acuity in the service of predation. For example, the absence of certain socialized emotions in the psychopath (Meloy 1988; Patrick 2006) appears to increase the accuracy of his observations of fear and distress in others and their vulnerability to victimization (Book et al. 2007). Bateman and Fonagy (2006) suggest that therapy in such individuals be focused on removing the gratification from their misuse of mentalization.

TRANSFERENCE-FOCUSED PSYCHOTHERAPY

TFP, developed in the United States by Kernberg and his colleagues, is a specific, empirically validated, manualized, two to three times weekly face-to-face individual psychoanalytic psychotherapy for patients with severe personality disorders; it is based on psychoanalytic object relations theory (Clarkin et al. 2006). In this model such patients suffer from a syndrome of identity diffusion, resulting from the failure of psychological integration, in which aggressive internalized object relations dominate and separate from idealized ones. The patient's ego is fixated at a primitive level (borderline or psychotic), and the use of primitive defensive operations such as projective identification, omnipotence, devaluation, and primitive idealization suffuses the personality and behavior of the borderline patient, resulting in poor impulse control, unstable relationships, and chaotic lifestyle. One of the main differences between this model of borderline personality disorder and the mentalization model is that the former sees borderline personality disorder as based on conflict, whereas the mentalization model is largely based on deficit.

The main strategy in TFP for borderline patients consists of facilitating the reactivation, in the treatment, of the patient's split-off internalized object relations as observed and interpreted in the transference. The technical instruments used in TFP are somewhat modified versions of the essential techniques of psychoanalysis (Gill 1954)—namely, interpretation, transference analysis, and technical neutrality—with the addition of countertransference analysis. Unlike MBT, TFP does not see early interpretation as damaging the patient and imposing mental contents on him that he does not experience consciously. It views such interpretations as helping the patient link mental states that he is dissociatively experiencing in his interactions with the therapist. The initial stages of TFP, however, are very similar to MBT.

Kernberg et al. (2008) recommend TFP as the treatment of choice for patients with borderline personality organization, which includes most patients with personality disorders functioning at a borderline level. Although they note that such patients who display antisocial behavior may be treatable by TFP, they exclude narcissistic patients with severe antisocial features and patients who are chronically dishonest, as well as "patients with an antisocial personality disorder proper" (p. 613). However, they recommend that "patients with aggressive, provocative, irresponsible social behavior, who, however, still are able to experience some degree of loyalty, investment in friendship and work, are optimal candidates for TFP" (p. 614). We suggest that Kernberg's definition of "antisocial personality disorder proper" is similar to our use of the term "severely psychopathic." His description of antisocial patients who could benefit from TFP, in our opinion, would include antisocial personality-disordered patients with mild to moderate levels of psychopathy.

Conclusion

A large meta-analysis of treatment outcome research for complex mental disorders, including patients with personality disorders, found that long-term psychodynamic psychotherapy showed significantly better results in overall effectiveness, target problems, and personality functioning when compared to shorter forms of treatment (Leichsenring and Rabung 2008). Antisocial personality disorder in the mild to moderate psychopathic range is a reasonable targeted problem for both psychodynamic researchers and clinicians. With careful diagnostic assessment, the consideration of psychodynamic principles, the application of psychodynamic techniques, and continuous observation of countertransference, there is room for therapeutic hope.

Key Clinical Concepts

- ◆ Measurement of the severity of psychopathy in any antisocial patient is critical to successful treatment and risk management.
- ◆ The modality of therapy (group, family, individual, milieu) is distinguished from the theoretical approach or model for treatment (CBT, MBT, TFP, psychodynamic psychotherapy).
- ◆ Countertransference understanding is critical to treatment success.
- ◆ Forensic psychotherapy presumes the treatability of certain mildly to moderately psychopathic patients, and this view is supported by the treatment outcome research when such patients are compared with the negative treatment outcome data for severely psychopathic patients.
- ◆ The setting for treatment must always be able to safely contain the psychopathology of the patient.

Suggested Readings

Meloy JR: Antisocial personality disorder, in Gabbard's Treatments of Psychiatric Disorders, 4th Edition. Edited by Gabbard GO. Washington, DC, American Psychiatric Publishing, 2007, pp 775–790

Meloy JR, Reavis J: Dangerous cases: when treatment is not an option, in Severe Personality Disorders: Everyday Issues in Clinical Practice. Edited by van Luyn B, Akhtar S, Livesley J. Cambridge, UK, Cambridge University Press, 2007, pp 137–195

References

Allen JG, Fonagy P, Bateman AW: Mentalizing in Clinical Practice. Washington, DC, American Psychiatric Publishing, 2008

Andrews DA, Bonta J, Hoge RD: Classification for effective rehabilitation: rediscovering psychology. Crim Justice Behav 17:19–52, 1990

Baron-Cohen S: The empathizing system: a revision of the 1994 model of the mindreading system, in Origins of the Social Mind: Evolutionary Psychology and Child Development. Edited by Ellis BJ, Bjorklund DF. New York, Guilford, 2005, pp 468–492

Bateman A: Narcissism and its relation to violence and suicide, in Psychoanalytic Understanding of Violence and Suicide. Edited by Perelberg R. London, Routledge, 1999, pp 109–124

Bateman A, Fonagy P: Psychotherapy for Borderline Personality Disorder: Mentalization-Based Treatment. Oxford, UK, Oxford University Press, 2004

Bateman A, Fonagy P: Mentalization-Based Treatment for Borderline Personality Disorder: A Practical Guide. Oxford, UK, Oxford University Press, 2006

Beech A, Fisher D, Beckett R: An Evaluation of the Prison Sex Offender Treatment Programme. London, HMSO, 1999

Beech A, Erikson M, Friendship C, et al: A Six-Year Follow-Up of Men Going Through Probation-Based Sex Offender Treatment Programmes. London, HMSO, 2001

Bion WR: Learning From Experience (1962). London, Karnac Books, 1984

Book A, Quinsey V, Langford D: Psychopathy and the perception of affect and vulnerability. Crim Justice Behav 34:531–544, 2007

Cartwright D: Psychoanalysis, Violence and Rage-Type Murder. New York, Brunner-Routledge, 2002

Clarkin JF, Yeomans FE, Kernberg OF: Psychotherapy for Borderline Personality: Focusing on Object Relations. Washington, DC, American Psychiatric Publishing, 2006

Cleckley H: The Mask of Sanity. St Louis, MO, Mosby, 1941

Cordess C, Cox M (eds): Forensic Psychotherapy: Crime, Psychodynamics and the Offender Patient. London, Jessica Kingsley, 1996

Cox M: Group psychotherapy in a secure setting. Proc R Soc Med 69:215–220, 1976

Davies R: Technique in the interpretation of the manifest attack on the analyst, in Psychoanalytic Understanding of Violence and Suicide. Edited by Perelberg R. London, Routledge, 1999, pp 125–144

Department of Health and Home Office: Managing Dangerous People With Severe Personality Disorder: Proposals for Policy Development. London, Home Office and Department of Health, 1999

Dolan B, Coid J (eds): Psychopathic and Antisocial Personality Disorders. London, Gaskell, 1993

Dowsett J, Craissati J: Managing Personality Disordered Offenders in the Community: A Psychological Approach. New York, Routledge, 2008

Fonagy P, Target M: Towards understanding violence: the use of the body and the role of the father, in Psychoanalytic Understanding of Violence and Suicide. Edited by Perelberg R. London, Routledge, 1999, pp 51–72

Foulkes S: Introduction to Group-Analytic Psychotherapy (1948). London, Karnac, 1983

Foulkes S: Therapeutic Group Analysis. London, George Allen & Unwin, 1964

Freud S: Some character types met with in psychoanalytic work, I: the exceptions (1916), in The Standard Edition of the Complete Psychological Works of Sigmund Freud, Vol 14. Translated and edited by Strachey J. London, Hogarth Press, 1957, pp 309–315

Friedman A, Lewak R, Nichols D, et al: Psychological Assessment With the MMPI-2. Mahwah, NJ, Erlbaum, 2001

Friendship C, Blud L, Erikson M, et al: An Evaluation of Cognitive Behavioural Treatment for Prisoners (Home Office Research Findings, No 161). London, Home Office, 2002

Gabbard GO: Psychodynamic Psychiatry in Clinical Practice, 4th Edition. Washington, DC, American Psychiatric Publishing, 2005

Gacono C, Meloy JR: Rorschach Assessment of Aggressive and Psychopathic Personalities. Hillsdale, NJ, Erlbaum, 1994

Gaddini E: A Psychoanalytic Theory of Infantile Experience. London, Routledge, 1992

Gendreau P, Ross R: Revivification of rehabilitation: evidence from the 1980s. Justice Quarterly 4:349–407, 1987

Gill M: Psychoanalysis and exploratory psychotherapy. J Am Psychoanal Assoc 2:771–797, 1954

Glasser M: Aggression and sadism in the perversions, in Sexual Deviation, 3rd Edition. Edited by Rosen I. Oxford, UK, Oxford University Press, 1996, pp 279–299

Gunn J: Introduction: what is forensic psychiatry? Crim Behav Ment Health 14 (suppl 1): S1–S5, 2004

Hare RD: Manual for the Psychopathy Checklist–Revised, 2nd Edition. Toronto, Ontario, Canada, Multi-Health Systems, 2003

Harris GT, Rice ME, Cormier CA: Psychopathy and violent recidivism. Law Hum Behav 5:625–637, 1991

Harris GT, Rice ME, Cormier CA: Psychopaths: is a therapeutic community therapeutic? Therapeutic Communities 15:283–299, 1994

Jones M: A Study of Therapeutic Communities. London, Tavistock, 1952

Kazdin AE: Conduct Disorders in Childhood and Adolescence. Thousand Oaks, CA, Sage, 1995

Kernberg OF: Severe Personality Disorders: Psychotherapeutic Strategies. New Haven, CT, Yale University Press, 1984

Kernberg OF, Yeomans FE, Clarkin JF, et al: Transference focused psychotherapy: overview and update. Int J Psychoanal 89:601–620, 2008

Klein M: Notes on some schizoid mechanisms, in Envy and Gratitude. London, Hogarth, 1946, pp 1–24

Leichsenring F, Rabung S: Effectiveness of long-term psychoanalytic psychotherapy: a meta-analysis. JAMA 300:1551–1565, 2008

Linehan MM: Cognitive-Behavioral Treatment of Borderline Personality Disorder. New York, Guilford, 1993

Livesley WJ: Practical Management of Personality Disorder. New York, Guilford, 2003

Livesley WJ: Introduction to the special feature on recent progress in the treatment of personality disorder. J Pers Disord 18:1–2, 2004

Main TF: The concept of the therapeutic community: its variations and vicissitudes, in The Evolution of Group Analysis. Edited by Pines M. London, Routledge & Kegan Paul, 1983

McGauley G, Adshead G, Sarkar S: Psychotherapy of psychopathic disorders, in The International Handbook of Psychopathic Disorders and the Law: Diagnosis and Treatment, Vol 1. Edited by Felthouse A, Sass H. New York, Wiley, 2007, pp 449–466

Meloy JR: The Psychopathic Mind: Origins, Dynamics and Treatment. Northvale, NJ, Jason Aronson, 1988

Meloy JR: Violent Attachments. Northvale, NJ, Jason Aronson, 1992

Meloy JR: Antisocial personality disorder, in Treatments of Psychiatric Disorders, 2nd Edition, Vol 2. Edited by Gabbard GO. Washington, DC, American Psychiatric Press, 1995, pp 2273–2290

Meloy JR (ed): The Mark of Cain: Psychoanalytic Insight and the Psychopath. Hillsdale, NJ, Analytic Press, 2001

Meloy JR: Pathologies of attachment, violence, and criminality, in Handbook of Psychology, Vol 11: Forensic Psychology. Edited by Goldstein A. New York, Wiley, 2002, pp 509–526

Meloy JR: Antisocial personality disorder, in Gabbard's Treatments of Psychiatric Disorders, 4th Edition. Edited by Gabbard GO. Washington, DC, American Psychiatric Publishing, 2007, pp 775–790

Meloy JR, Meloy MJ: Autonomic arousal in the presence of psychopathy: a survey of mental health and criminal justice professionals. Journal of Threat Assessment 2:21–33, 2002

Minne C: Psychoanalytic aspects to the risk of containment of dangerous patients treated in high security, in Lectures on Perversion and Delinquency: The Portman Papers. Edited by Morgan D, Ruszczynski S. London, Karnac, 2007

National Institute for Health and Clinical Excellence (NICE): Antisocial Personality Disorder: Treatment, Management, and Prevention. 2009. Available at: http://www.nice.org.uk/nicemedia/pdf/APSDFullVersionConsultation.pdf. Accessed October 6, 2009.

Norton K, McGauley GA: The counselling transaction, in Counselling Difficult Clients. Edited by Norton K, McGauley GA. London, Sage, 1998, pp 1–15

Ogloff JR, Wong S, Greenwood A: Treating criminal psychopaths in a therapeutic community program. Behav Sci Law 8:181–190, 1990

Parsons T: The Social System. Glencoe, IL, Free Press, 1951

Patrick C (ed): Handbook of Psychopathy. New York, Guilford, 2006

Pine F: Some impressions regarding conflict, defect, and deficit. Psychoanal Study Child 49:222–240, 1994

Salekin R: Psychopathy and therapeutic pessimism: clinical lore or clinical reality? Clin Psychol Rev 22:79–112, 2002

Saunders DG: Feminist-cognitive-behavioral and process-psychodynamic treatment for men who batter: interaction of abuser traits and treatment models. Violence Vict 11:393–414, 1996

Schlapobersky J: A group-analytic perspective: from the speech of hands to the language of words, in Forensic Psychotherapy: Crime, Psychodynamics and the Offender Patient. Edited by Cordess C, Cox M. Philadelphia, PA, Jessica Kingsley, 1996, pp 227–244

Skeem J, Monahan J, Mulvey E: Psychopathy, treatment involvement, and subsequent violence among civil psychiatric patients. Law Hum Behav 26:577–603, 2002

Steiner J: Patient-centered and analyst-centered interpretations: some implications of containment and countertransference. Psychoanalytic Inquiry 14:406–422, 1994

Sutker P, Bugg F, West J: Antisocial personality disorder, in Comprehensive Handbook of Psychopathology, 2nd Edition. Edited by Sutger P, Adams H. New York, Plenum, 1993, pp 337–369

Tyson P: Neurosis in childhood and in psychoanalysis: a developmental reformulation. J Am Psychoanal Assoc 44:143–165, 1996

Welldon E: Group-analytic psychotherapy in an out-patient setting, in Forensic Psychotherapy: Crime, Psychodynamics and the Offender Patient. Edited by Cordess C, Cox M. London and Philadelphia, Jessica Kingsley, 1996, pp 63–82

Winnicott DW: Ego distortion in terms of true or false self (1960), in The Maturational Processes and the Facilitating Environment. London, Karnac Books, 1990, pp 140–152

Winnicott DW: Transitional objects and transitional phenomena (1951), in Collected Papers: Through Paediatrics to Psycho-Analysis. London, Karnac Books, 1991, pp 229–242

Wong S, Gordon A: Violence Risk Scale. Saskatchewan, Canada, Department of Psychiatric Research, Regional Psychiatric Centre, Solicitor General of Canada, 2000

Wong S, Gordon A: Violence Risk Scale. Saskatchewan, Canada, Department of Psychiatric Research, Regional Psychiatric Centre, Solicitor General of Canada, 2004

Wong S, Hare R: Guidelines for a Psychopathy Treatment Program. Toronto, Ontario, Canada, Multi-Health Systems, 2005

Yakeley J: Psychoanalytic contributions to risk assessment and management, in Lectures on Perversion and Delinquency: The Portman Papers. Edited by Morgan D, Ruszczynski S. London, Karnac Books, 2007

Yang Y, Glenn A, Raine A: Brain abnormalities in antisocial individuals: implications for the law. Behav Sci Law 26:65–84, 2008

Young JE, Klosko JS, Weishaar ME: Schema Therapy: A Practitioner's Guide. New York, Guilford, 2003

CHAPTER 12

Cluster C Personality Disorders

Prevalence, Phenomenology, Treatment Effects, and Principles of Treatment

Martin Svartberg, M.D., Ph.D.
Leigh McCullough, Ph.D.

As defined by DSM-IV-TR (American Psychiatric Association 2000), the Cluster C personality disorders comprise the avoidant (AVPD), the dependent (DPD), and the obsessive-compulsive personality disorder (OCPD). As a group, they are the most prevalent personality disorders in the general population and in the outpatient clinical setting. In the largest and most recent and rigorous community survey of personality disorders, Torgersen et al. (2001) found that 9.4% of the population (Oslo, Norway) met DSM-III-R (American Psychiatric Association 1987) criteria for any of the Cluster C personality disorders. The specific prevalence rates were 5.0% for AVPD, 1.5% for DPD, and 2.0% for OCPD. Except for AVPD, these rates were largely in line with 10 previous surveys that found median rates to be 1.2%, 1.25%, and 2.15%, respectively. Torgersen et al. (2001) also found that OCPD was more frequently observed among men than among women and in those with more than less education.

In outpatient clinical samples, investigators have used semistructured interviews in three clinical surveys to diagnose DSM personality disorders. Among 298 patients in a general outpatient clinic in Oslo, Alnaes and Torgersen (1988) found that DSM-III (American Psychiatric Association 1980) prevalence rates were 55% for AVPD, 47% for DPD, and 20% for OCPD, whereas among 100 applicants for outpatient psychoanalysis in New York City, Oldham et al. (1995) found that 16% met DSM-III-R criteria for AVPD, 6% for DPD, and 10% for OCPD. Finally, in a large New England outpatient sample ($N=859$), Zimmerman et al. (2005) observed that 21.4% of the patients met DSM-IV (American Psychiatric Association 1994) criteria for any Cluster C personality disorder; rates for the specific disorders were 14.7% for AVPD, 1.4% for DPD, and 8.7% for OCPD.

Cluster C personality disorders tend to co-occur. Stuart et al. (1998) found that more than 50% of inpatients and outpatients with either DPD, OCPD, or passive-aggressive personality disorder also met DSM-III-R criteria for AVPD. However, Zimmerman et al. (2005) observed that AVPD and OCPD were much more strongly associated with schizoid personality disorder, whereas DPD was associated with borderline personality disorder rather than with any of the other Cluster C personality disorders. In that same survey, 1) the presence of generalized anxiety disorder was associated with significantly high rates of each of the Cluster C personality disorders, 2) panic disorder and social phobia were associated with significantly high rates of AVPD and OCPD, and 3) major depression was associated with significantly high rates of AVPD and DPD. In a study of anxiety disorders, Massion et al. (2002) observed high Axis I and Axis II comorbidity rates for generalized anxiety disorder (AVPD: 20%, DPD: 10%, OCPD: 9%) and social phobia (AVPD: 35%, DPD: 6%, OCPD: 7%) but lower rates for panic disorder (AVPD: 14%, DPD: 3%, OCPD: 3%). AVPD and social phobia are known to co-occur to a high degree, and debate has been ongoing for many years as to whether the two disorders are truly distinct. Hummelen et al. (2007) found that patients with social phobia without AVPD had higher levels of global functioning and lower levels of symptom distress and interpersonal problems than did AVPD patients without social phobia; however, the two groups were similar with respect to degree of social anxiety and introversion. AVPD was also more strongly associated with having an eating disorder, additional personality disorder criteria, and suicidality.

Diagnosis: Core Features, Clinical Course, and Psychodynamic Conceptualization

In a recent factor analytic study of the DSM-IV-TR personality disorder criteria, Fossati et al. (2006) found that the AVPD, DPD, and OCPD grouped together, sharing a common dimension often termed fearfulness. Core fears comprise fear of negative evaluation in the AVPD patient, fear of separation in the DPD patient, and fear of not having personal and interpersonal control in the OCPD patient.

AVOIDANT PERSONALITY DISORDER

Originally described and conceptualized in the tradition of trait psychology and interpersonal circumplexes within academic psychology (Millon et al. 1996), AVPD is characterized in DSM-IV-TR by a pervasive and enduring pattern of social inhibition, feelings of inadequacy, and hypersensitivity to negative evaluation indicated by specific diagnostic criteria such as interpersonal avoidance; fear of shame or ridicule; fear of criticism, rejection, or disapproval; and a view of self as inadequate, socially inept, inferior, or personally unappealing to others. As with most personality disorders, some of the diagnostic features can be understood as personality traits, whereas others can be seen as maladaptive behaviors assumed to be relatively stable over time.

Shea et al. (2002) found that 56% of 82 AVPD patients continued to meet full criteria 1 year after initial assessment and various treatments, whereas Grilo et al. (2004), who used different methodology in the same patient sample, found remission rates over 24 months to be 31%. Furthermore, McGlashan et al. (2005) observed in the same sample that the most prevalent and enduring features were views of self as inadequate or socially inept, whereas the least prevalent and enduring features were avoidance of interpersonal jobs or embarrassing situations. The former features were regarded as traitlike, linked to personality, and possibly to temperamental and genetic risk factors, whereas the latter features were regarded as more behavioral and reactive and were likely those that remitted in the Grilo et al. study. Both types of features were seen as key to defining AVPD. In another study of the stability and course of personality disorders, Lenzenweger et al. (2004) estimated that on average it would take about 11 years for a diagnosis of AVPD to decrease by one diagnostic criterion (0.09 criterion per year).

Because AVPD as a separate diagnostic entity is relatively new, was originally developed in academic psychology, and has been defined primarily in the DSM system, it has not been much conceptualized in the psychodynamic tradition. However, a high degree of overlap has been noted between the core diagnostic features of AVPD and avoidant attachment insecurity (Bartholomew et al. 2001). On the basis of internalized representations of the self with the attachment figure (structuralized as internal working models), AVPD can be conceptualized as a combination of a negative view of self (as inadequate, inferior, socially inept, or unappealing, and, by implication, unlovable) and a negative view of others (as critical, rejecting, or disapproving, and, by implication, uncaring and unavailable). This combination of negative views of self and others is commonly defined as fearful attachment (Bartholomew et al. 2001) and manifests subjectively as high attachment anxiety (fear of ridicule, rejection, or negative evaluation) and behaviorally as avoidance of closeness and keeping of a safe distance in interpersonal relationships (e.g., restraining and inhibiting oneself). Fearful attachment has been shown to be associated with early rejection by cold and unloving caregivers, unresolved loss, and childhood abuse (Bartholomew et al. 2001), leaving a strong desire in the average AVPD patient for unconditional love and acceptance within an intimate relationship. In the parlance of the more traditional psychodynamic conflict model, this desire or wish for love and acceptance in a close and intimate relationship has become conflicted and a source of anxiety and shame because its expression repeatedly has been associated with criticism, ridicule, rejection, or disapproval by significant others. Anxiety or shame, both then and now, gives rise to the characteristic defensive behaviors of interpersonal avoidance, social inhibition, and constriction of affect, the effects of which tend to diminish the wish for further closeness.

DEPENDENT PERSONALITY DISORDER

In DSM-IV-TR, the typical DPD patient is characterized by a pervasive and excessive need to be taken care of that leads to submissive and clinging behavior and fears of separation indicated by specific criteria that include dependency on a partner for everyday decision making and the taking of responsibility and initiatives; fears of being left to care for self and cope on one's own; and a prototypical interpersonal style characterized by compliant, docile, submissive, helpless, and clinging behaviors bordering in the extreme case on self-effacement and exploitability. Although the interpersonal dimension of dependency is well represented in DSM, the manual has been criticized for not endorsing the dimension of attachment strongly enough (Livesley et al. 1990). With respect to the stability and course of the diagnostic criteria, Lenzenweger et al. (2004) estimated that on average it would take about

11 years for a diagnosis of DPD to decrease by one diagnostic criterion (0.09 criterion per year), which is the same rate as for AVPD.

In light of the general DSM-IV-TR criterion of a pervasive and excessive need to be taken care of, DPD lends itself more easily than any other personality disorder to being conceptualized as an attachment disorder. The internalized representations of the self with the attachment figure can, in the typical DPD patient, be more specifically conceptualized as constituting a negative view of self (as instrumentally incompetent, lacking in self-confidence, needy, and helpless) (Benjamin 2003; PDM Task Force 2006), whereas the view of others is basically ambivalent, ranging from perceiving the other as a powerful and effective provider of security, nurturance, and support (when securely attached) to perceiving the other as an untrustworthy attachment figure (when attachment is threatened). When self and others are viewed together, DPD overlaps with the preoccupied attachment strategy or category (negative view of self, positive view of others) when attachment is not threatened and with the fearful strategy (negative views of self and others) when attachment is threatened (Bartholomew et al. 2001). Unlike the prototypical preoccupied strategy of the histrionic and borderline personality disorders, DPD patients, in response to an attachment threat, tend to deal with their attachment anxiety not in an active, demanding, and explicitly approach-oriented way but rather in a passive way through the display of helplessness, sulkiness, clinginess, and depressive affects.

In one of the few empirical investigations of pathological dependency, Bornstein (2005) found an association between overprotective or authoritarian parenting and dependency in the adult. In explaining this association, Benjamin (2003) maintained that the parents of the DPD patient failed to stop nurturing or wean when it became developmentally appropriate. Because it represents interpersonal control (Benjamin 2003), age-inappropriate nurturance may be perceived as degrading and humiliating in the growing child and fosters submissive behaviors and lack of competence and independence, which are typical in DPD patients.

In the language of a psychodynamic conflict model, the DPD patient's need and wish for care and protection are seen as invariably threatened in an ongoing close relationship, eliciting attachment anxiety, which gives rise to maladaptive attachment behaviors such as clinging and helplessness. Even though such behaviors may serve to dampen anxiety in the first place, they also may, over time, run the risk of alienating the partner, confronting the DPD patient with a serious attachment dilemma.

OBSESSIVE-COMPULSIVE PERSONALITY DISORDER

Once described by Wilhelm Reich (1933) as "living machines," typical OCPD patients are characterized in DSM-IV-TR by a pervasive pattern of preoccupation with orderliness, mental and interpersonal control, and perfectionism, indicated by specific criteria that include rigidity and strictness about morality, values, and rules; excessive concern with work and productivity, money spending, and the discarding of worthless objects; and reluctance to delegate tasks.

Shea et al. (2002) found that 42% of OCPD patients continued to meet full criteria 1 year after initial assessment, whereas Grilo et al. (2004), who used different methodology in the same patient sample, found remission rates over 24 months to be 38%. McGlashan et al. (2005) studied the same sample and found that the most prevalent and stable criteria were rigidity, problems delegating, and perfectionism (regarded as traitlike criteria), whereas the least prevalent and stable criteria were miserliness and strict morality (regarded as symptomatic behaviors). The authors speculated that the traitlike criteria contain "elements of withholding, resistance to change, and the need to control" and possibly relate to "the neurobiology of aggressive control." Furthermore, Lenzenweger et al. (2004) estimated that, on average, it would take about 8 years for a diagnosis of OCPD to decrease by one diagnostic criterion (0.12 criterion per year), which is somewhat faster than for AVPD and DPD. Finally, in a recent factor analytic study of all personality disorder criteria, Hummelen et al. (2008) found that the first dimension to emerge was *perfectionism*, represented by the OCPD criteria "preoccupation with orderliness" and "perfectionism," whereas the second dimension was termed *aggressiveness* and was represented by the two OCPD criteria "problems delegating" and "stubbornness and rigidity" as well as criteria from some other personality disorders. As can be seen, the three traitlike criteria found by McGlashan et al. (2005) (rigidity, problems delegating, and perfectionism) are also the OCPD criteria that constitute the first two dimensions in the Hummelen et al. study, pointing to the centrality of perfectionism and aggressive control in the OCPD patient.

Unlike AVPD and DPD, OCPD has for a long time been subject to psychodynamic conceptualizations in general and to conflict formulations in particular. Traditionally, conflicts over aggressive urges and feelings have been viewed as the most central (PDM Task Force 2006). If regarded as not legitimate by the individual, these feelings tend to be frightening and to evoke fears of losing self-control, making a mistake, or becoming the target of blame and guilt; these fears are easily associated with a sense of being not-nice, disobedient, improper, or poorly controlled. Such feelings of fear and guilt tend to give rise to defensive behaviors such as interpersonal distancing, excessive self-discipline, restraint of feelings, harsh self-criticism, and undoing. Many OCPD patients end up feeling lonely, isolated, and alienated, and with an impoverished emotional life. Despite that and because they tend to distance themselves from significant others and deny the effect of negative interpersonal experiences, they are usually able to maintain a positive sense of self (Bartholomew et al. 2001). In terms of their attachment style, many OCPD patients would be characterized as dismissing, in that they combine a positive view of self (as self-reliant, competent, righteous, proper) with a negative view of others (as potentially critical, blaming, dominant). As pointed out by Bartholomew et al. (2001), they tend to come across as overly independent and, when distressed, rely on themselves rather than the support of others. A dismissing attachment style may be considered "a successful form of adaptation" because research shows that it is associated with "high self-esteem and low levels of distress and depression," albeit at the cost of "low relationship satisfaction" (Bartholomew et al. 2001).

Effects of Psychodynamic Psychotherapy

The effects of individual psychodynamic psychotherapy with Cluster C patients have been examined empirically in only a handful of studies. They comprise two randomized controlled trials of Cluster C patients only (Emmelkamp et al. 2006; Svartberg et al. 2004), two randomized controlled trials of mostly Cluster C patients (Vinnars et al. 2005; Winston et al. 1994), one naturalistic study of AVPD and OCPD patients (Barber et al. 1997), and one randomized controlled trial, originally conducted to study the effect on depressed patients, of a subsample of Cluster C patients who were analyzed separately (Hardy et al. 1995).

Svartberg et al. (2004) compared the effectiveness of short-term dynamic psychotherapy (STDP) with that of cognitive therapy for 50 outpatients who received 40 weekly sessions of either treatment and met criteria for one or more Cluster C personality disorders and not for any other personality disorders. The most common Axis I diagnoses were major depression, generalized anxiety disorder, and social phobia, and AVPD was the most frequently diagnosed personality disorder (62%), followed by OCPD (34%) and DPD (20%). Approximately one-quarter of the patients met criteria for more than one personality disorder. McCullough-Vaillant's (1997) STDP model, which is discussed in detail later, was used. The cognitive therapy model was based on Beck and Freeman's (1990) book, which emphasizes initial work with coexisting Axis I problems, identification and evaluation of key negative automatic thoughts, use of guided imagery and homework assignments, and specific emotion-focused techniques to dispute and restructure core maladaptive beliefs. Therapists were experienced full-time clinicians who received manual-guided supervision. Patients in both conditions showed statistically significant improvements on measures of symptom distress, interpersonal problems, and core Cluster C personality functioning during treatment as well during a 2-year follow-up period. No statistically significant differences were seen between STDP and cognitive therapy on any measure during any period. However, only in patients receiving STDP did symptoms improve significantly after treatment, and significantly more STDP patients had improved in personality functioning at 2-year follow-up than at posttreatment, but this was not the case for patients who received cognitive therapy. In terms of clinically significant change, 54% of STDP patients and 42% of cognitive therapy patients had recovered symptomatically or returned to normal functioning at 2-year follow-up, whereas approximately 40% of patients in both conditions recovered with respect to interpersonal problems and personality functioning. In light of these results, both STDP modeled after McCullough-Vaillant and cognitive therapy modeled after Beck and Freeman have a place in the treatment of Cluster C personality disorders.

Emmelkamp et al. (2006) randomly assigned 62 patients with AVPD to either 20-session cognitive-behavioral therapy (CBT), 20-session brief dynamic therapy (BDT), or a wait-list control condition (WLC). CBT was modeled after Beck and Freeman (1990) and Emmelkamp et al. (1992). Informed by Malan's psychodynamic conflict model and the supportive module of Luborsky's (1984) supportive-expressive model, therapists in the BDT condition worked primarily to strengthen the alliance and restructure defenses and affects. All therapists had at least 5 years of postgraduate clinical experience.

Patients in both treatment conditions showed statistically significant improvements during treatment on measures of anxiety symptoms; avoidant behaviors; and core beliefs related to avoidance, dependency, and, for CBT patients only, obsessive-compulsiveness. For CBT, improvements were associated with large effect sizes (5 of 6), and for BDT, improvements were associated with small (2), medium (2), and large (2) effect sizes. The effects of CBT were superior to those of WLC in terms of avoidant beliefs and avoidant behaviors and to those of BDT on all measures, whereas the effects of BDT were not superior to those of WLC. I (the first author, M.S.) calculated between-group effects to be of medium size, implying that the average improvement rate among CBT patients was twice that of the improvement rate among BDT patients

(Rosenthal 1984). At 6-month follow-up, gains were generally maintained; however, the effects of CBT were superior to those of BDT for all types of core beliefs and AVPD remission rates. Of the BDT patients, 36% met AVPD criteria at 6-month follow-up, compared with only 9% of the CBT patients. These remission rates of 64% and 91%, respectively, are truly impressive and exceed greatly those found in studies of the disorder's natural course (Grilo et al. 2004; Shea et al. 2002). Note, however, that the diagnostician was not blind to treatment groups. Finally, only BDT patients showed significant change in obsessive beliefs during the follow-up period. The overall results led the authors to conclude that CBT was superior to WLC and BDT and that BDT was not superior to WLC.

In a randomized controlled trial, Winston et al. (1994) compared the effectiveness of STDP ($n=25$) with that of brief adaptive psychotherapy (BAP; $n=30$), which is a moderately confrontive form of dynamic therapy, and with wait-list control subjects ($n=26$). Of the patient sample, 77% had either a Cluster C personality disorder or a personality disorder not otherwise specified (PD NOS) with predominantly Cluster C features, and the remaining patients had mostly histrionic personality disorder or PD NOS. Based on principles developed by Davanloo (1980), STDP is characterized by very active confrontation of defenses, anxiety, and unconscious impulses as well as the eliciting of painful affect. Although the BAP therapist is also rather active, he or she focuses primary attention on cognitive aspects of the patient's core maladaptive pattern as manifested in past and present relationships. Patients in both conditions received 40 weekly sessions and were treated by experienced psychiatrists, psychologists, and social workers. Results showed that patients in both conditions made significant and equivalent improvements on measures of symptom distress, social functioning, and target complaints; that treated patients did significantly better than did control subjects; and that gains were maintained at 1.5-year follow-up.

Vinnars et al. (2005) randomly assigned 156 outpatients to 40-session supportive-expressive psychotherapy (Luborsky 1984) or 21-session community-delivered psychodynamic psychotherapy (with an emphasis on supportive techniques). Although one-fourth of the sample met criteria for borderline personality disorder and some met criteria for Cluster A and other Cluster B diagnoses, the great majority of patients had a diagnosis of either Cluster C or passive-aggressive and depressive personality disorders. In supportive-expressive psychotherapy, the therapist initially uncovers the patient's main unconscious wishes, response of the other, and response of self (i.e., the core conflictual relationship theme), which becomes the central focus of the therapist's interventions. Results showed that patients in both treatments made significant and equivalent improvements between pretreatment and 1 year posttreatment in terms of number of Axis II criteria, symptom distress, and global functioning. Improvements were associated with large and medium-large effect sizes. Remission rates for the sample as a whole were 33.6% and 46.8% at termination and 1-year follow-up, respectively, and were not significantly different between treatment groups.

In a naturalistically designed study, the effectiveness of a 52-session supportive-expressive psychotherapy (Luborsky 1984) was examined at posttreatment for 24 AVPD and 14 OCPD patients. Both categories of patients made significant improvements on measures of anxiety, depression, personality functioning, interpersonal problems, and global functioning. Additionally, remission rates for AVPD were 61% and for OCPD were 85% at termination. Finally, in a randomized controlled trial originally designed to study the effectiveness of 8- and 16-session psychodynamic-interpersonal psychotherapy and 8- and 16-session CBT for depressed patients, a subsample of 27 patients with Cluster C personality disorders was analyzed separately. The psychodynamic-interpersonal treatment approach "was a relationship-oriented treatment based on Hobson's Conversational Model" (Hobson 1985, p. 999), in which "the therapeutic relationship is used as a vehicle for understanding and modifying relationship disturbances" (p. 999). Results showed that patients in both conditions made significant and large-sized improvements between pretreatment and 1-year follow-up in terms of depression, general symptoms, self-esteem, and interpersonal problems. In addition, patients with a personality disorder had a significantly poorer outcome in psychodynamic-interpersonal psychotherapy than did those without a personality disorder, whereas patients with and without personality disorder fared equally well in CBT. Sixteen-session treatments were not more effective than 8-session treatments. The results led the authors to conclude that brief psychodynamic-interpersonal therapies were "relatively less effective in the presence of a personality disorder, whereas cognitive-behavioral therapies were similarly effective regardless of these Axis II diagnoses" (p. 1002).

To conclude, six studies of psychodynamic psychotherapy of brief duration (8–52 sessions), mostly based on principles originally developed by Malan and Luborsky, reported statistically and clinically significant improvements for Cluster C patients on a variety of outcome measures, and gains generally were maintained or increased after treatment. In one study, CBT was superior to 20-session psychodynamic psychotherapy in the treatment of AVPD. In another study, 8- and 16-session psychodynamic-interpersonal therapies did more poorly in the treatment of patients with than without personality disorder, whereas CBT did equally well with these two patient groups. The findings of these two studies must be replicated before any treatment recommendations can be made.

Principles of Psychodynamic Psychotherapy With Cluster C Patients

The therapy model presented in this chapter is the affect-focused and anxiety-regulating model of STDP that was developed by the second author (L.M.) and empirically examined in patients with Cluster C personality disorders by the first author (M.S.). This model was based on Malan's conceptual schema of the Two Triangles representing the "universal principle of psychodynamic psychotherapy" (i.e., defenses and anxieties block the expression of true feeling). Thus, McCullough's treatment model is fundamentally psychodynamic with a major emphasis on psychodynamic conflict, but psychotherapeutic change is conceptualized in learning theory terms, as desensitization of affect conflicts or "affect phobias"; and the main treatment goal is to improve a patient's "affective capacity" to resolve problems in living.

This STDP model and the affect phobia conceptualization of change have been described in great detail in other sources (e.g., McCullough and McGill 2009; McCullough et al. 1991, 2003; McCullough-Vaillant 1994, 1997). Therefore, we present an overview of the affect-focused model as specifically adapted to Cluster C, with annotated transcripts of cases to illustrate how theory is put into practice.

FOCUS ON AFFECT IN SHORT-TERM DYNAMIC PSYCHOTHERAPY

STDP theory hypothesizes that most patients' problems can be traced to conflicts or fears surrounding feelings (Davanloo 1980, 1988; Malan 1963, 1979; McCullough 1991, 1999; McCullough and Andrews 2001; McCullough et al. 2003). Psychodynamic conflict is hypothesized to result from a conflict between 1) feelings such as grief, anger, excitement, or compassion that *activate* a response and 2) feelings such as anxiety or guilt that *inhibit*, hinder, or impede responses. When these two affect or motivational systems are in conflict, defenses emerge as a "compromise response" (in psychodynamic language) or as a "phobic avoidance response" (in learning theory terms).

Thus, the concept of affect phobia is a translation of the concept of psychodynamic conflict into the language of learning theory and behavior therapy. For example, affect conflicts or affect phobias that underlie unresolved losses might be expressed as: "If I cry in front of you [activation], I'll look weak and disgusting [inhibition]!" The affect phobia underlying victimization or masochism might be: "I don't try to speak up [activation] because I don't deserve to [inhibition]." For the problem of loneliness or social isolation, an affect phobia could be: "I closed my heart years ago [defense] and will never love again [activation] because I can't bear that much pain [inhibition]." Even deficit pathology presents as an affect conflict or phobia resulting from shame; the problem of low self-esteem or poor self-worth may take the following form: "I feel too worthless and ashamed [inhibition] to feel good about myself [activation]." (For a full discussion of conflict and deficit pathology in affect phobias, see McCullough-Vaillant 1997, pp. 40–45.)

The term *desensitization* refers to the process of exposure and extinction to break the conditioned association of "activating" affects (sadness/grief, anger, closeness, self-regard) that have become "sensitized" because of their conditioned association with inhibitory affects (e.g., anxiety, guilt, shame, pain, disgust). Anger can be blocked by anxiety. Grief can be blocked by pain. Excitement can be blocked by shame. The main goal of STDP is to improve the patient's *affective capacity* so that, for example, patients will be activated or motivated to grieve a loss, speak up, open their heart, or feel deserving without crippling effects of shame, guilt, or anxiety.

SHORT-TERM DYNAMIC PSYCHOTHERAPY DEVELOPED FOR ALL AXIS I DISORDERS, NOT ONLY CLUSTER C

This STDP model was designed for a wide range of Axis I and Axis II disorders, with diagnostic-specific adaptations carefully detailed in several publications (McCullough et al. 2003, Chapters 3 and 11; McCullough-Vaillant 1997, Chapter 3). The special focus on Axis II Cluster C patients (in both the Winston et al. [1991, 1994] and the Svartberg et al. 2004 randomized controlled trials) came from a wish to submit this new and potentially powerful therapy to a substantial challenge by treating a sample that was then considered almost intractable to treatment. In the years that have followed, it has become increasingly clear that the STDP method of dealing with entrenched defenses, although useful with Axis I disorders, is particularly well suited for the entrenched defenses of the Cluster C patient. Indeed, preliminary analyses of the Svartberg et al. (2004) trial in our laboratory show that improvement in affective capacity (i.e., increase in the ratio of level of activating affects to level of inhibitory affects) is responsible for reduction in Millon Clinical Multiaxial Inventory Cluster C items at 2-year follow-up, with 11% of the variance accounted for, but is *not* significantly associated with improvement in Cluster A or B items.

MAIN OBJECTIVES OF THE AFFECT PHOBIA MODEL AS ADAPTED TO CLUSTER C DISORDERS

In this subsection we outline the three main objectives of this STDP model in resolving affect phobias and guiding patients toward an *optimal affective capacity* (i.e., affects are better tolerated, integrated, and regulated, as well as adaptively expressed). Each of the three objectives is made up of two sub-objectives.

1. *Restructuring defenses:* a) acquiring insight and motivation to change; b) identifying and giving up defensive, maladaptive, and affect-phobic behavior
2. *Restructuring affect through exposure and desensitization:* a) reducing the fear of experiencing and expressing conflicted affect; b) improving the affective capacity in and balance between activating and inhibitory affects
3. *Building an adaptive sense of a) self and b) others.*

Restructuring Defenses

The challenge in Cluster C disorders.   The first objective in the STDP model—defense restructuring—involves 1) identifying or gaining insight into defensive or maladaptive behavior patterns centered around avoidance of feelings or affect phobias and 2) becoming motivated to change them. The greatest challenges in treating Cluster C disorders include breaking through defenses (which are typically unconscious and ego-syntonic) and identifying the affect focus that will resolve the problem at hand.

Building motivation to change the affect phobia.   Giving up maladaptive patterns is an even greater challenge than identifying defensive patterns. The defenses would not have occurred in the first place if there had not been a strong need for them, and that need is often carried into the future. Cognitive interventions are very useful in building the desire to give up defenses; for example, disputing the patient's logic: "What's the worst thing that can happen?"; or pointing out catastrophizing:

"Aren't you expecting something horrible to happen if you stopped the passive withdrawal? Would it really be so bad?" Such interventions help to reduce anxiety and other inhibitory affects such as shame, guilt, and pain, which elicit avoidant or inhibitory responses. The following excerpt from a case shows some of these principles.

THE OFF-PUTTING WOMAN

A 48-year-old successful business manager came to therapy with problems of not being able to build a close relationship with a man. She had never had a relationship with a man that lasted for more than two or three weeks, yet she had friendships with women and was a capable manager. She was addicted to therapy for meeting the dependency needs that she was not able to fulfill in her relationships outside of treatment.

Her brusque and dismissive style was clearly a distancing mechanism that needed to be addressed, but confronting this defense caused a rupture in the therapeutic relationship. After much struggle and exploration, she was able to see this destructive defensive stance.

Confrontation of Defenses Against Closeness	Objective/Intervention
Patient: I have always had troubles being close to men. No relationship has ever worked out.	
Therapist: *(After much discussion about her capability as a manager, and good friendships, it seemed that her problems might be more specific to romantic and intimate relationships.)* I wonder if there is something you might be contributing to the interaction with men that could be pushing them away?	Confront defense of distancing
Pt: *[with irritation]* Why do you say that? I have great relationships with my friends—and my employees. Why are you trying to put that off on me?	Defensive reaction
Th: Well, it probably isn't all you. But I wanted to explore what you might be bringing…	Support; repeat of confrontation
Pt: *[interrupting]* I'm feeling attacked!	Defensive reaction
Th: It must feel awful to feel attacked by your therapist!	Validation, support

Confrontation of Defenses Against Closeness	Objective/Intervention
Pt: It sure does! I am beginning to wonder if I can trust you now. I thought you were on my side!	
Th: In fact, I feel very much on your side. But you have come to me to get help with this lifelong problem. I may be seeing things that you're doing that are getting in your way. If I don't tell you, who is going...?	Self-disclosure, attempt to build motivation
Pt: *[interrupting]* I don't know, but I don't like this. It makes me distrust you, and I was just getting to feel comfortable here.	Defense of projection
Th: We need to look at this feeling of distrust then. Why would my feedback make you distrust me? *(After some exploration...)*	Explore projection
Pt: You remind me of my father. He always attacked me. Everything I did. Nothing I did ever pleased him.	Link to past and father transference
Th: Do I seem like that? If I point out something you do, it feels like a global disapproval of you as a person?	Checking reality of patient-therapist relationship
Pt: Yes. Just like my father.	Transference persists
Th: Sounds awful.	Empathy, validation
Pt: Yes, it was then. And it feels bad now.	
Th: Tell me about it. *(We go into the painful times that her father lost his temper and explore this over several sessions.)*	Exploring painful memories
(Several sessions later, after seeing how jumpy and reactive she had become in response to her father's frequent temper outbursts)	
Th: Can we go back now to you and me? Do I really feel as attacking as your father? Is there anything I do that might seem different from your father?	Undoing projection
Pt: Well, at least you talk to me about it. And you don't seem to get mad.	Rebuilding trust

Confrontation of Defenses Against Closeness	Objective/Intervention
Th: Can you imagine what would happen if I didn't point out your brusqueness? If I kept my mouth shut…It would be abandoning you, wouldn't it?	Attempt to build motivation
Pt: *[silence]* Yeah…I'd never know what I was doing. *[silence]* I don't like hearing it, but I need to hear it.	
Th: Well, it's hard to hear these things.	Validation, support
Pt: Yeah, I can see I really jump at people. Just like my father did! I never saw that before.	Recognizes defensive pattern
Th: Well, it was so reflexive, that it would have been like second nature…and protective to you.	Validation, support
Pt: Yeah. It made me feel strong. But it also has probably pushed away a lot of people. Now I catch myself doing it all the time…and stop it!	Sees benefits and costs of defenses

Affect Restructuring

Exposure to and balancing of activation, inhibition, and expression.
The main objectives in affect restructuring are to expose the patient to the inner experience of underlying but conflicted "activating" affects (motivating approach, appetitive responses) until inhibitory affects (motivating withdrawal or avoidance) are reduced, and affects can be tolerated and expressed to others in a well-modulated and adaptive manner. The fundamental change agents involve 1) exposure to and transforming of the activating affects (the bodily experience of anger, grief, closeness, compassion, excitement, sexual desire, etc.) and 2) response prevention by reducing the amount of associated inhibitory affects (the bodily experience of anxiety, guilt, shame, or pain), as well as the related avoidant defenses. It is worth noting that the exposure is focused on the physiological arousal of the adaptive form of the activating affect. For a thorough desensitization to occur, exposure must not be *only* to thoughts about feelings, words about feelings, or general fantasies or images about feelings.

It is essential that the affect be experienced *in the body* for desensitization to occur, because the physiological arousal of the affect is often the most frightening and overwhelming experience. Our experience in coding affect on videotape has shown that therapists most often leave out the exposure to visceral experience (feelings are talked about but not felt) and thus do not fully desensitize the patient to the conflicted feeling. Examples later in this chapter demonstrate these procedures.

Important distinction between affect regulation and affective capacity. Affect regulation is an extremely popular concept today, but the danger of excessive attention to affect regulation is that it can increase affect phobias, defensive avoidance, and suppression of vital affects. An optimal affective capacity means that affects can be experienced fully and then—and *only* then—regulated appropriately. Many models of treatment are teaching a premature and not sufficiently nuanced version of affect regulation, without making clear that adaptive affects are the "missing capabilities" that need to be identified, and *fully experienced*, and well regulated.

Restructuring the Sense of Self and Others

Maladaptive inner images of self and others are altered by reduction of shame and guilt attached to self-image and increasing (through exposure) the positive self-feelings (such as care and compassion) as well as appropriate feelings toward others. Examples of building an adaptive and compassionate sense of self are interwoven throughout the excerpts of cases later in this chapter, which address specific Cluster C diagnoses. Increasingly we are using the therapist-patient relationship for in vivo exposure and the self-compassion as a means to work through long-standing personality issues.

AFFECT PHOBIAS IN AVOIDANT PERSONALITY DISORDER MODELS

The activating feelings that would resolve AVPD are the capacity for tenderness, care and compassion for others, and self-compassion and self-esteem. The inhibitory affects that hold the AVPD in place include anxiety over closeness, shame over sense of self, and possibly pain over losses or hurts in previous relationships.

THE SPIRITUAL CHEMIST

The patient met ample criteria for AVPD. She had one distant male friend but no female friends, she was being fired from her job as a laboratory technician because of her poor relationships with co-workers, she was divorced, and her son was choosing to live with his father. She was distrustful of others and did not feel like part of the human race. She had experienced extreme neglect in her childhood and constant criticism.

In the session we describe, her relationship with the therapist is explored: first focusing on defenses, then on reduction or regulation of anxieties, and then on exposure to feelings of closeness and sense of self with the therapist. This third session was a pivotal one, and the 35-session therapy was extremely successful, resulting in remarkable change in lifelong character pathology. She went on to a successful career as a service provider, married a loving man, and adopted a foster child. Ten-year follow-up by an independent interviewer (not the therapist) found her happy and high functioning.

The Spiritual Chemist (Session 3)	Objective/Intervention
(After a discussion of her difficulties feeling liked by people.)	
Therapist: Yeah. What's your sense of my feeling toward you?	
Patient: *[pause]* I haven't thought about that. But I think you care about me as a person. I think it's also your job.	Defense: distancing
Th: Well, how does that make a difference? It's my job to care about somebody? What a difficult job!	Confrontation of the defense
Pt: Yeah! *[laughs]* You can't make yourself care about somebody!	Sees point
Th: On demand? It's my job to care?	Further confrontation
Pt: I guess I feel that that's hard to judge because in a lot of ways it's a very one-sided relationship—the give and take isn't there.	More defensiveness
Th: It's one-sided how?	Trying to understand
Pt: Part of caring is sharing yourself?	Questioning
Th: Well…how much do you feel like I am sharing in listening to what you have to say? *(The therapist had felt very involved with and responsive to her.)*	Confront defense of distancing
Pt: *[pauses]* I don't know, I'm feeling uncomfortable with this conversation. *[laughs]*	Anxiety is provoked
Th: I was just going to ask you. You seem [uncomfortable] and your eyes went all around the room, and you seem like you're not wanting to look at me. What's the discomfort right now?	Explores anxiety Pointing out defenses
Pt: *[long pause]* I think it's hard for me to make a judgment, and I think you're asking for a judgment somehow.	Defense: distancing of closeness

The Spiritual Chemist (Session 3)	Objective/Intervention
Th: Hmm. So I'm asking you to perform and you don't know how, maybe, to do it?	Clarification
Pt: Yeah, maybe.	
Th: It becomes a demand again that you've got to do something right, even in here. So it kind of gets turned around in your head that you've got to do something for me. But really, I'm saying, "What have I done for you?" "What have you gotten from me?" That's something you could seem to focus on.	Clarification; refocus on feelings of avoidance between patient and therapist
Pt: When you said, "Do I think that you care about me?" *[long pause]* It's a hard question for me to answer. *[voice cracking]*	Anxiety is provoked
Th: Yeah. It's important though.	Hold on the focus
Pt: Umm. Because there's a difference between caring and liking.	Intellectualization
Th: Hmm. Maybe there is some intellectualization there? It makes you roll your eyes.	Pointing out defenses
Pt: *[laughs]*	Heightened anxiety?
Th: Is it difficult for you to talk with me about this?	Exploring anxiety
Pt: Yeah, it is.	Exploring anxiety
Th: What's the hardest part right now?	
Pt: I don't…Right now it's maybe realizing that it's hard for me to talk about…or think about someone caring for me. *[near tears]*	Brief exposure #1 to sorrow of unmet longing
Th: Yeah. It brings up some sadness.	Focus on sorrow about avoidance (builds motivation)
Pt: Mm-hmm.	
Th: And what's the sadness right now?	
Pt: *[long pause, sigh]* That it's sad that it's an area that would be hard for me to talk about or deal with.	Self-disclosure/shared affect
Th: Makes me sad as you say it. [Recalling] what you just said about your mother. The person who should be caring the most about you and you don't have that feeling.	Link to past Validation of sadness
Pt: Yeah.	

The Spiritual Chemist (Session 3)	Objective/Intervention
Th: How could it be otherwise for you?	Validation repeated
Pt: That thinking about someone caring about me? You're saying, "Why shouldn't it be hard if I don't have that from my mother?"	
Th: Yeah. Of course, it'll be hard…and sad. But, let's just stay with you and me…with this issue of closeness here. And how much resonance to you can you feel from me?	Empathic comment Refocus: another exposure to closeness with therapist
Pt: [sighs] Well, I think there's some because otherwise I wouldn't be as comfortable sharing the things that I shared with you.	Exposure #2: closeness
Th: Right, so you're more comfortable than you expected?	Assessing anxiety
Pt: Yeah, yeah. But again I think that at least recently being able to share feelings is something I've been able to do a lot more easily than I thought I could.	Improved affective capacity since beginning therapy
Th: It's been right under the surface.	Validation of feeling
Pt: Yeah.	
Th: It seems like a tremendous amount of feeling. Right there but…pushed away.	Refocus on feelings and defenses
Pt: Yeah. There is so much care I couldn't feel. [wipes away tears]	Exposure #3: to feeling
Th: And in here with me, I think it's going to be expectable, for you to kind of push away that experience between us…. Maybe…?	Validation of the avoidance
Pt: Yeah….? [looks questioning]	
Th: What's your question?	
Pt: Well, I was thinking on the way down here about talking to you today. And I had… [voice breaking] a scary feeling that somehow it was scary. And I was trying to figure out why. And I think that part of it…was a sense that I was going to be looking at some things that were uncomfortable for me. [big sigh] But I think part of it was [sighs] that I was afraid that things…that I would share with you…would…make you …think…less of me. [voice cracks] And it wouldn't be hard for me, if I didn't care.	Anxiety raises; exposure #4: closeness

Affect Phobias in Dependent Personality Components

The underlying feelings in dependent diagnoses can involve the sense of self-efficacy, self-mastery, or capacity for independence. The DPD category has been criticized for not endorsing the dimensions of attachment strongly enough. Indeed, the affect phobia approach would explore not only the problems in feelings of attachment to others but also the problems in sense of self in relation to others.

In looking for an underlying dependent "core affect phobia," more than one etiology is possible. Dependent disorders can arise from over-indulgence, which robs a child of crucial mastery experiences in living or, on the other end of the continuum, from too great independence or isolation early in life. Both attachment patterns can result in longing for dependence and clinging, as well as an insecure or overly burdened sense of self. The case examples later in this chapter involve the "Off-Putting Woman" who had distancing defenses.

The patient presented in the following case did not have a typical "dependent" personality disorder. However, she had dependent traits and problematic dependency issues indicated by her needs to be a life-long patient and avoid intimate relationships. She had been denied a healthy dependency as a child, and, although capably independent at work, she craved a dependent relationship with her therapist despite the financial hardship. She had been in therapy for more than 20 years because of her inability to have a relationship with a man.

The Off-Putting Woman (discussed above): Lengthy Dependence on the Therapist

After the patient began to recognize and work to improve her off-putting style, we began to focus on her fear of closeness and her defensive dependency on therapy as an externalization of her attachment longing and a way to avoid a healthy dependence in a relationship. The following excerpts show her working with unmet longings for closeness.

The Off-Putting Woman and Affect Phobia: "Love Means Nothing But Pain"

This patient had been in therapy her whole life but had never really opened emotionally, so her dependency needs had not been worked through. More than 60 sessions were needed to help this woman become comfortable with a healthy dependence on the therapist and her parents. In a pivotal and emotional session, she finally allowed herself to recall warm and caring moments with her mother and father, in which she could see that under their dismissal and brusqueness, they truly loved her. This exposure in memory had a powerfully desensitizing effect on her ability to allow herself to love and be loved. She finally realized that "Love meant nothing but pain for me before, and I would never let myself feel it." Thus, at age 50, following desensitization of her affect phobia (or "working through") of closeness and dependency with the therapist, as well as her mother and her father, she was able to build a relationship with a warm and loving man for the first time in her life. Therapy was needed during the beginning phases of the relationship to help her with her tendency to distance, and her fear of being vulnerable, and a few couples sessions helped both of them learn how best to understand and respond to each other. But so much work had been done on these issues previously in her therapy that she was well prepared to deal with them. After 2 years, they moved in together, and the relationship has continued very successfully for the past 5 years.

Focus on Affect Phobia	Objective/Intervention
Patient: I just have this image…Whenever I wanted my parents' attention, they would say: "Stop it. Go play. Leave us alone."	
Therapist: But isn't it typical for every child to cry out, "Mommy, mommy!" And tug at her…or try to crawl in her lap….	Validating longing for closeness
Pt: Yeah. I can remember doing that…and being pushed away.	
Th: And think about yourself as a little child. At that age, your heart is on your sleeve, and your little heart must have been broken. When you're so young and so open, there's such longing. So their distance could have been devastating.	Intensifying longing for closeness
Pt: [nods, looking as if in pain]	
Th: Yeah. Where in your body do you feel that?	Exploring feelings
Pt: A little here, but nowhere else… [points to throat area]	Bodily awareness, unclear
Th: OK. Let's just stay with that then. Do memories come up? Being pushed away or not responded to?	Continuing focus, exposure to feeling
Pt: It's still tight here. [points to neck again]	Inhibitory reaction
Th: Mmm, still tight. I wonder if you might have shut your mouth and swallowed your words? Because isn't there a force that wants to come out? Isn't it there, in all of us? It's tragic to think about how your silence kept you so alone.	Exploring reasons for inhibition. What's withheld? The costs of holding back.

Focus on Affect Phobia	Objective/Intervention
Pt: *[nods and pauses]* I'm just thinking. I never let them see me cry.	
Th: So you could never let that show?	
Pt: Right. They disapproved of crying.	Remembers disapproval
Th: But if your parents were disapproving of your need for them, you would have been hungry all the time…in a constant state of deprivation.	Validating defense and longing
Pt: If there was ever any praise from my parents, it was for achievement. Not for being needy, or helpless…	Links to pattern in the past
Th: No acceptance of dependency needs. [Pt: Right] That's so sad.	Validation, empathy
Pt: *[looks sad]* I have a headache…	Possible somatization?
Th: There must be so much in there that wants to come out. What would help, here with me, to let those feelings of need and longing come out here with me?	Focus on feeling and patient-therapist relationship
Pt: It would be so hard to really lean on you or anyone.	Fear of dependence
Th: It's been hard for you to cry in here with me. [Pt: Yeah.] Yet you have been in therapy for many years and often want to come more than once a week. I wonder if you might be hanging on to the physical presence of a therapist but not really letting yourself open up enough to really feel close.	Exploring anxiety about closeness or dependency Explore defenses about closeness
Pt: That would terrify me.	Anxiety increases
Th: We don't have to go into those feelings until you feel comfortable doing so. First, let's just look at what's the hardest or scariest part.	Anxiety regulation before beginning exposure

AFFECT PHOBIAS IN OBSESSIVE-COMPULSIVE PERSONALITY COMPONENTS

OCPD behaviors involve perfectionism; aggressive control; and fear of losing self-control, making a mistake, or becoming the target of blame and guilt. These fears are easily associated with a sense of being not-nice, disobedient, improper, or imperfect.

The following case involved a dramatic 12-session therapy that helped soften a hard-driving, perfectionistic medical student.

THE EXERCISE FANATIC: DEALING WITH DRIVEN DEFENSES

She came to therapy because she was miserable and exhausted but utterly driven to be perfect. She reported extreme levels of perfectionistic self-control, starvation to be thin (she weighed 99 pounds), perfect grades in a top university, 5 hours of exercise per day, and competition in a world-class-level gymnastics group. She had married a much more low-key medical student. She felt jealous of his ease in living but drove herself to be the perfect wife and was so tired each day that she had to fake enjoyment of sexual intercourse.

Exploration and Undoing of Self-Destructive Defenses (Session 4)	Objective/Intervention
Therapist: You think you might lose those things that make you so superhuman. Would Jeremy love you if you were low-key?	Confronting the costs of giving up perfectionistic defenses
Patient: I don't know how to be low-key.	
Th: Whooo...I'm just feeling the weight of it! Somehow you got programmed early on...being what other people want you to be...and maybe you don't know how to stop.	Self-disclosure by the therapist about seeing the burden of her defenses
Pt: If I only had the courage to care for myself.	Motivation to change
Th: What's scary about caring for yourself? Are you scared that people won't accept you as you are?	Exploring anxiety about change
Pt: Yes! Jeremy married me the way I am. And I wouldn't accept me another way.	Ego-syntonic defenses
Th: Would you demand this of your own children?	Trying to turn defenses against themselves
Pt: No! I hope not. I hope I figure it out so I don't do it to them. But I can't stop myself.	
Th: You're driving yourself in a way that is tragic to watch. Has anyone said that maybe you need to bottom out...before you stop doing this to yourself?	Wrestling with destructive defenses
Pt: [crying out] How much more bottom do I have to go!! I've been on the bottom for 6 months. I hate my life!	Defenses beginning to be ego-dystonic

Exploration and Undoing of Self-Destructive Defenses (Session 4)	Objective/Intervention
Th: I wonder what your parents did to set this in motion?	Exploring origins of defenses
Pt: It's hard to blame them. My father was very low-key.	

Her father was a successful doctor, but very easygoing, spending much time at home on the couch. But he was very loving toward his daughter. The mother had devalued him for being overweight and not being more ambitious. He died of a heart attack when the patient was 13. She was grief-stricken and became attached to a gymnastic coach who drove his team to inhuman levels of performance. In treatment she began to see that her escape to a driven, perfectionistic world helped her avoid her grief over the loss of her father and escape the easygoing and seemingly unhealthy lifestyle he lived.

The next 7 sessions dealt with her grief over the loss of her father and her anger toward the coach and her mother. She was able to talk to the mother very frankly, and her mother was deeply sorry for the pattern that had been established. This young woman made such rapid changes that the therapist needed to help her adjust to her new sense of self.

Help With Assimilation of Rapid Changes	Objective/Intervention
Therapist: If the coach had never come into your life, how'd you do today?	Changes in capacity to care for self have not yet become fully assimilated and accepted
Patient: I'd laugh more.... Actually...I feel happy these days. I'm too tired to go to the gym. I feel better and I enjoy lying on the couch with Jeremy and watching TV. I know this is a better life for me. But, I don't feel proud. I really respected myself when I was hard-driving. And I've also gained 30 pounds! Jeremy says I look sexier, but I am not used to this weight. I know it is healthier...but...	Struggling to accept new self-image
Th: Let's look at what you are losing by letting yourself eat and relax.	Exploring anxiety around self-care and vulnerability
Pt: I used to have supernatural powers. No one could touch me...and now I just don't want to feel so vulnerable.	

Help With Assimilation of Rapid Changes	Objective/Intervention
Th: It sounds like that perfectionistic drive was a shield around you.	Exploring defense and validation/empathy
Pt: It was! Now I feel naked.	
Th: What did it protect you from?	Exploring defense
Pt: Well, I saw what lying on the couch did to my father.	Anxiety about father's death
Th: Who do you feel gave you more? Your gentle, loving father or the hard-driving coach.	New perspectives
Pt: You're right. There is no comparison. I learned a lot from the coach, but he also hurt me so much.	Anxiety regulation and more acceptance of self-care

One year later the therapist contacted this patient and found her healthy and functioning well. She reported, "I'll never be as low-key as you might want for me, but I will never be as destructive to myself as I used to be. I am so much more compassionate and caretaking toward myself. And much to my surprise, that makes me much less critical and judgmental of other people!"

A RETURN TO THE CHALLENGE OF FINDING THE AFFECT FOCUS

The above examples are only a few of the many probable developmental patterns (or personality disorders) that can lead to Cluster C problems, and it is the challenge for the therapist to figure that out. However, our experience is that an affect phobia focus derived from Malan's Two Triangles (identifying defenses, activating feelings, and inhibitory feelings) can streamline the process. If one affect phobia focus does not lead to some behavioral improvement in a few weeks, then the patient and therapist can explore other possible affective etiologies or the secondary gain that might make the affect phobia highly rewarding and difficult to give up. But why do affect-focused therapies do no better than any other form?

Because preliminary research is showing that resolution of affect conflicts is associated with improvement across theoretical orientation, we suggest that all therapies may influence affective functioning to some moderate degree ("all have won and all shall have prizes"). The affect phobia approach has universality and high face validity: most of our patients are afraid to speak up, or afraid to grieve, or too ashamed to feel deserving. Most therapies focus on the resolution of these issues, and when they are improved, life functioning should then be improved. It may be that cognitive therapies have not focused on affect specifically in session, but cognitive therapists give homework that exposes the patient to new forms of affective responding. Psychodynamic therapies may have a greater focus on affect but may not work intensively enough in the session and tend not to have homework that might provide the exposure. These are testable hypotheses, and with methods available to test them.

Cluster C personality disorders are devastating to relationships, rob life of richness, and generate lifelong suffering. If the affect phobia approach offers the potential to reduce this suffering in weeks or months, rather than in decades, then we believe that such a method merits further attention.

Key Clinical Concepts

- ◆ As a group, the Cluster C personality disorders are the most prevalent personality disorders in the general population and in the outpatient clinical setting.

- ◆ Cluster C personality disorders tend to group together, sharing a common dimension often termed fearfulness—that is, fear of negative evaluation in the avoidant personality disorder, fear of separation in the dependent personality disorder, and fear of losing personal and interpersonal control in the obsessive-compulsive personality disorder.

- ◆ There is growing empirical evidence that shows brief psychodynamic psychotherapy is effective and patients are able to maintain treatment gains over time.

- ◆ The underlying affect conflicts for each personality disorder must be identified and focused on in treatment to desensitize the conflicts; activating affects should be enhanced and inhibitory affects regulated.

- ◆ Exposure to the core affect must be experienced in the body for desensitization to occur, because the physiological arousal of the affect contributes most to the affect phobia. However, coding affect on videotapes has shown that therapists most often leave out the exposure to visceral experience (i.e., feelings are talked about but not felt) and thus do not fully desensitize the patient to the conflicted feeling.

Suggested Readings

Benjamin LS: Interpersonal Diagnosis and Treatment of Personality Disorders, 2nd Edition. New York, Guilford, 2003. [Provides an in-depth understanding of personality disorders based on the interactive nature of the actions of the self and the other as well as intrapsychic ramifications.]

McCullough L, Kaplan A, Kuhn N, et al: Treating Affect Phobias: A Manual for Short Term Dynamic Psychotherapy. New York, Guilford, 2003. [A treatment manual for the affect phobia model of Short Term Dynamic Psychotherapy. Twelve chapters describe the basic theory and treatment interventions. At the end of each chapter are exercises to provide the reader with practice for acquisition of skills.]

McCullough Vaillant L: Changing Character: Short-Term Anxiety-Regulating Psychotherapy for Restructuring Defenses, Affects and Attachments. New York, Basic Books, 1997. [An in-depth discussion of the theory and background of Short Term Dynamic Psychotherapy, integrating psychodynamic theory with Tomkins affect theory and learning-theory principles of change. Descriptions of the three main objectives of treatment make up the body of the book, with many transcripted examples of interventions.]

References

Alnaes R, Torgersen S: DSM-III symptom disorders (Axis I) and personality disorders (Axis II) in an outpatient population. Acta Psychiatr Scand 78:348–355, 1988

American Psychiatric Association: Diagnostic and Statistical Manual of Mental Disorders, 3rd Edition. Washington, DC, American Psychiatric Association, 1980

American Psychiatric Association: Diagnostic and Statistical Manual of Mental Disorders, 3rd Edition, Revised. Washington, DC, American Psychiatric Association, 1987

American Psychiatric Association: Diagnostic and Statistical Manual of Mental Disorders, 4th Edition. Washington, DC, American Psychiatric Association, 1994

American Psychiatric Association: Diagnostic and Statistical Manual of Mental Disorders, 4th Edition, Text Revision. Washington, DC, American Psychiatric Association, 2000

Barber JP, Morse JQ, Krakauer ID, et al: Change in obsessive-compulsive and avoidant personality disorders following time-limited supportive-expressive therapy. Psychotherapy 34:133–143, 1997

Bartholomew K, Kwong MJ, Hart SD: Attachment, in Handbook of Personality Disorders: Theory, Research, and Treatment. Edited by Livesley WJ. New York, Guilford, 2001, pp 196–230

Beck AT, Freeman A: Cognitive Therapy for Personality Disorders. New York, Guilford, 1990

Benjamin LS: Interpersonal Diagnosis and Treatment of Personality Disorders, 2nd Edition. New York, Guilford, 2003

Bornstein RF: The Dependent Patient: A Practitioner's Guide. Washington, DC, American Psychological Association, 2005

Davanloo H (ed): Short-Term Dynamic Psychotherapy. New York, Jason Aronson, 1980

Davanloo H: The technique of unlocking of the unconscious. Part I. International Journal of Short-Term Psychotherapy 3:99–121, 1988

Emmelkamp P, Bourman T, Scholing A: Anxiety Disorders. Chichester, UK, Wiley, 1992

Emmelkamp PM, Benner A, Kuipers A, et al: Comparison of brief dynamic and cognitive-behavioural therapies in avoidant personality disorder. Br J Psychiatry 189:60–64, 2006

Fossati A, Beauchaine TP, Grazioli F, et al: Confirmatory factor analyses of DSM-IV Cluster C personality disorder criteria. J Pers Disord 20:186–203, 2006

Grilo CM, Shea MT, Sanislow CA, et al: Two-year stability and change of schizotypal, borderline, avoidant, and obsessive-compulsive personality disorders. J Consult Clin Psychol 72:767–775, 2004

Hardy GE, Barkham M, Shapiro DA, et al: Impact of Cluster C personality disorders on outcomes of contrasting brief psychotherapies for depression. J Consult Clin Psychol 63:997–1004, 1995

Hobson RF: Forms of Feelings: The Heart of Psychotherapy. London, Tavistock, 1985

Hummelen B, Wilberg T, Pedersen G, et al: The relationship between avoidant personality disorder and social phobia. Compr Psychiatry 48:348–356, 2007

Hummelen B, Wilberg T, Pedersen G, et al: The quality of the DSM-IV obsessive-compulsive personality disorder construct as a prototype category. J Nerv Ment Dis 196:446–455, 2008

Lenzenweger MF, Johnson MD, Willett JB: Individual growth curve analysis illuminates stability and change in personality disorder features: the longitudinal study of personality disorders. Arch Gen Psychiatry 61:1015–1024, 2004

Livesley WJ, Schroeder ML, Jackson DN: Dependent personality disorder and attachment problems. J Pers Disord 4:131–140, 1990

Luborsky L: Principles of Psychoanalytic Psychotherapy: A Manual for Supportive-Expressive Treatment. New York, Basic Books, 1984

Malan DM: A Study of Brief Psychotherapy. New York, Plenum, 1963

Malan DM: Individual Psychotherapy and the Science of Psychodynamics. London, Heinemann-Butterworth Press, 1979

Massion AO, Dyck IR, Shea MT, et al: Personality disorders and time to remission in generalized anxiety disorder, social phobia, and panic disorder. Arch Gen Psychiatry 59:434–440, 2002

McCullough L: Davanloo's short-term dynamic psychotherapy: a cross-theoretical analysis of change mechanisms, in How People Change: Inside and Outside of Therapy. Edited by Curtis RC, Stricker G. New York, Plenum, 1991, pp 59–79

McCullough L: Short-term psychodynamic therapy as a form of desensitization: treating affect phobias. In Session: Psychotherapy in Practice 4:35–53, 1999

McCullough L, Andrews S: Assimilative integration: short-term dynamic psychotherapy for treating affect phobias. Clinical Psychology: Research and Practice 8:82–91, 2001

McCullough L, McGill M: Affect-focused short-term dynamic therapy: empirically-supported strategies for resolving affect phobias, in Evidence-based Psychodynamic Psychotherapy. Edited by Levy R, Ablon S (Clinical Currents in Psychiatry; Rosenbaum J, series ed.). New York, Humana, 2009, pp 249–277

McCullough L, Kuhn N, Andrews S, et al: Treating Affect Phobia: A Manual for Short-Term Dynamic Psychotherapy. New York, Guilford, 2003

McCullough-Vaillant L: The next step in short-term dynamic psychotherapy: a clarification of objectives and techniques in an anxiety-regulating model. Psychotherapy 31:642–654, 1994

McCullough-Vaillant LM: Changing Character. New York, Basic Books, 1997

McGlashan TH, Grilo CM, Sanislow CA, et al: Two-year prevalence and stability of individual DSM-IV criteria for schizotypal, borderline, avoidant, and obsessive-compulsive personality disorders: toward a hybrid model of Axis II disorders. Am J Psychiatry 162:883–889, 2005

Millon T, Davis RD, Millon CM: Disorders of Personality: DSM-IV and Beyond. New York, Wiley, 1996

Oldham JM, Skodol AE, Kellman HD, et al: Comorbidity of Axis I and Axis II disorders. Am J Psychiatry 152:571–578, 1995

PDM Task Force: Psychodynamic Diagnostic Manual (PDM). Silver Spring, MD, Alliance of Psychoanalytic Organizations, 2006

Reich W: Character Analysis. New York, Farrar, Straus & Giroux, 1933

Rosenthal R: Meta-Analytic Procedures for Social Research. Beverly Hills, CA, Sage, 1984

Shea MT, Stout R, Gunderson J, et al: Short-term diagnostic stability of schizotypal, borderline, avoidant, and obsessive-compulsive personality disorders. Am J Psychiatry 159:2036–2041, 2002

Stuart S, Pfohl B, Battaglia M, et al: The cooccurrence of DSM-III-R personality disorders. J Pers Disord 12:302–315, 1998

Svartberg M, Stiles TC, Seltzer MH: Randomized, controlled trial of the effectiveness of short-term dynamic psychotherapy and cognitive therapy for Cluster C personality disorders. Am J Psychiatry 161:810–817, 2004

Torgersen S, Kringlen E, Cramer V: The prevalence of personality disorders in a community sample. Arch Gen Psychiatry 58:590–596, 2001

Vinnars B, Barber JP, Noren K, et al: Manualized supportive-expressive psychotherapy versus nonmanualized community-delivered psychodynamic therapy for patients with personality disorders: bridging efficacy and effectiveness. Am J Psychiatry 162:1933–1940, 2005

Winston A, McCullough L, Trujillo M, et al: Brief psychotherapy of personality disorders. J Nerv Ment Dis 179:188–193, 1991

Winston A, Laikin M, Pollack J, et al: Short-term dynamic psychotherapy of personality disorders. Am J Psychiatry 151:190–194, 1994

Zimmerman M, Rothschild L, Chelminski I: The prevalence of DSM-IV personality disorders in psychiatric outpatients. Am J Psychiatry 162:1911–1918, 2005

CHAPTER 13

Psychodynamic Approaches Integrated Into Day Treatment and Inpatient Settings

William E. Piper, Ph.D.
Paul I. Steinberg, M.D., F.R.C.P.C.

In this chapter we primarily focus on the psychodynamic day treatment of patients with personality disorders (PDs). We consider to a lesser degree psychodynamically informed inpatient treatment as a precursor to day treatment or as a treatment outlet for patients who seriously regress during day treatment. It is well known, and amply documented in this volume, that PDs are one of the most important sources of long-term impairment in psychiatric populations (Merikangas and Weissman 1986). The costs of care of PD patients are associated with high levels of unemployment, substance abuse, hospitalization, suicide, marital difficulties, and family discord (Pilkonis et al. 1999). Persons with PDs are frequent users of health and social services (Bender et al. 2001). Because many of the troublesome characteristics associated with PDs are interpersonal in nature, the costs to society involve many people in addition to the patients themselves (e.g., family, friends, and work associates). Significant others often spend considerable time and resources in attempting to help persons with PDs. Unfortunately, such efforts often turn out to be disappointing and only create additional tensions between the parties.

The characteristics of PDs that create difficulties for patients who receive PD diagnoses and for others with whom they interact appear to be stable, resistant to change, and difficult to treat. No single treatment intervention is likely to address and modify the diverse set of troublesome characteristics. Most patients whose symptoms meet criteria for a PD meet the criteria for other PDs as well (Dolan et al. 1995). They also frequently have symptoms that meet criteria for one or more Axis I disorders. The clinician is frequently faced with the formidable task of treating multiple disorders and deciding which to address first.

Terminology

Because of extensive comorbidity, patients with PDs often require diverse and intensive interventions. Gunderson et al. (2005) have distinguished four levels of intensity of care for patients with PDs. In these authors' conceptualization, intensity is largely defined in terms of the number of hours of treatment received by the patient. Beginning with the least intensive approach, *outpatient care* involves 1–5 hours of treatment per week. In contrast, *intensive outpatient care* involves 3–6 hours of integrated therapies per week. Next, *day treatment* involves 2–8 hours of treatment per day, 3–5 days per week, of mostly group therapies. Finally, full *hospitalization* (24 hours per day) represents the most intensive form of care.

Gunderson et al. (2005) believe that the best care for the patient is the least intensive alternative that works. On this principle, the patient is encouraged to rely on his own resources, generalize to the challenges presented by the specific problem, and avoid regressive behavior. Thus, one would expect that outpatient care (either regular or intensive) would serve as the treatment of choice over day treatment and inpatient care. This is true. However, it is also true that most participants in day treatment have previously had one or more unsuccessful courses of outpatient treatment. Unfortunately, outpatient care that lasts for several months or even years may not be sufficient to bring about significant and lasting positive change for many patients. In such cases, a course of day treatment may be indicated.

A difficulty for those who refer patients to day treatment programs is that what is included in day treatment programs varies considerably in the literature. The variability involves the number of hours the program operates each day and week, the types of activities (treatment and non-treatment) that patients experience, the degree of support and confrontation provided, and the overarching theoretical orientation of the program. Referral sources may be unaware of important features of a program (e.g., daily participation in a large group) that may be quite intimidating to some patients. Because of the diversity of features, carefully informing referral sources about the specific nature of the program to which the patient is being referred is essential. If referral sources are well informed, they can assist in preparing the patient for what to expect.

Another impediment to understanding the nature of day treatment programs is the presence in the literature of additional terminology that is similar to *day treatment* but refers to programs with quite different objectives. Examples are *day hospital, day care,* and *partial hospitalization.* To avoid confusion, we suggest using the following distinctions. In contrast to day treatment programs, *day hospital* programs are concerned primarily with treatment of acute illness. They are appropriate for individuals who would otherwise be treated as inpatients (e.g., a decompensated patient with a borderline personality disorder [BPD]). They also may assist patients in transition from inpatient to outpatient care. *Day care* programs are concerned primarily with maintaining the stability of patients with chronic debilitating mental disorders such as schizophrenia. Treatment occupies only a small role in such programs. The term *partial hospitalization* is used to refer to any of these intensive programs (day treatment, day hospital, or day care) currently under consideration. For that reason, and because it involves no amount of full (24-hour) hospitalization, we do not find it to be a very useful concept. Thus, day treatment programs differ in their objectives by attempting to achieve the successful treatment and rehabilitation of patients. They appear to have unique advantages in treating PDs. They offer intensive ambulatory services within a stable therapeutic milieu.

Psychodynamic Foundation

All of the programs described in this chapter use psychodynamic theory as the conceptual foundation of their treatment approach. By *psychodynamic theory,* we mean a system of basic concepts, and processes indicating how the concepts are related to one another, that originated in the writings of Sigmund Freud, his contemporaries, and those who followed the early figures and who continued to refine and develop various aspects of the theory. Examples of psychodynamic concepts are structures of the mind (e.g., id, ego, superego), goal-oriented behavior, and the unconscious. Examples of psychodynamic processes are functions of the mind (e.g., wish fulfillment, transference, and resistance), repression, and conflict resolution. Within general psychodynamic theory, a growing number of specific schools of psychodynamic theory can be distinguished. The schools differ in how much they emphasize some of the basic concepts and processes. They also differ in terms of additional concepts and processes that they have introduced to the field. The schools use concepts from drive psychology, ego psychology, object relations psychology, self psychology, relational psychology, and attachment psychology. In addition to the basic psychodynamic concepts and processes, and concepts and processes that are unique to each school, other concepts and processes distinguish day treatment approaches. These are concepts and processes associated with group therapy, milieu therapy, systems theory, and biological psychiatry. Definitions of psychodynamic concepts and descriptions of schools are succinctly presented by Piper et al. (2002) and Yeomans et al. (2005).

Day treatment programs may or may not include individual psychotherapy as part of their treatment approach. They also may or may not be time-limited from the perspective of the individual patient. If they are time-limited, each patient enters and departs the program after a set period of time (e.g., 18 months). Some time-limited programs delineate specific phases that each patient is believed to pass through (Piper et al. 1996). The specific combination of groups provided for the patient is selected to highlight issues that are relevant to each phase (e.g., a discharge group just prior to termination of day treatment).

Power of Group Therapies

Although individual therapy is optional in day treatment programs, group therapy is not. Patients almost always participate in a variety of therapy groups. Group therapies are capable of mobilizing strong forces of change, such as peer pressure. They are sometimes referred to as *social microcosms* (Yalom and Leszcz 2005). They can exert considerable social pressure on patients to participate. They often are capable of eliciting the typical maladaptive behaviors of each patient. The other patients can observe, provide feedback, and offer suggestions for change. Subsequently, the patient can practice adaptive behavior. This entire process is referred to as *interpersonal learning*. Some patients may learn through observation and imitation, simply recognizing that other patients have difficulties similar to their own (universality) and helping other patients with their problems (altruism). These processes have been regarded as powerful therapeutic factors (Yalom and Leszcz 2005). Several other features contribute to making group therapy a powerful treatment. First, patients participate in several different groups each day. Second, the groups vary in size, structure, objectives, and processes, which provides a comprehensive approach. Third, the different groups are integrated and synergistic. Fourth, patients benefit from working with multiple staff members and many other patients.

Characteristics of Therapeutic Communities

If a day treatment program is running well (i.e., patients are working and appear to be making outcome gains), the program takes on characteristics that traditionally have been attributed to the therapeutic community or milieu therapy. Four such characteristics highlighted by Rapoport (1980) are democratization, permissiveness, communalism, and reality confrontation. These characteristics are believed to strengthen cohesion and assist patients in enduring difficult periods of treatment without missing sessions or dropping out. *Democratization* indicates that each patient should share equally in the exercise of power in decision making about affairs of the program. *Permissiveness* indicates that all patients should tolerate a wide degree of behaviors on the part of other patients in the program. *Communalism* indicates that the functioning of the program should be characterized by tight-knit and intimate sets of relationships. *Reality confrontation* indicates that patients should be continually presented with interpretations of their behavior as it is seen by most others in the program.

Systems theory refers to a set of assumptions and concepts that view the program as a whole organic entity that is composed of hierarchical levels of groups (E.J. Miller and Rice 1967; J.G. Miller 1978). *Biological psychiatry* concerns the physical condition of the patients in the program. Most of the time this pertains to the use of psychotropic medication. Most of the patients in a day treatment program commonly use such medication (e.g., antidepressants).

Although psychodynamic day treatment programs have received strong clinical endorsements, evidence for the efficacy and effectiveness of such programs is very limited. We found only two studies that had used a randomized clinical trial design and methodology.

Outcome Research

Bateman and Fonagy (1999) reported on a randomized clinical trial of a day treatment program for patients with BPD. They compared the effectiveness of a psychoanalytically oriented day treatment program, which later was conceptualized as and labeled *mentalization treatment*

(Bateman and Fonagy 2006), with standard psychiatric care for these patients. The day treatment program consisted of psychoanalytically oriented individual psychotherapy once per week, group analytic psychotherapy three times per week, expressive psychotherapy oriented toward psychodrama techniques once per week, and a community meeting once per week. Therapies and informal patient-staff contact were organized in accordance with a psychoanalytic model of BPD as a disorder of attachment, separation tolerance, and capacity to think of oneself in relation to others. Patients attended the program 5 days per week for a maximum of 18 months. The day program was able to accommodate up to 30 patients. Standard care consisted of medication; meetings with a psychiatrist, as necessary (average=twice per month); inpatient admission, if necessary (admission rate=90%, average stay= 11.6 days), preferably with discharge to nonpsychoanalytic, psychiatric partial hospitalization focusing on problem solving (72% of the sample were partially hospitalized, average stay=6 months); and outpatient and community follow-up (every 2 weeks). Patients in the standard care group received no formal psychotherapy.

Forty-four patients with BPD were randomly assigned to either day treatment or standard care. Outcome measures included the frequency of suicide attempts and acts of self-mutilation, the number and duration of inpatient admissions, and the use of psychotropic medication (i.e., the need for medication), as well as self-report measures of depression, anxiety, general symptomatic distress, interpersonal function, and social adjustment.

The authors found that patients who participated in the day treatment program showed significant improvements on all measures, in contrast to those in the standard care group, who showed limited change and even deterioration over the same period. Improvement for those in the day program began after 6 months in treatment and continued until the end of treatment at 18 months. Bateman and Fonagy (1999) concluded that psychoanalytically oriented day treatment was superior to standard psychiatric care for patients diagnosed with BPD and may be a more cost-efficient alternative to inpatient care and general psychiatric treatment for these individuals.

Bateman and Fonagy (2008) conducted a follow-up study with 41 patients with BPD from the original trial. This assessment was 8 years after the initial assessment was conducted and treatment began. They found that mentalization-based treatment by partial hospitalization continued to show superiority to treatment as usual for suicidality, diagnostic status, service use, medication use, global functioning, and vocational status. Thus, once again after 8 years, the mentalization-based treatment by partial hospitalization resulted in greater improvement than did treatment as usual.

Our research group also conducted a prospective controlled trial of day treatment (Piper et al. 1993). As in the Bateman and Fonagy study, we attempted to avoid the problems associated with previous studies of day treatment, including small sample size, lack of randomization, minimal control of variables such as diagnosis or medication, lack of standard outcome measures, and poorly defined programs. We used a randomized treatment versus control (delayed treatment) design to examine a day treatment program for psychiatric outpatients with mood disorders and PDs.

Sixty matched pairs of patients completed the treatment and control conditions. Of the 120 patients, 60% had a PD. The most frequent DSM-III-R (American Psychiatric Association 1987) Axis II diagnoses were dependent PD and BPD. The program was time-limited (18 weeks), psychodynamic, and group-oriented. Patients admitted to the program were expected to attend 7 hours per day, 4.5 days per week. The program consisted of a large variety of groups, including psychotherapy, role-play, television feedback, skills training, and peer government. In addition, all patients participated in weekly social-recreational activities, and some took part in academic or work-training groups. No individual therapy was offered. The program was designed to accommodate 40 patients at any one time. Treatment outcome was determined in several areas, including interpersonal functioning, psychiatric symptoms, self-esteem, life satisfaction, defensive functioning, and personalized target objectives. Assessments were conducted before and after therapy and at follow-up an average of 8 months posttherapy.

The study showed that treated patients had significantly better outcomes than did control subjects on seven outcome variables: social dysfunction, family dysfunction, interpersonal behavior, mood level, life satisfaction, self-esteem, and severity of disturbance with respect to personalized target objectives. These findings could not be accounted for by use of medication. Analyses were not conducted for specific PD categories because of the small number of patients in each diagnostic group. Benefits were maintained over the 8-month follow-up period. Overall, the study supports the efficacy of an intensive day treatment program for patients who manifest significant difficulties associated with PDs.

Wilberg et al. (1998) conducted a comprehensive study of day treatment for patients with a PD diagnosis. The study was naturalistic and prospective, not a randomized clinical trial, and involved 183 patients admitted to a day treatment program. Eighty percent of the patients received a PD diagnosis. The most frequent PD diagnoses were borderline and avoidant PDs. The 18-week program could accommodate 24 patients. It consisted of a combination of analytically oriented groups and cognitive-behavioral groups. Patients attended the program for 5 hours per day, 5 days per week. A total of 138 patients completed the program. Outcome variables included health or sickness status, general psychiatric symptomatology, unemployment, social isolation, and suicide attempts. Improvement on some of the outcome variables indicated favorable change over the treatment period. In addition, a 1-year follow-up of these patients (Wilberg et al. 1999) indicated that improvements were maintained in the follow-up period. The investigators also found that patients who participated in outpatient group therapy after finishing day treatment had better outcomes than patients who did not (Wilberg et al. 2003).

Case Studies

Two cases of patients who participated in the Edmonton Day Treatment Program are presented next. They represent a successful outcome and an unsuccessful one.

THE CASE OF MR. M

This case is that of a typical "difficult" patient with a PD who participated in the Edmonton Day Treatment Program. To preserve patient anonymity, the specific information about this case has been taken from several patients.

Background

Mr. M, a 41-year-old unemployed man, abused drugs and lived with a common-law partner. He presented to the local hospital emergency department stating that he was going to shoot himself. He faced a few long-term problems and precipitating events. His drug abuse and financial debt were escalating. He had lost his driver's license after driving while intoxicated, and his partner was threatening to leave him. It was not surprising that he was agitated and depressed. Mr. M had received counseling for his problems on several occasions in the past, but he had never been able to maintain an ongoing therapeutic relationship and currently was without a therapist. Given the circumstances, he was admitted to an adult care psychiatric unit for additional observation and evaluation on a certificate of involuntary admission.

Inpatient Behavior

On most inpatient units, patients are not treated with formal psychodynamic therapy. However, as is the case for day treatment programs, psychodynamic theory can serve as a useful foundation (Shur 1994; Stanton and Schwartz 1954) by providing understanding and direction for individual patients and the group as a whole.

> During the first few days, Mr. M was very demanding if not threatening in his attempt to obtain medication for his symptoms. On one occasion he made threatening gestures, and on another he knocked over pills on the medication cart, for which he was placed in seclusion. He constantly made special requests and tested the resolve of the staff. He was noted by staff to be particularly vulgar, argumentative, and hostile toward female patients. Female staff reported that he seemed to invade their personal space. He seemed oblivious to their stepping back and indicating their discomfort with his standing so close to them. Despite his aggravating behaviors, he succeeded in winning the compassion of some staff members, who viewed him as wounded and hurt. The ability to split staff over their evaluation of his actions is common among such patients.
>
> The inpatient unit ran a supportive therapy group that was psychodynamically informed. The day after Mr. M was placed in seclusion, he was informed by the group leader that both patients and staff were concerned about him and that his behavior of the day before could not be tolerated. Some of the patients reinforced these comments, and some added that they were afraid of him. He momentarily seemed affected by this feedback but soon dismissed the comments of the patients with the exception of one: Mrs. Q, who was 20 years older than he. She described her son, who was also a drug abuser. She described how she had not been the mother that he needed. With tears in her eyes, she told Mr. M that she did not want to see him on skid row, eventually dying of an overdose as her son had. This seemed to move him.
>
> Mr. M's certificate of involuntary admission was lifted after 6 days. He had been hospitalized for a total of 13 days. On discharge, he appeared in generally better health and had not used illicit drugs for more than 2 weeks. He grudgingly accepted his psychiatrist's referral to the day treatment program but appeared skeptical about what good it might do for him. His referring psychiatrist believed that without intensive treatment he would indeed revert to his self-destructive patterns of behavior. His discharge diagnosis was PD not otherwise specified with narcissistic, borderline, and antisocial traits.

Day Treatment Behavior

Admission to the day treatment program, as presented to Mr. M by the day treatment staff, was contingent on his not drinking alcohol, not using illicit drugs, and not behaving in a threatening or violent manner. Violations of these basic conditions would result in his discharge. He agreed but seemed to have a casual attitude toward the conditions.

Having the entire day treatment program staff involved in the admission process helps the staff cope with a patient's behavior problems and deal with their countertransference reactions.

> During the first week, after an outburst of temper in a group, Mr. M was prescribed quetiapine to help him control his temper. During his third week, Mr. M arrived late one morning. He was unshaven, appeared generally disheveled, and had a bruise and cut on his face. He had been drinking and fighting the night before. The staff asked him what he thought had triggered this occurrence. He virtually told the staff to mind their own business. Mr. P, a 28-year-old man in his sixteenth week of the program, confronted Mr. M. He reminded others that he too had a history of drinking and fighting and also knew he could avoid these behaviors. He said that in day treatment he had learned what triggered such behaviors and how to control them. Part of the solution for him was learning that he needed to confront the person he was angry with directly and discuss things in a calmer way. Mr. P also said that he had seen patients discharged from the program for the type of behavior violations Mr. M had engaged in. Mr. M asked if he would be discharged. After consultation with the staff, the psychiatrist in the program informed Mr. M that the staff was prepared to allow him to stay if he recognized the seriousness and destructiveness of his behavior and if he was committed to stopping it. He agreed.
>
> During a small group session, Mr. M was again asked what had precipitated his drinking and fighting. He deflected the question once again by simply claiming that he didn't know. Ms. S, a 25-year-old patient, reminded him that in the small group session that preceded this episode, several patients, including Ms. S, had confronted him about his lack of concern for others. She pointed out how this attitude put people off and disclosed how as an adolescent she had assumed a similar attitude of not caring about her mother, which prevented her from having the kind of relationship she had longed for. She joked about the similarity between the two of them—being tough guys with soft insides. Mr. M claimed that he was surprised to hear that he was regarded as uncaring and said that he appreciated their concern for him.

A notable and important feature of the Edmonton Day Treatment Program is a weekly staff relations group (O'Kelly and Azim 1993). It provides staff with an opportunity to examine their feelings and other reactions to difficult patients such as Mr. M. Sometimes staff feel guilty about their negative reactions and view them as a sign of unprofessional behavior. Patients with PDs often succeed in splitting staff in regard to their reactions, which makes it difficult to arrive at a consensus about what realistically should be expected of such patients. Staff members had to deal with their countertransference reactions toward Mr. M, who was prepared to assume little responsibility for his use of alcohol and illicit drugs. Other staff seemed more tolerant and sympathetic about the difficulties that Mr. M experienced. For example, one staff member (Mr. T) appeared to allow Mr. M to dominate the discussion in several groups. Another staff member, who was closest to Mr. T, gently suggested that Mr. T himself had a rather dominant personality, which may have made it difficult for him to recognize the negative effects of Mr. M's behavior. This confrontation took place over several staff relations group sessions before it was constructively resolved. Mr. T agreed that he was giving Mr. M "too much slack" and brought himself more in line with the approach taken by other staff. Another staff member, Mr. U, found himself intimidated by Mr. M to the point that he found himself not looking forward to coming to work. After some discussion, he was able to link his current predicament to his situation as a child with a brother who was intimidating and somewhat bullying. Mr. U received support from other staff members, who encouraged him to continue discussing his difficulties with Mr. M in staff relations meetings. He found this to be very helpful.

Mr. M completed the 18 weeks of the day treatment program. He appeared to have benefited considerably, particularly in terms of his relationships with others. Toward the end of his stay in the program, he was actually supporting staff in confronting patients and telling them about his own experiences in the day treatment program. The day treatment staff believed that the combination of support and confrontation offered by both staff and patients on an intensive basis enabled Mr. M. to respond well to psychodynamic group therapy. Mr. M ended with cordial relationships with most of the staff and patients. The last 4 weeks of his treatment were characterized by no outbursts of temper whatsoever and by his actively involving himself in groups in a constructive way.

After participating in the day treatment program, Mr. M was referred to a once-weekly follow-up group. The group consisted of patients who had completed the program and who wished to continue treatment for a commitment of at least 1 year. The staff believed that the follow-up group would facilitate Mr. M's involvement and positive interactions with other people. Staff believed that his ability to benefit from a once-weekly group was only made possible by his experience in the day treatment program. Had he been offered a similar group rather than the day treatment program, it is doubtful that he would have been able to benefit and he probably would have dropped out.

A day treatment patient occasionally is admitted to a psychiatric inpatient unit by way of the emergency department. It usually occurs when clinicians have a significant concern about suicide risk. It also might occur if psychotic symptoms persist or if a patient appears dangerous to others (Steinberg and Duggal 2004; Steinberg et al. 2008).

THE CASE OF MRS. R

In the case of Mrs. R, concerns about suicide precipitated hospitalization. As in the previous case, information was taken from several patients.

Background

Mrs. R, a 57-year-old divorcée, was raised in a rural village, the youngest of seven siblings. Her mother was neglectful and at times physically abusive. The mother did not work outside the house. She abused alcohol on a regular basis and was not consistent in maintaining sanitary standards in the house or even in providing regular meals. Mrs. R's older siblings often "threw something together" when they came home from school if their mother was incapacitated by alcohol or was "in a bad mood." From an emotional point of view, Mrs. R was largely raised by her oldest brother, who was 10 years older. He was friendly and at times supportive but understandably busy with his own concerns. Her father, a manual laborer, worked many hours of overtime, apparently to avoid his wife. He also was friendly but often was not available and did not protect Mrs. R from her mother. Mrs. R learned from a young age that she could get some attention from her oldest brother, and sometimes from her father, by behaving flirtatiously with them. She often "told on" her older siblings to her eldest brother, informing him of their misbehavior.

Day Treatment Behavior

Mrs. R presented herself in a rather dramatic way that often attracted the attention of men. In the day treatment program, she soon became friendly with Mr. W. She flirted with him, and he responded with a host of chivalrous behaviors. Mr. W became enamored with her and wished to spend time with no one else. Mrs. R experienced difficulty engaging in the program. Patients were irritated with her attention-seeking manner and her neglect of others. Staff found her affective style to be superficial.

During her fourth week, Mrs. R was confronted by other patients, presumably because of inconsistencies in her history of intimate relationships. Subsequently, she was accused of spreading malicious gossip. The group leader attempted to modulate the intensity of the confrontation but was handicapped by his own negative transference toward her. She denied their allegations and fled to another room. Mr. W came to the rescue by expressing his concern about her suicidal comments to the staff. He took her side and was critical of the staff, who allegedly allowed events to escalate. As is routine in such circumstances, the psychiatrist and several other staff members met with her to assess suicide risk.

Although the staff believed that her intent to "do away with myself" was unconvincing, the psychiatrist had her evaluated by the emergency psychiatry consultation team. She was ultimately admitted to the psychiatric ward, where she stayed for 1 night. Her admission to the psychiatric ward coincided with her discharge from the day treatment program. In retrospect, the staff believed that she was never committed to the psychotherapeutic work of the day treatment program and at some level wished to be discharged. Unfortunately, her manner of discharge left some of the patients who had confronted her feeling guilty and responsible for her discharge. Her discharge diagnosis was histrionic PD with dependent traits.

As this case illustrates, inpatient treatment is usually prompted by a crisis of some sort. The main objective is to provide support and observation in an effort to stabilize the patient until outpatient care can be arranged or resumed. Although group treatment is usually a regular part of the ward regimen, it may represent only a small part. It is not likely to be aimed at modifying long-standing personality traits. In North America, the lengths of stay in hospitals or residential centers have been decreasing significantly in response to escalating costs. Thus, in many cases, inpatient treatment is often a short-term treatment of 1 week or less. Exceptions include prison systems that include a strong rehabilitative objective for inmates who have antisocial disorders or traits. A psychodynamic approach to working with patients in residential treatment groups is described by Kibel (2003). If inpatient settings and day treatment settings share a common theoretical foundation, work within each setting and, when appropriate, patient movement from one to the other are facilitated.

Patient Suitability for Day Treatment

The fact that Mr. M appeared to have a successful course of day treatment, whereas Mrs. R did not, raises the question about whether suitability for day treatment can be accurately assessed before treatment. Usually, numerous potential predictors of success are available from a formal study of outcome. Typical predictors include demographic variables, historic variables, diagnostic variables, disturbance variables, and personality variables. To identify significant predictors from past outcome studies over a 25-year period (1968–1993), we conducted a review of outcome for 16 large-scale studies (Piper et al. 1994). We had hoped to find a set of consistent predictors of outcome but did not. Several reasons may have accounted for this lack of consistency.

◆ There was much variability in the types of programs.
◆ Prediction of outcome was of secondary interest.
◆ Determination of favorable outcome in comparisons between control and treatment conditions was primary.
◆ Predictor variables were chosen by theory or previous findings.
◆ Many variables were studied.
◆ The fact that only a small number of predictor variables were used, relative to the total number of variables studied, increased the chances of statistical error.

Predictor Research

Several prospective studies have been conducted to identify predictors of clinical outcome, such as whether patients remain in, work in, and benefit from day treatment. The practical value of such investigations lies in their ability to provide clinicians with information that will allow them to direct the most appropriate patients into day treatment.

Perhaps one of the most comprehensive examinations of day treatment success was conducted with the Edmonton Day Treatment Program by our research group (Piper et al. 1994). We were interested in determining whether pretreatment characteristics of the patients could predict whether they would remain in the program and achieve favorable outcome. Five predictor variables (age, marital status, previous psychiatric hospitalization, presence of a PD, and level of initial disturbance) were chosen on the basis of significant findings of previous research. Two other variables, quality of object relations (QOR) and psychological mindedness, were selected on the basis of previous research (McCallum and Piper 1990a; Piper et al. 1990) and theory.

Quality of object relations (QOR) is defined as an individual's enduring tendency to establish certain kinds of relationships with others (Azim et al. 1991). It refers to a lifelong pattern. It is measured by a semistructured interview with explicit scoring criteria. Its psychometric properties have been strong (Piper and Duncan 1999). Scores range along a 9-point dimension from primitive to mature. At the primitive end of the 9-point scale, the person tends to react to perceived separation from or loss of the object, or to disapproval or rejection by the object, with intense anxiety and affect. An inordinate dependence on the object provides a sense of identity. At the mature end of the scale, the person tends to enjoy equitable relationships characterized by love, tenderness, and concern for objects of both sexes. There is a capacity to mourn and tolerate intolerable relationships.

Psychological mindedness is defined as the ability to identify dynamic (intrapsychic) components and relate them to a person's difficulties (McCallum and Piper 1990b). The components (wishes, fears, and defenses) are often in conflict with one another. Thus, psychological mindedness also represents an understanding of certain basic assumptions associated with psychodynamic theory. Psychological mindedness is assessed in a 15-minute semistructured interview during which the patient comments about a videotaped scenario of an actress patient talking to her therapist. Ratings range from a score of 1 to 9. At the low end of the scale, the patient merely recognizes the existence of internal states and their motivational qualities. At the high end of the scale, the patient recognizes defense mechanisms and the fact that they are only partially successful. Psychological mindedness also has had promising psychometric properties (McCallum and Piper 1997).

Overall, the strongest predictors found in our study (Piper et al. 1994) were the personality characteristics psychological mindedness and QOR. Psychological mindedness was directly related to favorable outcome on three of the four outcome factors (general symptoms, social maladjustment, and pathological dependency). The ability to identify conflictual components and relate them to a person's difficulties represents a valuable skill in a psychodynamic day treatment program. The degree to which patients worked in therapy also was assessed in the study. Psychological mindedness was found to be directly associated with patient work. QOR was directly related to remaining in the program and to favorable outcome on two of the outcome factors (general symptoms, social maladjustment). The lesser ability to establish mature, give-and-take, relationships may not have allowed patients to tolerate the daily interpersonal demands and stresses of the program. Three other predictors made significantly independent contributions to patient success. Older patients, who had greater life experience and possibly greater motivation to work, tended to remain. Married patients, who may represent those who are willing to enter into a serious intimate relationship, also tended to remain. Finally, patients with previous psychiatric hospitalization improved more on interpersonal functioning. The reason for this finding is not clear.

Wilberg et al. (1998) also explored personality predictors of the course of treatment in their day treatment program. The 128 patients studied over a 3.5-year period were divided into two groups: those with a Cluster A or B personality disorder and those with a Cluster C personality disorder or no PD; the latter group had better outcome on global functioning and health sickness. Clinical experience suggests that the number of patients with certain diagnoses and behavior problems should be limited. These include patients with antisocial behaviors, organic dysfunction, psychotic symptoms, active substance abuse, pending criminal charges, or a history of repeated failures in treatment. Most day treatment programs can tolerate the presence of some patients in these exclusion categories. The optimal composition of patients for day treatment programs is yet to be discovered.

Summary of Research Findings

Research that has focused on the outcome of psychodynamic day treatment for patients with PDs has consistently positive findings, but few studies have been done. Studies found that day treatment led to significant reductions in psychiatric symptoms and improvements in social and interpersonal functioning. Follow-up assessments have indicated that improvements for many patients have been maintained for months, or years, after the completion of the day treatment. Particularly notable were significant improvements for patients with BPD. This patient group is often very difficult to treat. Thus, day treatment should be considered an effective alternative for individuals with a PD, including those with BPD.

Studies of day treatment also have identified significant predictors of patients remaining in the program compared with those of patients dropping out prematurely. In addition to having a history of mature relationships, patients who are more likely to remain in day treatment are older and married. Patients with previous psychiatric hospitalization improve more on interpersonal functioning.

In addition to these research findings, clinical experience suggests that patients with certain traits do not do well in day treatment programs. These include antisocial traits, psychotic symptoms, organic dysfunction, recent substance abuse, and criminal behavior. These criteria are usually associated with severe PDs.

Problems of Implementation

Successful implementation of day treatment involves avoiding certain pitfalls that have historically plagued many programs. These include 1) attempting to treat inappropriate patients in day treatment (e.g., those who are too acutely disturbed or too chronically disabled to engage in therapeutic tasks); 2) attempting to treat a mixture of patients with conflicting needs in the same program (e.g., those who would benefit from intensive treatment and those who require support and management); and 3) alternating between leadership that is characterized by abdication of authority and by abuse of power.

No program can continuously adhere to ideal principles and completely avoid difficult problems. Programs must have ongoing opportunities for staff members to reflect on the multilevel processes of the program and make adjustments that support the principles and that attempt to overcome the difficulties. Staff members must be willing to examine their own interactions with patients and with one another. This can be done in a regular staff relations group. Essential qualities of a staff member include humility, containment of narcissistic needs, capacity to contain projections of patients, and, above all, a willingness to learn. These qualities require time to develop, which underscores the importance of maintaining a stable staff over time.

Findings from predictor studies should be regarded as tentative. Prediction is never perfect. Some patients regarded as high risk on the basis of their selection characteristics inevitably surprise us and do well. Excluding all persons who do not meet selection criteria means that such individuals would be prevented from receiving beneficial treatment. Clearly, we do not want to deprive all high-risk patients of an opportunity to benefit, even though we know that some of them will not. Researchers can inform clinicians about selection and risk factors, and then clinicians can decide how much risk or how many high-risk patients to accept for their program. Having a few high-risk patients in a day program is far different from having many.

Conclusion

More than 10 years ago, we concluded our book on time-limited day treatment (Piper et al. 1996) by highlighting nine themes that we believed characterized the field at that time. We have touched on a few of them in this chapter. They include the intransigent nature of PDs, the intensity and power of day treatment programs, the positive contribution of attributes of therapeutic communities, the efficacy of day treatment, and the time-effective quality of day treatment. These positive attributes have remained in effect but have not seemed to result in a proliferation of day treatment programs. Unfortunately, another theme that we identified in our book—inequitable funding and possible bias—is a likely contributor to what appears to be underuse of day treatment programs.

Historically, funding patterns of third-party payers for day treatment have tended to show inequalities. Financial support for day treatment has been less than that for inpatient care. In addition to higher copayment costs for patients, fees for psychiatrists have been lower. Other factors that have probably contributed to underuse are lack of clarity about what day treatment involves, less control of patient management, concern about malpractice actions, and less training of potential staff. If valid, all of these factors tend to favor the use of inpatient care, which may indicate a bias.

To be fair, however, the personnel costs for a day treatment program are considerable. An entire team must be employed. For example, although the Edmonton Day Treatment Program can treat as many as 40–45 patients simultaneously, it requires a part-time psychiatrist, a full-time coordinator, a secretary, and five full-time therapists. In the current uncertain and recessionary financial climate that most countries are facing, this type of financial investment may seem daunting. Nevertheless, overcoming the inequalities that we have identified is a necessary step if we want day treatment to be accessible. Otherwise, therapists and patients with PDs will be deprived of an effective treatment. We hope that the field can improve during the next decade.

Key Clinical Concepts

- ◆ Progress in developing and studying day treatment programs has been hampered by inconsistent and confusing terminology. Day treatment, day hospital, day care, and partial hospitalization should be clearly distinguished.

- ◆ Staff relations groups are an important component of day treatment programs. They help maintain a consistent and constructive management approach.

- ◆ Clinicians must be especially aware of their countertransference reactions, which may become quite intense in day treatment programs. Clinicians inevitably are pulled into enactments with patients in day treatment programs. They need to identify the enactments and find ways to convert the experiences into those that can be reflected on with patients as opposed to acted on. Often patients in inpatient care and patients in day treatment programs are more receptive to feedback from other patients than from staff members.

- ◆ Group therapies integrated into day treatment programs provide a powerful form of treatment for patients with personality disorders.

- ◆ Although few in number, large-scale outcome studies have found that day treatment is a cost-effective treatment for patients with personality disorders.
- ◆ Quality of object relations and psychological mindedness are among the best predictors of success in day treatment programs.
- ◆ Historically, day treatment has been provided with fewer resources and funds compared with inpatient care. This has contributed to underuse of day treatment.

Suggested Readings

Bateman A, Fonagy P: 8-Year follow-up of patients treated for borderline personality disorder: mentalization-based treatment versus treatment as usual. Am J Psychiatry 165:631–638, 2008. [These investigators reported on the follow-up status of patients with borderline personality disorder, who had participated in a randomized clinical trial that compared a psychoanalytically oriented day treatment program with a treatment-as-usual condition. The follow-up assessment occurred 8 years after the initial assessment.]

Gunderson JG, Gratz KL, Neuhaus EC, et al: Levels of care in treatment, in The American Psychiatric Publishing Textbook of Personality Disorders. Edited by Oldham J, Skodol AE, Bender DE. Washington, DC, American Psychiatric Publishing, 2005, pp 239–255. [These authors present a useful system that distinguishes among levels of intensity for treatments of personality disorders. Intensity of treatment is mainly defined by the number of hours of treatment. Day treatment occupies the third level of intensity.]

Piper WE, Rosie JS, Joyce AS, et al: Time-Limited Day Treatment for Personality Disorders: Integration of Research and Practice in a Group Program. Washington, DC, American Psychological Association, 1996. [This book presents a historical perspective of day treatment, research findings associated with a randomized clinical trial involving the Edmonton Day Treatment Program, and ideas about future directions that day treatment may take in the field of treating personality disorders. It attempts to integrate research and practice.]

References

American Psychiatric Association: Diagnostic and Statistical Manual of Mental Disorders, 3rd Edition, Revised. Washington, DC, American Psychiatric Association, 1987

Azim HFA, Piper WE, Segal PM, et al: The Quality of Object Relations Scale. Bull Menninger Clin 55:323–343, 1991

Bateman A, Fonagy P: Effectiveness of partial hospitalization in the treatment of borderline personality disorder: a randomized controlled trial. Am J Psychiatry 156:1563–1569, 1999

Bateman A, Fonagy P: Mentalization-Based Treatment for Borderline Personality Disorder: A Practical Guide. Oxford, UK, Oxford University Press, 2006

Bateman A, Fonagy P: 8-Year follow-up of patients treated for borderline personality disorder: mentalization-based treatment versus treatment as usual. Am J Psychiatry 165:631–638, 2008

Bender DS, Dolan RT, Skodol AE, et al: Treatment utilization by patients with personality disorders. Am J Psychiatry 158:295–302, 2001

Dolan B, Evans C, Norton K: Multiple Axis-II diagnoses of personality disorder. Br J Psychiatry 166:107–112, 1995

Gunderson JG, Gratz KL, Neuhaus EC, et al: Levels of care in treatment, in The American Psychiatric Publishing Textbook of Personality Disorders. Edited by Oldham J, Skodol AE, Bender DE. Washington, DC, American Psychiatric Publishing, 2005, pp 239–255

Kibel HD: Interpretive work in milieu groups. Int J Group Psychother 53:303–329, 2003

McCallum M, Piper WE: A controlled study of effectiveness and patient suitability for short-term group psychotherapy. J Consult Clin Psychol 40:431–452, 1990a

McCallum M, Piper WE: The Psychological Mindedness Assessment Procedure. Psychol Assess 2:412–418, 1990b

McCallum M, Piper WE: The Psychological Mindedness Assessment Procedure, in Psychological Mindedness: A Contemporary Understanding. Edited by McCallum M, Piper WE. Mahwah, NJ, Erlbaum, 1997, pp 27–58

Merikangas KR, Weissman MM: Epidemiology of DSM-III Axis II personality disorders, in Psychiatry Update: The American Psychiatric Association Annual Review, Vol 5. Edited by Frances AJ, Hales RE. Washington, DC, American Psychiatric Press, 1986, pp 258–278

Miller EJ, Rice AK: Systems of Organization: The Control of Task and Sentient Boundaries. New York, Tavistock, 1967

Miller JG: Living Systems. New York, McGraw-Hill, 1978

O'Kelly JG, Azim HF: Staff-staff relations group. Int J Group Psychother 43:469–483, 1993

Pilkonis PA, Neighbors BD, Corbitt EM: Personality disorders, in Cost-Effectiveness of Psychotherapy. Edited by Miller NE, Magruder KM. New York, Oxford University Press, 1999, pp 279–290

Piper WE, Duncan SC: Object relations theory and short-term dynamic psychotherapy: Findings from the Quality of Object Relations Scale. Clin Psychol Rev 19:669–685, 1999

Piper WE, Azim HF, McCallum M, et al: Patient suitability and outcome in short-term individual psychotherapy. J Consult Clin Psychol 58:475–481, 1990

Piper WE, Rosie JS, Azim HF, et al: A randomized trial of psychiatric day treatment for patients with affective and personality disorders. Hosp Community Psychiatry 44:757–763, 1993

Piper WE, Joyce AS, Azim HF, et al: Patient characteristics and success in day treatment. J Nerv Ment Dis 182:381–386, 1994

Piper WE, Rosie JS, Joyce AS, et al: Time-Limited Day Treatment for Personality Disorders: Integration of Research and Practice in a Group Program. Washington, DC, American Psychological Association, 1996

Piper WE, Ogrodniczuk JS, Duncan SC: Psychodynamically oriented group therapy, in Comprehensive Handbook of Psychotherapy, Vol 1: Psychodynamic/Object Relations. Edited by Kaslow FW, Magnavita JJ. New York, Wiley, 2002, pp 457–479

Rapoport RN: Community as Doctor. New York, Arno, 1980

Shur R: Counter-transference Enactment: How Institutions and Therapists Actualize Primitive Internal Worlds. Northvale, NJ, Jason Aronson, 1994

Stanton AH, Schwartz MS: The Mental Hospital: A Study of Institutional Participation in Psychiatric Illness and Treatment. New York, Basic Books, 1954

Steinberg PI, Duggal S: Threats of violence in group-oriented day treatment. Int J Group Psychother 54:5–22, 2004

Steinberg PI, Duggal S, Ogrodniczuk J: Threats of violence to third parties in group psychotherapy. Bull Menninger Clin 72:1–18, 2008

Wilberg T, Friis S, Karterud S, et al: Outpatient group psychotherapy: a valuable continuation treatment for patients with borderline personality disorder treated in a day hospital? A 3-year follow-up study. Nord J Psychiatry 52:213–221, 1998

Wilberg T, Urnes O, Friis S, et al: One-year follow-up of day treatment for poorly functioning patients with personality disorders. Psychiatr Serv 50:1326–1330, 1999

Wilberg T, Karterud S, Pedersen G, et al: Outpatient group psychotherapy following day treatment for patients with personality disorders. J Pers Disord 17:510–521, 2003

Yalom IE, Leszcz M: The Theory and Practice of Group Psychotherapy, 5th Edition. New York, Basic Books, 2005

Yeomans FE, Clarkin JF, Levy KN: Psychodynamic psychotherapies, in The American Psychiatric Publishing Textbook of Personality Disorders. Edited by Oldham J, Skodol AE, Bender DE. Washington, DC, American Psychiatric Publishing, 2005, pp 275–287

CHAPTER 14

Treatability of Personality Disorders

Possibilities and Limitations

Michael H. Stone, M.D.

One of the enduring paradoxes of analytically oriented psychotherapy is that personality disorders are, from a dynamic standpoint, often easy to understand yet uncommonly difficult to correct. The same may be said for certain persistent personality traits that fall short of amounting to an identifiable "disorder" but are challenging to remediate.

When Freud and his colleagues were developing psychoanalysis a century ago, most of the patients they described and treated had a character disorder (the word *personality* was not much used at the time). The various disorders were arrayed along a developmental track according to the supposition that there was a natural progression from an oral-cannibalistic stage in the earliest months of infant life, through later anal stages and finally a genital stage (representing the healthiest of the stages). If the latter were attained, one graduated, as it were, from the earlier neuroses, ending up as a relatively nonneurotic, psychologically intact individual. Broadly speaking, the generation of the pioneers tended to equate a particular character disorder with each successive stage: depressive (with the oral stage), obsessive-compulsive (anal stage), and hysteric (genital stage). Here we can make a generalization; namely, that the patients who exemplified these disorders showed inhibitions—particularly in the sexual realm. Even the "healthiest" of the neurotic patients—the hysteric—was pictured as a seductive, emotionally expressive yet sexually frightened and inhibited person (a woman, usually) who sought treatment for the conflict between her yearning for adequate sexual fulfillment and her fear of sexual intimacy. A generation later, some psychoanalysts added subdivisions to the original developmental scale. Wilhelm Reich (1929/1994), for example, described a *phallic-narcissistic* stage, proximate to the genital stage, the features of which were similar in some respects to the current narcissistic personality disorder. Yet Reich's patients, even those with what he called an "aristocratic" character, also were troubled primarily by inhibitions.

Dynamic psychiatry, when dealing with inhibited patients, often has good results. Inhibitions, especially in the sexual realm, typically center on a conflict in which a patient has a socially acceptable desire that happens to run counter to parental or cultural approval. As these patients gradually become aware that their desires are not inappropriate, let alone "sinful," they are able to make bolder steps into the hitherto forbidden areas. Many inhibited patients enjoy another advantage, vis-à-vis the demands of dynamic therapy: their problematic traits are egodystonic; they *suffer*—and thus have enhanced motivation to endure the rigors of therapy and see the process through to its conclusion.

Patients whose personality disorders lie largely in the noninhibited realm present problems of a quite different nature. Rather than the anxious and self-effacing attributes of inhibited persons, one sees entitlement, often of a grossly exaggerated quality, along with a dismissive attachment style. Entitlement and dismissiveness are defining characteristics of narcissistic personality disorder. These characteristics are often ego-syntonic, hence more impregnable to the forces of dynamic psychotherapy and more likely to be accompanied by poor motivation. Such a combination poses a stumbling block in the path of establishing a therapeutic alliance. Abrupt termination of therapy is common in such patients. Yet their psychodynamics may be as transparent as are those of their inhibited counterparts. The paradox alluded to earlier—dynamics easily understood but successful therapy difficult to achieve—is commonly encountered in patients of this sort. The personality disorders with strong narcissistic traits can in fact be well ordered along a spectrum, each component representing more severe and deeply embedded narcissistic traits and more powerful roadblocks in amenability to therapy. The spectrum may be pictured as beginning with narcissistic personality disorder, followed by malignant narcissism (as described by Kernberg [1992]), antisocial personality, and finally psychopathy and psychopathy with sadistic personality. Psychopathy, as described according to the criteria of either Robert Hare (Hare et al. 1990) or David Cooke (Cooke and Michie 2001), is simply not amenable to psychotherapy (Stone 2006).

If we view amenability to dynamic psychotherapy with a wide-angle lens, we see at the more favorable end the disorders of the so-called anxious cluster (obsessive-compulsive, dependent, and avoidant) and the aforementioned severe narcissistic disorders at the opposite end. One would have to add "hysteric character" as originally described in the earlier psychoanalytic literature to the more amenable types. In between the extremes are borderline and histrionic disorders (the other entities of the dramatic cluster) and the eccentric cluster disorders: schizoid, schizotypal, and paranoid. Histrionic personality disorder (HPD), as depicted in DSM, is a conflation of the older (and milder) hysteric attributes and other traits similar to those of borderline personality. Histrionic patients tend to be more chaotic and at times more irritable or hostile than are the "classical" hysteric patients (Stone 2005). Difficulties in applying dynamic therapy to histrionic patients come not so much from entitlement as from their tendency to be irresponsible about appointments, flighty, and prone to acting out (rather than dealing verbally with) the transference. A conceptual overlap is seen between the patients who satisfy DSM-IV-TR (American Psychiatric Association 2000) criteria for HPD and those described by Kernberg (1967) under the heading of infantile personality. The capacities for entering into a genuine therapeutic alliance and for self-reflection are not well developed in such patients.

The problems posed by patients in the eccentric cluster likewise center less on entitlement than on other factors, such as mistrustfulness (with its accompanying dismissive attachment style) in paranoid patients, lack of motivation in schizoid patients, and peculiarities in communication in schizotypal patients.

Some schizotypal patients are maddeningly concrete in their thinking. As a result, they have a hard time understanding the analogies a therapist may make relating a distortion in one area of thought or behavior to similar areas of thought or behavior. Thus, I once requested that a patient not leave apple cores on the waiting room table (as being unpleasant for the next patient); she left a banana peel on the table before her session a few days later. She challenged my admonition about leaving such material on the table with the comment, "You didn't say anything about bananas!" Other schizotypal patients may show idiosyncratic, not to say solipsistic, speech patterns that, albeit deeply meaningful to the patient, are quite baffling to the therapist. One such patient announced to me, for example, that "I was walking down your hall in a 'Ray Milland' way this morning, Dr. Stone; it's really all a matter of *ahimsa!*" I had no idea what was special about that movie actor's "way of walking," let alone what she meant to convey about her copying his gait. *Ahimsa* is the practice of "no harm" (to living creatures) advocated by certain Hindu sects. But what she hoped to communicate to me by this obscure metaphor remained unclear. It need hardly be said that speech patterns of this sort create impediments, often insuperable, in the path of dynamic psychotherapy.

Favorable Versus Unfavorable Attributes

A review of one's successes and failures within the roster of patients treated by dynamic psychotherapy helps create a catalog of qualities—some primarily cognitive, others primarily behavioral—that affect prognosis. By prognosis, I mean the amenability to success with a specifically dynamic approach. Prognosis in the larger sense of ultimate outcome may of course be favorable via other approaches even when a dynamic approach may have run aground. Hints of this were discernible in Wallerstein's *Forty-Two Lives in Treatment* (1986), based on an earlier study at the Menninger Clinic: some borderline patients did well (as judged by their outcome 5 or 10 years later) by a purely or predominantly psychodynamic therapy; others had done well when their treatment was switched to a more supportive approach. The same contrasts were noted in the long-term (10- to 25-year) follow-up studies of McGlashan (1986) and Stone (1990a) that concentrated on formerly hospitalized patients with severe personality disorders: mostly borderline but also narcissistic, schizotypal, and others.

The catalog of qualities or personality attributes affecting amenability to dynamic therapy can be arrayed as a series of spectra, each with a favorable attribute at one end and an unfavorable attribute at the other. Table 14–1 includes a list of these favorable and unfavorable attributes in relation to dynamic therapy (the list is not exhaustive but focuses on the main features).

When speaking about amenability to dynamic psychotherapy for the various personality disorders, we encounter a particular difficulty stemming from the tendency to rely on category-based definitions of personality. One implication of this tendency is to assume that the "anxious cluster" disorders, as alluded to earlier, by virtue of their representing the inhibited personality types, would indeed respond better to

TABLE 14–1.　Favorable versus unfavorable attributes in relation to dynamic therapy

Favorable	Unfavorable
Good reflective capacity; psychological mindedness	Poor reflective capacity; concreteness
Good empathic capacity	Poor empathic capacity
Cooperativeness; ability to form a therapeutic alliance	Uncooperativeness
Calmness	Action-proneness; chaotic impulsivity
Psychological strength; unflappability	Fragility; extreme fearfulness
Openness; capacity for insight	Dismissiveness; contemptuousness
Honesty; integrity	Deceitfulness
A history of being raised in a mostly loving environment, with a minimum of traumata	A history of overwhelming traumatization; a gross lack of humanizing influences (such as parental—especially maternal—affection)

dynamic therapies than would the other disorders recognized by DSM-IV-TR. But this is clearly not the case. Clinical experience makes us aware of two related phenomena that put an end to this simplistic assumption. First, few personality disorders (such as those of DSM) are seen in "pure form"—free of traits belonging to one of the other categories. Second, because personality disorders are almost invariably admixtures of traits from two or even more categories, the nature of the associated traits figures importantly in both amenability and ultimate prognosis. Hence a dimensional approach is more helpful as a guide to what to expect regarding response to therapy and the likelihood of eventual success. As an example, if the predominant personality configuration is *obsessive-compulsive*, amenability and prognosis for dynamic therapy will be greater if the next-most-prominent traits are *avoidant* and poorer if those secondary traits are *paranoid* or *schizoid*. A combination such as obsessive-compulsive with secondary *narcissistic* traits might occupy an intermediate position. But even here, one must pay attention to *which* narcissistic traits: "requires excessive admiration" and "preoccupied with fantasies of brilliance and beauty" are less worrisome than some of the other, more malignant narcissistic traits—namely, "exploitative" and "lacking in empathy" (which overlap with psychopathic personality).

Some combinations of predominant and associated types are quite common, and others are distinctly rare. Figure 14–1 shows an approximation of what therapists will encounter clinically. In this figure, I have arrayed the DSM categories, along with five other types not currently in DSM (hysteric, passive-aggressive, depressive, hypomanic, and psychopathic), in a matrix; the predominant personality type is aligned along the vertical axis, and the next-most-prominent type is aligned along the horizontal axis. The numbers refer to the relative frequency or rarity of the various combinations. Few, if any, epidemiological studies have focused on the actual comorbidities of these 225 combinations. If traits of a less prominent or "tertiary" significance were included, then the matrix would expand to a bewildering 3,375 varieties: something highly resistant to statistical analysis yet something clinicians assess automatically as they become familiar with their patients.

The figure highlights the comparative rarity of encountering an obsessive-compulsive person with hysteric traits because conceptually these disorders are diametrically opposite. McCann (2009), alluding to an earlier work by Pfohl and Blum (1995), mentioned that considerable comorbidity is found between obsessive-compulsive personality disorder (OCPD) and other disorders, such as "paranoid, histrionic, borderline, narcissistic, and avoidant" (p. 673). But he added that persons with OCPD "tend to be restrained in the expression of emotion, unlike the emotionally expressive histrionic and borderline personalities" (p. 673), which would support my point that the combination of OCPD and HPD is not as common as OCPD and, for example, narcissistic or paranoid personality disorders.

A small proportion of persons with a predominantly narcissistic personality disorder are also psychopathic, whereas the predominantly psychopathic person is invariably narcissistic (hence the "5" in the psychopathic × narcissistic box in Figure 14–1). Patients with borderline personality disorder (BPD) may show secondary characteristics of almost any other disorder, with the exception of *schizoid*. In the case of BPD the secondary traits assume great importance vis-à-vis response to dynamic therapy. Thus, BPD × histrionic or depressive traits will tend to have much greater amenability and much better prognosis than does BPD × paranoid or antisocial traits. Something similar has already been suggested in relation to the broader domain of borderline personality organization by Clarkin et al. (1999). In their book is a diagram (p. 6) showing the realm of borderline personality organization—in which malignant narcissism and antisocial personality disorder are placed, appropriately, at the bottom of the diagram, and histrionic is placed at the upper level.

	sz	pr	st	hi	na	bp	as	oc	dn	av	hy	pg	dp	hm	pp
SZ	–	3	3	1	2	1	2	4	1	1	1	2	1	1	2
PR	2	–	2	1	4	3	3	3	2	3	1	4	1	3	2
ST	3	4	–	1	3	3	2	3	3	3	2	3	3	1	1
HI	1	3	2	–	4	4	4	1	4	1	3	3	3	3	3
NA	2	4	2	2	–	4	3	3	3	3	3	3	2	3	3
BP	1	4	2	4	4	–	3	2	4	3	2	3	4	4	2
AS	2	4	1	3	5	3	–	1	1	2	1	4	1	2	4
OC	2	4	1	1	3	2	1	–	2	3	1	4	3	2	1
DN	2	1	2	3	2	3	1	3	–	4	3	2	4	1	1
AV	2	4	3	2	2	3	1	3	3	–	3	2	4	1	1
HY	1	1	1	1	4	1	1	1	4	4	–	1	4	3	1
PG	2	4	1	1	4	3	3	3	3	3	1	–	4	2	3
DP	2	2	1	2	2	3	1	3	4	4	2	2	–	1	1
HM	1	3	1	3	5	3	3	2	1	1	2	2	2	–	2
PP	2	3	1	3	5	2	5	2	1	1	1	3	1	2	–

FIGURE 14–1. Matrix of approximate frequencies of personality type combinations.

Vertical axis, uppercase: predominant personality type.
Horizontal axis, lowercase: secondary (accompanying) personality type.

SZ=schizoid; PR=paranoid; ST=schizotypal; HI=histrionic; NA=narcissistic; BP=borderline; AS=antisocial; OC=obsessive-compulsive; DN=dependent; AV=avoidant; HY=hysteric; PG=passive-aggressive; DP=depressive; HM=hypomanic; PP=psychopathic.

Frequency of various combinations:
1 = rare; 2 = occasional; 3 = fairly often; 4 = common; 5 = very common to universal.

The numbers assigned in this chart reflect the author's own experience, both from private practice and from participation in research groups devoted to the study of patients with borderline personality disorder.

Reflective Function

A good capacity for reflective function has been shown to be a favorable prognostic factor in dynamic therapy for patients with personality disorders, particularly those with BPD (Diamond et al. 2003; Levy et al. 2006). Others have noted a conceptual overlap among concepts such as reflective function and mentalization (the latter emphasized by Fonagy and Bateman) and mindfulness, psychological mindedness, empathy, and affect consciousness (Choi-Kain and Gunderson 2008). A connection between impairment in early mother-infant attachment, later traumatic experiences, and the development of BPD has been suggested by the research of Fonagy and Bateman (2008). The capacity for mentalization was hampered in such a context. Many borderline patients, nevertheless, showed improvement in their reflective function after a year of transference-focused psychotherapy (Levy et al. 2006). These encouraging results reflect averages over a fairly large number of patients. In the randomized controlled study of three modes of therapy carried out at the Personality Disorder Institute of Kernberg and colleagues, the 90 BPD patients were assigned randomly, with 30 in each group, to transference-focused psychotherapy, dialectical behavior therapy (DBT), or supportive therapy (Clarkin et al. 2007). However, therapists who have worked with many BPD patients over long periods are aware that some with good reflective function (either at the start or as therapy progresses) fail to show much improvement. In others, the initially poor reflective function remains poor no matter how long therapy continues. Still other BPD patients have a meager capacity for this function, yet the patients ultimately do surprisingly well.

Borderline patients with pronounced paranoid tendencies often fail to improve in reflective function over time and do not show much at the outset. The difficulty in putting oneself in the mindset of the other person— that is, the incapacity to "mentalize"—was apparent in a 29-year-old man in his fourth year of twice-weekly therapy. He related to me an incident that took place while he was reading his newspaper on the subway.

> A young woman was sitting next to him. When he had finished with one section of the paper, she asked if she might borrow that section for a bit to read it. The patient found this "intrusion" irritating and told me that he scowled at her and said, sharply, "No, you may not!" As the woman exited at the next stop, she muttered in his direction a highly uncomplimentary epithet.

I tried to explain to him that her request seemed quite innocent, and if he really did not want to share the paper with her, he could have said something to the effect, "Oh, I'm so sorry, ma'am, but I really need both parts of the paper, and I have to get off soon; otherwise, I would have been glad to." Then she would not have cursed at him. He told me, "The bitch didn't deserve it!" He simply could not grasp that it was his own rudeness that provoked her "bitchiness," which was probably not characteristic of her personality at all.

Another example of a patient with remarkably poor reflective function was a successful financial officer in a large corporation. The son of an upper-class English family, he had been sent to boarding school from age 6, after which he rarely saw his parents. He defined his problem as one of

marital difficulties. His wife at the time—his third—had been a man originally, a transsexual who had undergone surgery to create an artificial va-
gina. I was curious about what made such an alliance attractive to my
patient. Had there been an underlying interest in homosexual relationships at some point earlier in his life? Had he wished to avoid parenthood
in a "fail-safe" way by marrying someone anatomically incapable of having children? Thinking about the psychological meanings that might underlie his unusual choice of mate proved quite beyond this man. His
major complaint about his wife was that he—or she—was a "gold dig-
ger." My patient professed to not being averse to having children,
although, now in his 40s, he had had none by his first two wives and
certainly would have none by the current one. Even in a year's time in
therapy, he could come no closer to discovering any unconscious meanings to marrying a transsexual wife, as though it were not a matter of
choice but merely (as he put it) the luck of the draw. Ultimately, he did di-
vorce and some months later dated and then married a woman whom he
regarded as much sweeter and devoted than the previous three. Feeling
contented with his life, he left therapy at this point. It remained unclear
whether the therapy had been beneficial in any way, despite the absence
of any unearthing of dynamics or any insight, or whether his more har-
monious choice this time also was merely the luck of the draw.

At the opposite end of the spectrum are patients with severe personality disorders whose reflective function is excellent yet whose ability to
make positive gains in dynamic therapy is sharply limited. One factor
predisposing to this otherwise paradoxical situation is a firmly entrenched symptom disorder. I had occasion to work, for example, with a
mental health professional who hoarded canned food. The accumulation
grew to such proportions that his small apartment was nearly uninhab-
itable. His hoarding was a defense ostensibly against the possibility of either a natural disaster or an enemy invasion that would suddenly
denude grocery stores of their supplies. But underneath that unlikely
scenario was the dynamic, of which he was clearly cognizant, that his
cruel mother frequently punished him as a child by making him go to
bed without his supper. Even on good days she doled out his food in the
most exiguous portions, such that he was almost always hungry. The obsessive-compulsive disorder that eventually developed may have been
driven in large part to an inherited tendency to an anxiety disorder, but
the form it took, as he himself was aware, was shaped by the starvation
regimen of his early years. The symptom did not yield even to maximal
doses of fluoxetine. He also found the alternative task—of walking *past*
the grocery shop while writing down the anxious thoughts that emerged
as he steeled himself not to go inside and purchase anything—quite

impossible. Hence there was nothing more we could learn about the psychodynamics of his condition beyond what was already apparent.

Importance of Individual Traits

I have discussed the inadequacy of adhering to a strictly category-based approach when evaluating amenability to dynamic psychotherapy and suggested that we would be better served by regarding the various types in a dimensional model (much as is done in the Minnesota Multiphasic Personality Inventory), which permits finer distinctions. However, adding that step will not really suffice to address all the relevant particularities we see routinely in our clinical work with actual patients. As I have suggested elsewhere (Stone 1993, 2006), we need to pay attention also to the *lexical* level; that is, to the level of single personality traits. Included among the 10 DSM-IV-TR personality disorders are several dozen traits (as well as descriptors such as "suicidal gestures" or "frantic efforts to avoid abandonment," which are behaviors rather than traits). Such a catalog is briefer by several orders of magnitude compared with the list of significant traits in everyday language. I enumerated some 500 negative traits and 100 positive traits, which, taken together, constitute an irreducible minimum, irrespective of one's primary language. The number of combinations of these traits is mindbogglingly large, pointing to the uniqueness of the personality of each human being—akin to the uniqueness of our fingerprints.

Fortunately for psychotherapists, it is not necessary to grapple with 6 billion combinations or even the 600 important traits. Some are more important than others, whether as stumbling blocks to therapy or as facilitators. As for facilitators, Freud (1904/1953) said long ago that a precondition to the success of psychoanalytic treatment is having *good character*. Good character is composed of the traits mentioned in my list of the factors into which the 100 positive traits can be compartmentalized. Not each person with "good character" will have the same combination. However, people will show an assortment of traits from factors (or subcategories) such as friendly, attentive, serene, self-assured, kind (which would include compassionate and forgiving), respectful, assertive, conscientious, honest, open, and affiliative (Stone 1993, p. 111). The stumbling blocks are larger: as social creatures, we pay more attention to qualities in others that annoy, disgust, or threaten us than we do to the "expected" and favorable qualities we assume (until proven otherwise) are present in those with whom we interact. In my analysis of the negative traits, most were bothersome to others; some were troublesome to the person in question (such as anxious or shy). For didactic purposes I divided the many negative traits into some three dozen factors, including (alphabetically) *aggressive, angry/irritable*...down to *unfair* and *unsympathetic* (Stone 1993, p. 108). Later, I submitted a list of three dozen personality traits whose presence "if intense, create severe problems for psychotherapy, even in the absence of a definable personality disorder" (referring to the DSM categories) (Stone 2006, p. 195). These were all negative traits we view as troublesome to others and include qualities such as *abrasive, bigoted, bitter, humiliating, envious, maudlin, prudish, quarrelsome, spiteful, unforgiving, vindictive,* and *vicious*.

Traits troublesome primarily to the self usually constitute less serious impediments to dynamic therapy than is the case with the aforementioned obnoxious traits. Those who, for example, are oversensitive, overly scrupulous, or shy offend other people less; have less stormy interpersonal relationships; are often more introspective; and end up more responsive to the demands of dynamic, psychoanalytically oriented therapy. A few traits in this latter category are troublesome mostly to the self but do create formidable hurdles to any attempt at dynamic therapy. One example is that of "infantile personality," as described by Kernberg (1967). Although not included in some of the latest compendia of personality disorders (namely, Livesley 2001; Oldham et al. 2005), infantile personality is mentioned by Millon and Davis (2000) as a variation of HPD (p. 240). Their description shows an association between infantile personality and BPD and mentions traits such as labile, volatile, prone to childlike hysteria and nascent pouting, demanding, and clinging. It is characteristic of infantile persons to seek reassurance—in a most insistent and petulant manner—from others, including their therapists. Passivity is marked, one facet of which is that the infantile patient wants the therapist to do all the work.

Another impediment, belonging to the realm of inhibited or anxious types, and one seldom mentioned in the literature, is that of religious fundamentalism—when the latter is pressed into service to justify avoidance of sexual exploration and intimacy. Because certain fundamentalists rely on culturally sanctioned and, to their way of thinking, God-commanded prohibitions, theirs often becomes an impregnable (literally and figuratively) defense against overcoming sexual inhibitions.

Problems Arising Out of the Diversity in the Borderline Domain

Therapists concentrating on working in a dynamic mode with borderline patients sometimes fall into the trap of assuming that because certain forms of therapy have been recommended for patients with borderline personality organization (Kernberg 1967), or even with the narrower concept of BPD, these recommendations are applicable to all patients whose clinical descriptors fit within these definitions. Nowhere in the realm of the personality disorders is the fallacy of *one label/one therapy* more visible. This is so for two interrelated reasons. First, the diversity of clinical varieties that fall within these broad categories is much greater than is found with the other personality disorders. I noted earlier how BPD can be admixed with almost all the other disorders, yielding a heterogeneity that spans the spectrum from BPD and depressive (or "depressive-masochistic") personality disorder—with its relatively good amenability to dynamic therapy—to BPD and antisocial personality disorder—with its poor amenability and gloomy prognosis. Second, within the borderline domain, great diversity exists with regard to the life course leading up to the time of initial diagnosis. Some borderline patients have been fortunate enough to have suffered little in the way of traumata (verbal, physical, sexual, neglect-related) in their early years. A fair proportion, especially among female borderline patients, have been molested sexually, whether incestuously or by persons outside the family (Stone 1990b; Zanarini et al. 2002). In the incest cases, the worse the abuse, the less was the likelihood for remission of BPD via treatment (Zanarini et al. 2005); similarly, the earlier the abuse began, the worse the life course tended to be (and the greater the overlap with the diagnosis of posttraumatic stress disorder) (McLean and Gallop 2003). But this does not quite tell the whole story. Borderline patients who have been incest victims, especially before age 10 years, are already a fairly fragile group, not always readily amenable to psychoanalytically oriented therapy, but in a subset of such patients (almost all women), the degree of trauma was extraordinarily severe and their subsequent behavior was so catastrophic as to create insuperable hurdles to the task of conducting dynamic therapy.

Even in these situations, a proportion of therapists remain committed to the idea that because their patient is borderline, transference-focused psychotherapy or the mentalization-based treatment advocated by Bateman and Fonagy (2004) would be appropriate. During a visit to a European clinic specializing in dynamic psychotherapy, I learned recently about a whole roster of extremely traumatized borderline patients. One woman, living alone in her 40s, had been an incest victim for many years while growing up. A short while back, she had disemboweled herself (only the worst in a long string of severe self-cutting episodes) and then fingered her own intestines. The staff members of the clinic were highly trained and devoted professionals who, correct in their appraisal of this woman as "borderline," were persisting in their efforts to help her via a dynamic therapy, despite the many indications that she was beyond its reach. To the unrelenting horrors of her early life were now added poverty, solitude, meager capacities for self-support through work, and the advance of years—all of which imposed serious limits on her ability to improve. Added to these drawbacks was the intensity of her rage, first at the incest perpetrator, later at her own self—all collapsed together in the unprecedented nature of her self-destructiveness (this was not a Japanese person committing *seppuku*). There may well have been a psychotic core behind the otherwise BPD-like psychopathology, given the rarity of her symptom. That would impose even more stringent limits on the efficacy of dynamic, as opposed to supportive, psychotherapy.

Symptoms that are at once bizarre and unique often point to a psychotic core in patients who appear at first glance as borderline.

> I saw in consultation a black high school senior. She had been adopted at birth by a white professional family with two children of their own. They had hoped to give her opportunities she would not have enjoyed had she remained in her own community. She felt estranged from her black classmates, who rejected her because she had grown up in a well-to-do white family; she felt alienated from white people because she was black. Her ego fragility was such that she felt great shame because of her race, and this had led to her symptom of defecating on the bathroom floor—because she felt her body would somehow befoul the toilet seat for the rest of the family were she to use it.

She was referred to me as a patient with BPD, but I believed that her symptom, along with other signs of a more serious illness, pointed to schizophrenia, for which a psychoanalytically oriented therapy would have been contraindicated.

In general, as is mentioned in Table 14–1, a history of overwhelming traumatization should serve as a cautionary note in relation to the efficacy of dynamic psychotherapy, granted that patients of course differ in their resiliency: those blessed with the strongest constitutions and the best combination of modulating ("protective") genes may flourish despite their traumatic history and may manifest a good degree of reflective function that justifies a dynamic approach. As Mitton and coworkers (1997) suggested, although many sexually abused borderline patients ultimately made good recoveries at long-term follow-up, the recovery process often took 5–10 years longer than was the case with nonabused borderline patients (p. 200). Meanwhile, the less hardy (and maximally traumatized) will require a more supportive and educative approach.

Effect of Narcissistic Traits

A burgeoning literature indicates the difficulties in carrying out psychotherapy, especially of a dynamic type, with narcissistic patients. Those who function at the borderline level in Kernberg's model of psychic organization often present still more formidable challenges; greater still are those we encounter when dealing with patients meeting criteria for both BPD and narcissistic personality disorder (as described in DSM-IV-TR). Several authors have drawn attention to common countertransference problems. Arnold Cooper (1986) mentioned that the therapist is "more likely to find himself bored, or angry...or generally uneasy with the feeling of lifelessness presented in treatment." He added that the patient's cold grandiosity may arouse a retaliatory anger in the therapist or that the therapist's interventions are ignored or denigrated, and no indications are perceptible that any tie exists between the two parties (pp. 140–141). Glen Gabbard (1998) sounded a similar note, underlining the common feelings of boredom and of being distanced by the narcissistic patient, adding that therapists are prone to react negatively to the patient's contemptuous attitude, conveyed often enough in comments to the effect that the therapist has nothing new or useful to say (p. 136). Other comments of a denigrating nature "tend to erode the therapist's confidence and feelings of effectiveness" (p. 137). In patients with BPD and narcissistic personality disorder, one often encounters a grandiosity that is spread thin over a deeper layer of inadequate feelings and envy (the latter being the most corrosive of the seven deadly sins [Schimmel 1997]).

In the context of dynamic therapy, a conflict will emerge in narcissistic-borderline patients in which their attitude will shift between two extremes. At one end, the patient will feel comfortably superior to the therapist (in intelligence, social standing, wealth) but therefore hopeless about getting better (because the therapist has "nothing to offer" that the patient has not already thought of)—*and will break off treatment.* At the other end, the patient will feel a measure of hope in the treatment on the grounds that the therapist may be superior in certain ways. Yet the patient consequently will feel consumed with envy about this very painful disparity—*and will break off treatment.* This paradox-ridden situation helps account for the dismissiveness of narcissistic patients, a side effect of which is the premature rupture of the therapeutic relationship.

Borderline patients do have a high quit rate, compared with many other types of patients with personality disorders (apart from their equally dismissive antisocial counterparts). Waldinger and Gunderson (1984) reported a 40% rate of premature quitting in their analysis of several samples of borderline patients—a figure that corresponds to my own experience over the years. Methodical surveys focusing on the comparative quit rates among the various subtypes of BPD patients are lacking. In my experience, more of the BPD–narcissistic personality disorder patients I have worked with over the years have broken off treatment prematurely than has been the case with other subtypes, except for the even higher quit rate for BPD–antisocial personality disorder patients.

Most of the predominantly narcissistic patients (some with borderline features as well) have been male; their most striking trait was contemptuousness. In a few others their main trait was a peacock-like self-absorption and grandiosity: they were highly successful and affluent men still obsessed with dating runway models, lamenting only that, as they approached their 50s, they still "hadn't found the right one." These men entertained some hope that I might magically (meaning: quickly) help them find the "right one"—but they were no more committed to me and the therapy than they were to the pretty "bimbos" they courted, who served mostly as "arm candy" to inflate their egos. None stayed for any appreciable length of time. The narcissistic patients whose main trait was contemptuousness had been more motivated for therapy but quit for the reason I outlined earlier: ambivalence about my being a professional of some repute in the community. After a short while, their competitiveness and envy rose to the surface. It was no consolation that I was 40 years older. This may in the transference have moved me from a more successful "older brother" to an even more threatening father figure, given that their fathers had been arrogant and dismissive. Contempt became the antidote to envy, and they left treatment. These narcissistic patients, via their own dismissiveness, could now continue to maintain the illusion that I could not help them, no one else could either, and therefore they were "superior" after all, albeit lonely. In the psychological calculus of the narcissist, it is safer to sever relations with someone who (like one of their dismissive parents) might turn out to be a carbon copy of the disappointing parent than to risk continuing in therapy and face the (in their minds) inevitable disappointment head on.

The overall picture with narcissistic traits is not as gloomy as these remarks suggest: in many patients, including those with borderline features, their narcissistic traits are 1) not as pronounced as in the patients I have described and 2) not composed of the more malignant qualities of low empathy, exploitativeness, and arrogance. Kernberg (1992) has written about these more therapy-receptive narcissistic patients, offering suggestions about how best to approach the challenges they present.

Effect of Antisocial Traits

Thanks to the polythetic criteria sets for the Axis II personality categories, considerable diversity is already built into the system, which gives it a measure of dimensionality, limited of course to the confines of each supposed category. Figure 14–1 reflects a broader dimensionality because it asks the clinician to record the next-most-prominent group of traits after the most significant one. To do full justice to the evaluation of personality disorder, ideally all noteworthy traits would be included, but this task requires the addition of a lexical approach. To do even fuller justice to our evaluations, we would also want to pay attention to the intensity (in scalar terms, the amplitude) of each trait. Mental exercises of this sort are particularly important when dealing with patients who show antisocial traits.

With this in mind, I have shown via a graph in Figure 14–2 the contrasting intensities of the seven DSM-IV-TR criteria for antisocial personality disorder. The intensities are reflected in the comparative heights of the X's for each item of the DSM criteria set. Currently DSM-IV-TR requires only three of the seven items, allowing for some 210 combinations—within the antisocial personality disorder criteria set itself and not taking into account the myriad admixtures with the traits of other disorders.

Both of the patients in Figure 14–2 were chosen from the 23 antisocial patients (14 male; 9 female) seen in my private practice over the past 43 years. Both patients were women in their late 20s and had been referred to me for analytically oriented therapy. Patient 1 was the only female patient who remained in treatment for an appropriate length of time. Her antisocial traits were less prominent than were those of Patient 2 (who manifested antisocial personality disorder proper, endorsing all seven items). Both came from upper-middle-class families whose other members were solid, responsible persons.

> Patient 1's problems included stalking a former boyfriend via multiple means, including sending him letters as if written by other acquaintances (all penned by Patient 1 herself, using different e-mail addresses, different stationery, etc.), reprimanding him for his "outrageous mistreatment" of his girlfriend. She showed no reflective capacity and externalized blame entirely onto the boyfriend. I urged her, not without some vehemence, to stop the stalking behavior, but it was to no avail. She lied to me that she had not tried to communicate with him any longer, but I was certain she had done so. With her permission, I contacted the young man and had him e-mail me whenever she sent him e-mails, made "hang-up" calls, or wrote letters. Because her deceptive-

1	2	3	4	5	6	7	<<	>>	1	2	3	4	5	6	7
							J	J							X
							I	I	x						
	X						H	H			x	x		x	
							G	G	x				x		
x							F	F							
		x					E	E							
							D	D							
					X		C	C							
			x			x	B	B							
					x		A	A							

············Patient 1············   ············Patient 2············

FIGURE 14–2. Contrasting profiles of two borderline patients with antisocial traits (as evaluated according to DSM criteria for antisocial personality disorder).

1=failure to conform to social norms; repeated acts that are grounds for arrest; 2=deceitfulness (repeated lying, use of aliases; conning others); 3=impulsivity or failure to plan ahead; 4=irritability and aggressiveness (namely, fights and assaults); 5=reckless disregard for the safety of others; 6=consistent irresponsibility (in work, in honoring debts); 7=lack of remorse (for acts hurtful to others).

A=not present or negligible; C=present to a fair degree; E=present to a moderate degree; G=a very prominent characteristic; J=present to an extreme degree.

X=intensity level of criterion for each patient; larger X's indicate greater intensity.

ness was now exposed, she eventually desisted. The several suicide gestures she had made while still dating the boyfriend also ceased. She did stalk yet another boyfriend, briefly, but he pressed charges—because of which she spent one night in detention. The judge allowed the offense to be expunged if she would refrain from a repeat of such activity for the next year. This was the turning point in her eventual recovery. She later married, maintained a good work record, and has been more open and honest with me during the past several years. She would no longer meet the DSM-IV-TR criteria for antisocial personality disorder.

Patient 2, also referred because of a "mood disorder," was bipolar. This may have heightened the risk for antisociality because a proportion of bipolar manic persons are highly irritable and aggressive, grandiose, contemptuous of the law, and prone to substance abuse (which further leads to impaired self-control and to dangerous behaviors). Patient 2's most noticeable characteristic was malice. Fancying herself a great beauty and actress, whose strivings for the fame to which she was surely entitled had been thwarted by the attention her parents bestowed on her sister rather than herself, she now devoted her efforts to avenge herself of their (in her words) heinous neglect. She sought ways to get back at each family member. She called her mother, "informing" her that she had "solid evidence" that her father was having an affair with his secretary. At first this caused a serious rift in her parents' relationship, but when it eventually became clear that the story was a tissue of lies, her parents reunited and kicked her out of the house. Morbidly envious of her sister, who had made a successful marriage, Patient 2 tried to poison her brother-in-law against her sister by "informing" him of "rumors" that her sister had cheated on him. After a half-dozen sessions, Patient 2 told me that since Plan 1 (the malicious rumors) was without effect, she was moving to Plan 2: traveling to where her sister and her husband lived and hiring someone to kill the sister. At this point I informed all her relatives of the plan and dismissed the patient from treatment.

The case of Patient 2 serves to explain the reason that dynamic therapy would be ineffective with such a patient. Psychodynamic therapy deals with conflicts between different mental agencies—customarily, between a strong desire and the voice of conscience. With an amoral patient, this situation is not relevant: no conscience, no conflict. Patient 2 was more than merely antisocial; she was what Robert Hare (1993) has called the "white-collar psychopath," further examples of which I have provided in a recent book (Stone 2009). Unlike psychopathic persons (most of whom will be men) from disadvantaged social circumstances, who show the typical behavioral attributes of the psychopathic patient (e.g., early conduct disorder, juvenile delinquency, revocation of conditional release), psychopathic persons from more affluent families show fewer of those "criminological" attributes. Instead, their personality aberrations are confined mostly to the extreme narcissistic items of Hare's factor #1 in the Psychopathy Checklist—Revised (Hare et al. 1990). These consist of glibness, grandiosity, deceitfulness, conning and manipulativeness, callousness, lack of remorse, and inability to acknowledge responsibility for one's actions. Unlike the behavioral items that are usually quite visible to outsiders (assaults, arrest records, inability to hold a job), the narcissistic items can more easily be kept hidden for a long time, even from therapists with analytic training, with whom such persons may on occasion end up in treatment focusing on dynamics. Of the 23 patients I identified in my practice as antisocial, four of the women (including Patient 2) and seven of the men also met criteria for this white-collar psychopathy (with high scores on factor #1 and no more than modest scores on the behavioral items of factor #2). Only two of the 23 patients remained in treatment long enough for some important goal to be achieved. These two had antisocial features but were not psychopathic; Patient 1 was one of these, and the other was an alcoholic man in his 20s who had done several dramatically hostile acts aimed at getting his wealthy parents in trouble. Once he joined Alcoholics Anonymous, under my persuasion, he made rapid improvement, but the therapy was supportive rather than dynamic.

Summary of the Main Impediments to Dynamic Therapy

Thus far I have enumerated the major attributes of personality and of general mental state that render the task of carrying out a successful psychodynamically oriented therapy either difficult or impossible. These attributes constitute the limitations of treatability by this method. Some of these were already listed in Table 14–1. The list can now be broadened to include some of the traits of antisocial or psychopathic disorders, as well as others not previously highlighted. This fuller list is detailed in Table 14–2.

I have not yet drawn attention to *sadistic traits,* such as those outlined in Appendix A of DSM-III-R (American Psychiatric Association 1987). My colleagues and I at the New York State Psychiatric Institute recently compartmentalized the eight items mentioned in DSM-III-R into three main factors, to which we gave the names *gleeful cruelty, super control,* and *soul murder* (Stone et al. 2009). The first of these captures the main prototypical sadistic trait: taking pleasure in inflicting suffering on others. The second focuses on the sadist's quest for absolute domination and control; the subjugation of one's will to the will of the sadist. The third addresses the tendency of sadistic persons to humiliate others, especially when the victims are surrounded by an "audience"—whose presence will necessarily add to the embarrassment of the victims. Sadists of the gleefully cruel type are encountered mostly in forensic work, especially among those who physically torture their victims. The closet sadists, who are rarely encountered in private practice or clinics, make a living hell for their sexual partners or spouses, children, or subordinates at work by virtue of their domineering interactions and extreme unfairness (the super-control group, which also includes workplace bullies) or by making humiliating comments, imposing degrading tasks, and so forth (the soul-murder group).

Sadistic personality is no longer included in the more recent editions of DSM, which is unfortunate for two reasons: 1) sadistic persons continue to exist in impressive numbers, and 2) the defining criteria are distinct from those of either antisocial personality disorder or psychopathy

Table 14–2.   Limiting factors in the treatment of personality disorders

1. Diminished reflective capacity, especially one that resists amelioration with one of the dynamic therapy approaches; marked concreteness of thought

2. Marked ego fragility (because of factors such as proneness to psychotic disorganization or overwhelming past traumatization)

3. Poor empathic capacity (because of marked narcissistic personality structure, as noted in narcissistic personality disorder, antisocial personality disorder, and psychopathy, or Asperger's-type autistic spectrum disorder)

4. Chaotic impulsivity (with corresponding tendency to "act out," especially if aggravated by substance abuse: alcohol, cocaine, methamphetamine, and the like)

5. Narcissistic traits or full-blown narcissistic personality disorder in which envy, arrogance, grandiosity, contemptuousness, entitlement, and exploitativeness are the dominant features; the syndrome of malignant narcissism

6. The "narcissistic" traits within the domain of antisocial personality disorder or psychopathy, especially lying, deceitfulness, callousness, conning, and lack of remorse

7. A predominantly dismissive attachment style

8. Other personality traits not readily subsumed under the criteria sets of the current Axis II disorders: bitterness, indiscretion, abrasiveness, shallowness (with lack of firm values), spitefulness, vindictiveness, marked sensation-seeking, malice

9. Sadistic traits: a strong penchant for humiliating others, subjugating others to one's will, and taking pleasure in the suffering of others

10. Marked rigidity of personality, as noted, for example, in believers of fundamentalist religions

and therefore (if only because of their importance in forensic psychiatry) deserve separate designation. Sadistic persons rarely if ever seek psychiatric help and are not amenable to it (the milder forms and rare exceptions aside). This means that sadists, like psychopathic persons, are beyond the reach not just of the dynamic therapies but also of all forms of treatment. One can make an even more compelling case for this when contemplating the overlap group; namely, the *sadistic psychopaths*, such as those whom forensic psychiatrists are called on to evaluate in cases of recidivist rapists, serial killers, and the like (Stone 2009). We fare no better with the more "genteel," less sadistic, psychopathic persons encountered among corrupt politicians, dodgy entrepreneurs, Ponzi-scheme swindlers, and the like.

Religious Fundamentalism as a Barrier to Treatability

In the Western world religious freedom is considered, both literally and figuratively, sacrosanct. Believers in all the major religions exist on a spectrum: at one end are believers who are not particularly observant and whose daily lives are affected only to a modest extent by the rules and pronouncements of their professed faith; at the other end are believers who, paradoxically, use their religious freedom to curtail greatly the ordinary freedoms and liberties taken by their less devout counterparts in the ways they live their day-to-day lives. Their self-imposed limitations, because they are not troubled by biblical injunctions against theft and murder, are expressed chiefly in the *sexual* sphere. Masturbation remains problematic for some, but constraint is more often honored in the breach in today's generation. However, premarital sexual intercourse continues to inspire major conflicts in the religiously devout, especially in those whose rigidity and insistence on the strictest of moral codes place them in the ranks of what we can call *fundamentalists*. By this term I do not mean zealotry of a sort that seeks to impose their faith on others; I refer, rather, to an iron-clad severity of observance that is confined to their personal lives. Sometimes this severity is simply the product of having been raised in a similarly strict religious household and community. But in recent years I have seen increasing numbers of patients, in their late teens or early adult life, who either have been influenced by fundamentalist teachers or have gravitated of their own accord to very strict religious groups or cults. Thus men with fears about sexual performance or about "commitment" to a lasting relationship and women with fears about sexual relations in general (and premarital sexual intercourse in particular) or about pregnancy and motherhood are able to submerge one arm of the sexual conflict underneath the patina of religious injunction. "I would really like to" is papered over by "Thou shalt not."

Because sexual urges have a way of trumping even these moral strictures, some fundamentalist persons eventually seek help from psychiatry. From the standpoint of personality, obsessive-compulsive and avoidant traits are usually quite prominent. Because these traits belong to the realm of *inhibition*, the underlying conflicts should be resolvable by any of the currently popular approaches: psychodynamically oriented (especially because of its focus on conflict resolution), cognitive-behavioral, or supportive. But the more rigid the personality structure, the less amenable to therapy these sexual conflicts are. What I have noted instead in some patients is a tendency to engage repeatedly in behaviors that externalize the problem, as though the trouble is really "out there" rather than within themselves. One such patient—a woman with marked anxieties about self-image and about intimacy, both psychological and sexual—had begun to affiliate with a small religious group that was of the same denomination as that of her parents but far more strict. This allowed her to rationalize her problem along the lines that even the mildest of premarital sexual behaviors such as kissing or petting were sinful; her avoidance therefore was not a reflection of inhibitions within her. The invitation to consider the possibility that internal conflicts might be the driving force behind her avoidant behavior did not meet with relief and subsequent exploration in therapy; it led instead to her abruptly quitting treatment. Along similar lines, a young man who had admired certain classmates from afar, but who had never dated, spent a year abroad, during which time he got swept up in a religious cult far stricter in its prohibitions against any forms of premarital sexual play than was the case with his observant but not fanatical parents. In his personality the prominent features were obsessive-compulsive and also a kind of compensatory narcissism that hid underlying feelings of inferiority. Subject to mood swings that were probably the harbinger of incipient bipolar disorder, he spent inordinate amounts of time on the Internet searching for the "right" combination of medications that would cure him. Once in treatment, he dwelt endlessly on the subject of these magical combinations. He avoided all reference to his personal life. As for the dating problem, he also resorted to the Internet, looking at dating Web sites pertinent to his newfound religious order. He found a few young women from faraway places. But he was reluctant to accept that any meetings that might grow out of such searches were doomed from the start because he could never get to know any of them as one does those in one's own area. His religion, albeit of new vintage, served as a shield protecting him from trying his luck with sexual performance and with testing the merits of any girlfriends to discover which ones might be suitable as a long-term mate. When this interpretation was made, he broke off treatment. In these examples, religion rendered traits and attitudes *ego-syntonic* that would better have remained *ego-dystonic* to provide the necessary impetus and motivation for completing the therapeutic task.

Conclusion

In the realm of personality disorders the literature on treatability is vast; that dealing with the limitations of treatment is scant. Recommendations regarding treatability bespeak optimism; talk of limitations or outright untreatability reaches less receptive ears.

I mentioned at the beginning of this chapter that inhibited personality types are generally responsive to dynamic therapy approaches, which require good character and rely on adequate motivation and perseverance. Other currently available approaches are also likely to succeed with patients who show these basic characteristics. Dynamic approaches still may be useful with milder instances of, say, narcissistic, histrionic, borderline, or even paranoid traits.

In confronting patients with significant admixture of antisocial traits, the efficacy of dynamic therapy begins rapidly to fade; cognitive approaches have greater likelihood of being effective, at least to some degree, so long as the patient stops short of outright psychopathy. Beck and Freeman (1990) made a useful statement: "Rather than attempting to build a better moral structure through the induction of affect such as anxiety or shame, cognitive therapy of ASPD [antisocial personality disorder] can be conceptualized as improving moral and social behavior through enhancement of cognitive functioning" (p. 152). In a more optimistic note than I would have offered, they even stated that "psychopaths have been shown to learn from experience when the contingencies are immediate, well-specified, tangible, and personally relevant" (p. 151). Recognizing that antisocial and psychopathic persons (except perhaps those with the mildest expression of these tendencies) are less prone to anxiety and shame than are healthy persons, Beck and Freeman made a good argument for moving toward a cognitive mode oriented toward better *cost-benefit* analysis in the social milieu. It would indeed be better (as they recommend), if presented with a last-minute assignment at work on a late Friday afternoon, to grumble a bit under one's breath and to do the work rather than tell the boss to go to hell and get fired. Such recommendations have no relevance, however, in dealing with violent criminal psychopaths who are notoriously adept at conning prison and hospital personnel that they have "turned over a new leaf" and are "truly" now ready for reintroduction to life in the community. Among the ranks of serial killers, for example, premature release from institutions or prisons, with subsequent commission of even worse crimes, occurs in more than a quarter of the cases (Stone 2009).

Contemporary research, including that of prospective follow-up, suggests that the currently used methods for treating BPD are about equally effective in remediating the common symptom component of self-cutting and other types of self-harm (de Groot et al. 2008). However, those most closely associated with each particular method argued for the superiority of their method (see Linehan 1993, for DBT; Bateman et al. 2007, for mentalization-based treatment; Clarkin et al. 2007, for transference-focused psychotherapy; Davidson et al. 2006, for cognitive therapy). John Livesley (2007) suggested the adoption of an *integrated* approach for BPD therapy, in which one is free to choose from the different approaches those elements of particular utility to each BPD patient, given the particularities of each patient as the therapist becomes familiar with these over time. Therapists must remain well grounded in the treatment approach in which they were trained while simultaneously remaining open to certain advantages that other approaches may confer at various points during the (usually rather lengthy) course of therapy for BPD. This flexible treatment philosophy is embodied also in the recommendations of Judd and McGlashan (2003) in their excellent treatise on borderline patients.

Supportive therapy, many elements of which (e.g., reassurance, sympathy, exhortation, education, limit-setting, advice) constitute the bedrock on which the more specialized techniques rest, is particularly indicated for all but the mildest instances of the eccentric cluster disorders. Supportive therapy is often the mainstay for patients with other personality disorders, for whom some of the specialized approaches are out of reach because of disadvantages in economic circumstances, deficiencies in intellectual capacity, or peculiarities of cognitive style.

Admittedly, the most severe limitations in working therapeutically with patients with personality disorders pertain more to the domain of forensic than of conventional psychiatry. Every therapist's roster will include a percentage of scarcely treatable, or even untreatable, patients. For forensic psychiatrists, this percentage will be considerably greater. It is always valuable to be aware of the limitations inherent in our field, so that our energies are spent more wisely and (especially in the forensic domain) our decisions vis-à-vis the community are similarly wise.

Key Clinical Concepts

- ◆ The treatability of personality disorders depends greatly on the admixture, in any given patient, of favorable versus unfavorable traits.
- ◆ In the domain of borderline personality disorder, accompanying traits, symptoms, and cognitive patterns are very diverse; amenability to psychotherapy will be affected by the nature and mixture of these factors.
- ◆ The patient's attachment style is an important factor influencing treatability: those with a predominantly dismissive style will be more difficult to treat; those with secure, entangled, fearfully preoccupied, or other styles generally will be more amenable to therapy (Levy et al. 2005).

- One must often pursue an integrated approach to therapy for borderline patients in particular; only a minority can be treated successfully by just one of the widely recognized treatment approaches from the very beginning to the end of treatment.
- Not all personality disorders fall within the realm of treatability: those with severe antisocial personality or with psychopathic or sadistic personalities lie largely outside this realm.

Suggested Readings

Clarkin JF, Yeomans FE, Kernberg OF: Psychotherapy for Borderline Personality. New York, Wiley, 1999. [This book gives the reader an excellent grasp of what transference-focused psychotherapy for BPD patients is and the guidelines for carrying out this type of treatment.]

Gabbard GO: Gabbard's Treatments of Psychiatric Disorders, 4th Edition, Part 10: Personality Disorders. Gunderson JG, Section Editor. Washington, DC, American Psychiatric Publishing, 2007, pp 757–854. [This section contains useful guidelines about the treatment of all the personality disorders recognized in DSM.]

Judd PH, McGlashan TH: A Developmental Model of Borderline Personality Disorder. Washington, DC, American Psychiatric Publishing, 2003. [A highly readable text with many informative clinical illustrations and sensible suggestions about psychotherapy for borderline patients.]

Millon T, Davis R (eds): Personality Disorders in Modern Life. New York, Wiley, 2000. [This book covers not only the DSM-listed disorders but also some of the other important disorders, including the sadistic personality. The book contains rich material about both diagnosis and therapy.]

Stone MH: Personality-Disordered Patients: Treatable and Untreatable. Washington, DC, American Psychiatric Publishing, 2006. [A comprehensive look at which types of personality disorders are amenable to psychotherapy.]

References

American Psychiatric Association: Diagnostic and Statistical Manual of Mental Disorders, 3rd Edition, Revised. Washington, DC, American Psychiatric Association, 1987

American Psychiatric Association: Diagnostic and Statistical Manual of Mental Disorders, 4th Edition, Text Revision. Washington, DC, American Psychiatric Association, 2000

Bateman A, Fonagy P: Psychotherapy for Borderline Personality Disorder: Mentalization-Based Treatment. Oxford, UK, Oxford University Press, 2004

Bateman A, Ryle A, Fonagy P, et al: Psychotherapy for borderline personality disorder: mentalization-based therapy and cognitive analytic therapy compared. Int Rev Psychiatry 19:51–62, 2007

Beck AT, Freeman A: Cognitive Therapy of Personality Disorders. New York, Guilford, 1990

Choi-Kain LW, Gunderson JG: Mentalization: ontogeny, assessment, and application in the treatment of borderline personality disorder. Am J Psychiatry 165:1127–1135, 2008

Clarkin JF, Yeomans FE, Kernberg OF: Psychotherapy for Borderline Personality. New York, Wiley, 1999

Clarkin JF, Levy KN, Lenzenweger MF, et al: Evaluating three treatments for borderline personality disorder: a multiwave study. Am J Psychiatry 164:922–928, 2007

Cooke DJ, Michie C: Refining the concept of psychopathy: toward a hierarchical model. Psychol Assess 13:171–188, 2001

Cooper AM: Narcissism, in Essential Papers on Narcissism. Edited by Morrison AP. New York, New York University Press, 1986, pp 112–143

Davidson K, Norrie J, Tyrer P, et al: The effectiveness of cognitive behavior therapy for borderline personality disorder: results from the Borderline Personality Disorder Study of Cognitive Therapy (BOSCOT) trial. J Pers Disord 20:450–465, 2006

de Groot ER, Verheul R, Trijsburg RW: An integrative perspective on psychotherapeutic treatments for borderline personality disorder. J Pers Disord 22:332–352, 2008

Diamond D, Stovall-McClough C, Clarkin JF, et al: Patient-therapist attachment in the treatment of borderline personality disorder. Bull Menninger Clin 67:227–259, 2003

Fonagy P, Bateman A: The development of borderline personality disorder: a mentalizing model. J Pers Disord 22:4–21, 2008

Freud S: On psychotherapy (1904), in The Standard Edition of the Complete Psychological Works of Sigmund Freud, Vol 7. Translated and edited by Strachey J. London, Hogarth Press, 1953, pp 257–268

Gabbard GO: Transference and counter-transference in the treatment of narcissistic patients, in Disorders of Narcissism. Edited by Ronningstam EF. Washington, DC, American Psychiatric Press, 1998, pp 125–135

Hare RD: Without Conscience: The Disturbing World of the Psychopaths Among Us. New York, Pocket Books, 1993

Hare RD, Harper TJ, Hakstian AR, et al: The revised Psychopathy Checklist: reliability and factor structure. Psychol Assess 2:238–241, 1990

Judd PH, McGlashan TH: A Developmental Model of Borderline Personality Disorder. Washington, DC, American Psychiatric Publishing, 2003

Kernberg OF: Borderline personality organization. J Am Psychoanal Assoc 15:641–685, 1967

Kernberg OF: Aggression in Personality Disorders and Perversions. New Haven, CT, Yale University Press, 1992

Levy KN, Meehan KB, Weber M, et al: Attachment and borderline personality disorder: implications for psychotherapy. Psychopathology 38:64–74, 2005

Levy KN, Meehan KB, Kelly KM, et al: Change in attachment patterns and reflective function in a randomized control trial of transference-focused psychotherapy for borderline personality disorder. J Consult Clin Psychol 74:1027–1040, 2006

Linehan MM: Cognitive-Behavioral Treatment of Borderline Personality Disorder. New York, Guilford, 1993

Livesley WJ (ed): Handbook of Personality Disorders. New York, Guilford, 2001

Livesley WJ: An integrated approach to the treatment of borderline personality disorder. Lecture presented at the Zon and Schild Hospital, Amersfoort, The Netherlands, September 17, 2007

McCann JT: Obsessive-compulsive and negativistic personality disorders, in Oxford Textbook of Psychopathology, 2nd Edition. Edited by Blaney PH, Millon T. New York, Oxford University Press, 2009, pp 671–691

McGlashan TH: The Chestnut Lodge Follow-Up Study, III: long-term outcome of borderline patients. Arch Gen Psychiatry 43:20–30, 1986

McLean LM, Gallop R: Implications of childhood sexual abuse for adult borderline personality disorder and complex posttraumatic stress disorder. Am J Psychiatry 160:369–371, 2003

Millon T, Davis R (eds): Personality Disorders in Modern Life. New York, Wiley, 2000

Mitton MJ, Links OS, Durocher G: A history of childhood sexual abuse and the course of borderline personality disorder, in Role of Sexual Abuse in the Etiology of Borderline Personality Disorder. Edited by Zanarini MC. Washington, DC, American Psychiatric Press, 1997, pp 181–202

Oldham J, Skodol AE, Bender DS (eds): Textbook of Personality Disorders. Washington, DC, American Psychiatric Publishing, 2005

Pfohl B, Blum N: Obsessive-compulsive personality disorder, in The DSM-IV Personality Disorders. Edited by Livesley WJ. New York, Guilford, 1995, pp 261–276

Reich W: Character Analysis (1929). New York, Farrar, Straus, and Giroux, 1994

Schimmel S: The Seven Deadly Sins: Jewish, Christian and Classical Reflections on Human Psychology. New York, Oxford University Press, 1997

Stone MH: The Fate of Borderlines. New York, Guilford, 1990a

Stone MH: Incest in the borderline patient, in Incest-Related Syndromes of Adult Psychopathology. Edited by Kluft RP. Washington, DC, American Psychiatric Press, 1990b, pp 183–204

Stone MH: Abnormalities of Personality: Within and Beyond the Realm of Treatment. New York, WW Norton, 1993

Stone MH: Borderline and histrionic personality disorders: a review, in Personality Disorders (WPA Series: Evidence and Experience in Psychiatry, Vol 8). Edited by Maj M, Akiskal HS, Mezzich JE, et al. Chichester, UK, Wiley, 2005, pp 201–276

Stone MH: Personality-Disordered Patients: Treatable and Untreatable. Washington, DC, American Psychiatric Publishing, 2006

Stone MH: The Anatomy of Evil. Amherst, NY, Prometheus Books, 2009

Stone MH, Butler JR, Young K: Sadistic personality disorder, in Oxford Textbook of Psychopathology, 2nd Edition. Edited by Blaney PH, Millon T. New York, Oxford University Press, 2009, pp 651–670

Waldinger RJ, Gunderson JG: Completed psychotherapies with borderline patients. Am J Psychother 38:190–202, 1984

Wallerstein RS: Forty-Two Lives in Treatment: A Study of Psychoanalysis and Psychotherapy. New York, Guilford, 1986

Zanarini MC, Yong L, Frankenburg FR, et al: Severity of reported childhood sexual abuse and its relationship to severity of borderline psychopathology and psychosocial impairment among borderline inpatients. J Nerv Ment Dis 190:381–387, 2002

Zanarini MC, Frankenburg FR, Reich DB, et al: Adult experiences of abuse reported by borderline patients and Axis II comparison subjects over six years of prospective follow-up. J Nerv Ment Dis 193:412–416, 2005

PART III

RESEARCH AND FUTURE DIRECTIONS

CHAPTER 15

Evidence for Psychodynamic Psychotherapy in Personality Disorders

A Review

Falk Leichsenring, D.Sc.

In this chapter, first I discuss briefly the procedures of evidence-based medicine and empirically supported treatments. Then I review the available evidence for psychodynamic psychotherapy in personality disorders. The major focus is on randomized controlled trials (RCTs). In addition, I report the results of quasi-experimental studies. Finally, I discuss the current state of research in psychodynamic psychotherapy for personality disorders, including duration of therapy necessary for the treatment of personality disorders and open questions of research.

Evidence-Based Medicine and Empirically Supported Treatments

Experts continue to discuss which type of research design—RCTs or effectiveness or observational studies—provides the best evidence that a treatment works (Benson and Hartz 2000; Chambless and Hollon 1998; Chambless and Ollendick 2001; Concato et al. 2000; Pocock and El-bourne 2000; Rothwell 2005; Seligman 1995; Westen et al. 2004). RCTs are carried out under controlled experimental conditions. Thus, their strength lies in the control of factors influencing outcome external to the treatments in question, and they ensure high internal validity of the study. However, their clinical representativeness (external validity) can be limited by strict experimental control (Rothwell 2005). In contrast, effectiveness studies are carried out under the conditions of clinical practice. Consequently, they ensure clinically representative results (i.e., high external validity; Shadish et al. 2002). However, they cannot control for factors influencing outcome apart from the treatment to the same degree that RCTs can (threats to internal validity).

From the perspective of philosophy of science, however, *efficacy* and *effectiveness* studies refer to different intended applications (Leichsenring 2004): RCTs examine the efficacy of a treatment under controlled experimental conditions, whereas effectiveness studies address the effectiveness under clinical practice conditions (Leichsenring 2004). Thus, they address different research questions. As a consequence, the results of an efficacy study cannot be directly transferred to clinical practice and vice versa (Leichsenring 2004). From this perspective, a distinction is required between methodology of empirically supported therapies and that of RCTs (Leichsenring 2004; Westen et al. 2004). The relation between RCTs and effectiveness studies should not be considered rivalrous; rather, it is complementary.

Evidence for Psychodynamic Psychotherapy in Personality Disorders

Evidence for the efficacy of psychodynamic psychotherapy in mental disorders in general was reviewed, for example, by Fonagy et al. (2005) and Leichsenring (2005, 2009). A review of psychotherapy for personality disorders was given by Bateman and Fonagy (2000). In this chapter, I review the currently available evidence for psychodynamic psychotherapy in personality disorders. Here, the criteria proposed by the Task Force on Promotion and Dissemination of Psychological Procedures (1995) of the American Psychological Association, modified by Chambless and Hollon (1998) to define efficacious treatments, were applied. These criteria focus on RCTs. In addition to RCTs, results of quasi-experimental studies are reported here.

Quasi-experimental studies may or may not include control groups but do not randomly assign patients to treatments (Shadish et al. 2002).

PSYCHODYNAMIC PSYCHOTHERAPY

Psychodynamic psychotherapy operates on an interpretive-supportive continuum. The use of more interpretive or supportive interventions depends on the patient's needs (Gabbard 2004; Wallerstein 1989). Gabbard (2004) has suggested that therapies of more than 24 sessions or lasting longer than 6 months should be regarded as long-term. In this chapter, the definitions of short-term psychodynamic psychotherapy (STPP) and long-term psychodynamic psychotherapy (LTPP) given by Gabbard (2004) are applied. With regard to STPP, different models have been developed, which were reviewed, for example, by Messer and Warren (1995). Gabbard's definition of LTPP is the working model of this chapter (Gabbard 2004, p. 2): "a therapy that involves careful attention to the therapist-patient interaction, with thoughtfully timed interpretation of transference and resistance embedded in a sophisticated appreciation of the therapist's contribution to the two-person field." LTPP has no generally accepted "standard" duration. Lamb (2005) compiled more than 20 definitions given by experts in the field. They ranged from a minimum of 3 months to a maximum of 20 years. In our recent meta-analysis, we defined psychodynamic psychotherapy lasting for at least 1 year, or 50 sessions, as long-term (Leichsenring and Rabung 2008). This criterion is consistent with the definition given by Crits-Christoph and Barber (2000, p. 456) and other experts in the field.

Psychodynamic psychotherapy focuses on patients' conflicts or personality organization rather than on their symptoms. For this reason, psychodynamic psychotherapy was the first form of psychotherapy that addressed the treatment of personality or personality disorders. Some of the most important contributions are from the pioneering work of Karl Abraham (1924/1969), Wilhelm Reich (1933/1970), Otto Fenichel (1945), Heinz Kohut (1971), and Otto Kernberg (1967).

Two meta-analyses of psychodynamic psychotherapy for personality disorders are currently available (Leichsenring and Leibing 2003; Leichsenring and Rabung 2008). Both of these meta-analyses included RCTs and observational studies. The first meta-analysis addressed the effects of psychodynamic psychotherapy and cognitive-behavioral therapy (CBT) in personality disorders. It reported large effect sizes for both psychodynamic psychotherapy and CBT. Large effect sizes for psychodynamic psychotherapy in personality disorders were found not only for comorbid symptoms but also for core personality pathology (Leichsenring and Leibing 2003). The overall pre- to posttreatment effect size for psychodynamic psychotherapy for personality disorders was 1.46, which is a large effect size according to Cohen (1988). For core personality pathology, psychodynamic psychotherapy achieved an effect size of 1.56. With regard to specific types of personality disorders, psychodynamic psychotherapy yielded an overall effect size of 1.31 in patients with borderline personality disorder (BPD). In the studies included in this meta-analysis, the mean number of sessions was 23.17, and mean duration of therapy was 37.18 weeks. Thus, this meta-analysis included short- to medium-term forms of psychodynamic psychotherapy.

A 2008 meta-analysis addressed the outcome of LTPP in complex mental disorders. *Complex mental disorders* were defined as personality disorders, multiple mental disorders, or chronic mental disorders (Leichsenring and Rabung 2008). In this meta-analysis, large and stable effect sizes for LTPP in personality disorders were found regarding overall effectiveness (posttherapy=1.16; follow-up=1.21), target problems (posttherapy=1.58; follow-up=1.65), general symptoms (posttherapy=0.98; follow-up=0.92), personality functioning (posttherapy=0.95; follow-up=1.04), and social functioning (posttherapy=0.82; follow-up=1.13) (Leichsenring and Rabung 2008). In the total sample of studies including personality disorders and other mental disorders, the treatment effects of LTPP increased significantly between posttherapy assessment and follow-up assessment (Leichsenring and Rabung 2008). This meta-analysis did not find significant differences in pre- to posttherapy effect sizes between RCTs and observational studies (Leichsenring and Rabung 2008). This is consistent with other meta-analyses not only of psychotherapy but also of medical interventions (Benson and Hartz 2000; Concato et al. 2000; Shadish et al. 2000).

Currently 11 RCTs addressing the efficacy of psychodynamic psychotherapy in personality disorders are available. With regard to specific personality disorders, RCTs are available for borderline and avoidant personality disorders. In addition, several studies examined the efficacy of psychodynamic psychotherapy for Cluster C personality disorders. For CBT, the available research is comparable, with efficacy studies being available for BPD, avoidant personality disorder, and Cluster C personality disorders (Leichsenring et al. 2006; Nathan and Gorman 2002).

BORDERLINE PERSONALITY DISORDER

At this writing, seven RCTs have addressed the efficacy of psychodynamic psychotherapy for BPD. Except for one study (Munroe-Blum and Marziali 1995), LTPP was examined. The results can be summarized as follows. In an RCT conducted by Munroe-Blum and Marziali (1995),

STPP yielded significant improvements on measures of borderline-related symptoms, general psychiatric symptoms, and depression and was as effective as an interpersonal group therapy (Table 15–1). Bateman and Fonagy (1999, 2001, 2003) studied psychoanalytically oriented (mentalization-based) partial hospitalization treatment for patients with BPD. The major difference between the treatment group and the control group was the provision of individual and group psychotherapy in the former. The treatment lasted a maximum of 18 months. LTPP was significantly superior to standard psychiatric care, both at the end of therapy and at the 18-month follow-up (Bateman and Fonagy 1999, 2001). This was true even 5 years after discharge from (mentalization-based) partial hospitalization treatment (Bateman and Fonagy 2008). Costs of partial inpatient care were offset by less psychiatric inpatient care and reduced emergency department treatment. The trend for costs to decrease in the follow-up period was not apparent in the treatment-as-usual group (Bateman and Fonagy 2003). The average annual cost of monitored health care for the partial hospitalization group was one-fifth that of the treatment-as-usual group. Thus, specialist partial hospitalization treatment for BPD is no more expensive than treatment as usual and shows considerable cost savings after treatment. In an RCT by Bateman and Fonagy (2009), mentalization-based treatment (MBT) was superior to an active treatment (Structured Clinical Management) in borderline outpatients. MBT was superior with regard to several outcome measures, including suicidal attempts and hospitalization.

Giesen-Bloo et al. (2006) compared LTPP (transference-focused psychotherapy; TFP) based on the model of Kernberg and colleagues (Clarkin et al. 1999) with schema-focused therapy (SFT). Treatment duration was 3 years with two sessions a week. The authors reported statistically and clinically significant improvements for both treatments. However, SFT was found to be superior to TFP in several outcome measures. Furthermore, a significantly higher dropout risk for TFP was reported. However, this study had serious methodological flaws. The authors used scales for adherence and competence for both treatments for which they adopted an identical cutoff score of 60 to indicate competent application. According to the data published by the authors (p. 651), the median competence level for applying SFT methods was 85.67. For TFP, a value of 65.6 was reported. The competence level for SFT clearly exceeded the cutoff, whereas the competence level for TFP just surpassed it. Furthermore, the competence level for SFT was clearly higher than that for TFP. Accordingly, both treatments were not equally applied in terms of therapist competence. For this reason, the results of that study are questionable. The difference in competence was not taken into

TABLE 15–1. Randomized controlled studies of psychodynamic psychotherapy in personality disorders

Study	Disorder	n (psychodynamic psychotherapy)	Comparison group	Concept of psychodynamic psychotherapy	Treatment duration
Abbass et al. 2008	Heterogeneous personality disorders	14	Minimal contact ($n=13$)	Davanloo	27.7 sessions (mean)
Bateman and Fonagy 1999, 2001, 2003, 2008	Borderline personality disorder	19	Treatment as usual ($n=19$)	Bateman and Fonagy	18 months
Bateman and Fonagy 2009	Borderline personality disorder	71	Structured clinical management ($n=63$)	Bateman and Fonagy	18 months
Clarkin et al. 2007	Borderline personality disorder	30	Dialectical behavior therapy ($n=30$); supportive therapy ($n=30$)	Kernberg and Clarkin	12 months
Doering et al. (in press)	Borderline personality disorder	52	Treatment by experienced community psychotherapists	Kernberg and Clarkin	12 months
Emmelkamp et al. 2006	Avoidant personality disorder	23	CBT ($n=21$); wait list ($n=18$)	Malan; Luborsky; Luborsky and Mark; Pinsker et al.	20 sessions
Giesen-Bloo et al. 2006	Borderline personality disorder	42	CBT ($n=44$)	Kernberg and Clarkin	3 years; 2 sessions per week

TABLE 15–1. Randomized controlled studies of psychodynamic psychotherapy in personality disorders

Study	Disorder	*n* (psychodynamic psychotherapy)	Comparison group	Concept of psychodynamic psychotherapy	Treatment duration
Gregory et al. 2008	Borderline personality disorder	15	Treatment as usual (*n*=15)	Gregory et al.	12–18 months
Hellerstein et al. 1998	Heterogeneous personality disorder	25	Brief supportive psychotherapy (*n*=24)	Davanloo	40 sessions
Munroe-Blum and Marziali 1995	Borderline personality disorder	31	Interpersonal group therapy (*n*=25)	Kernberg	17 sessions
Muran et al. 2005	Cluster C personality disorders	22	Brief relational therapy (*n*=33); CBT (*n*=29)	Pollack et al.	30 sessions
Svartberg et al. 2004	Cluster C personality disorders	25	CBT (*n*=25)	Malan; McCullough-Vaillant	40 sessions
Vinnars et al. 2005	Heterogeneous personality disorders	80	Community-delivered psychodynamic therapy (*n*=76)	Luborsky	40 sessions
Winston et al. 1994	Heterogeneous personality disorders	25	Brief adaptive psychotherapy (*n*=30); wait list (*n*=26)	Davanloo	40 weeks (mean)

Note.   CBT=cognitive-behavioral therapy.

account by the authors in data analysis or in the discussion of results. Thus, this study raises serious concerns about an investigator allegiance effect (Luborsky et al. 1999b). In addition, most patients had not completed their treatments when outcome assessments were made (Leichsenring and Rabung 2008).

Another RCT (Clarkin et al. 2007) compared psychodynamic psychotherapy (TFP), dialectical behavior therapy (DBT), and psychodynamic supportive psychotherapy. Patients who received all three modalities showed general improvement in the study. However, TFP produced improvements not shown with either DBT or supportive psychotherapy. Those participants who received TFP were more likely to move from an insecure attachment classification to a secure one. They also showed significantly greater changes in mentalizing capacity and narrative coherence compared with the other two groups. TFP was associated with significant improvement in 10 of the 12 variables across the 6 symptomatic domains, compared with 6 for supportive psychotherapy and 5 for DBT. Only TFP made significant changes in impulsivity, irritability, verbal assault, and direct assault. TFP and DBT reduced suicidality to the same extent. In a recent RCT, TFP was compared to a treatment carried out by experienced community psychotherapists in borderline outpatients (Doering et al., in press). TFP was superior with regard to borderline psychopathology, psychosocial functioning, personality organization, inpatient admission, and dropouts.

Another RCT compared psychodynamic psychotherapy ("dynamic deconstructive psychotherapy") with treatment as usual in patients with BPD and co-occurring alcohol use disorder (Gregory et al. 2008). In this study, psychodynamic psychotherapy, but not treatment as usual, achieved significant improvements in outcome measures of parasuicide, alcohol misuse, and institutional care (Gregory et al. 2008). Furthermore, psychodynamic psychotherapy was superior with regard to improvements in borderline psychopathology, depression, and social support. No difference was found in dissociation. This was true even though treatment-as-usual participants received higher average treatment intensity.

In an open quasi-experimental study, patients with BPD achieved significant improvements and large effects. *Improvements* refers to the number of criteria for BPD, psychiatric symptoms, and other measures of outcome after a 1-year psychodynamic treatment (Stevenson and Meares 1992). Korner et al. (2006) confirmed these results and reported superiority of psychodynamic psychotherapy over a quasi-experimental comparison group (treatment as usual).

AVOIDANT PERSONALITY DISORDER

Avoidant personality disorder is a Cluster C personality disorder. In an RCT, Emmelkamp et al. (2006) compared CBT with STPP and a wait-list control condition in the treatment of avoidant personality disorder. The authors reported CBT as more effective than wait-list control or STPP. However, the study had several methodological shortcomings (Leichsenring and Leibing 2006). Design, statistical analyses, and the reporting of the results raise serious concerns about an investigator allegiance effect (Luborsky et al. 1999b).

In an open quasi-experimental study, Barber et al. (1997) evaluated psychodynamic psychotherapy (supportive-expressive therapy; Luborsky 1984, 1999a) for patients with avoidant personality disorder and obsessive-compulsive personality disorder. After 1 year of treatment, 61% of the patients with avoidant personality disorder no longer fulfilled the criteria for avoidant personality disorder. For patients with obsessive-compulsive personality disorder, this was true for 85% of the patients.

CLUSTER C PERSONALITY DISORDERS

Evidence indicates that psychodynamic psychotherapy has efficacy in the treatment of Cluster C personality disorders. In an RCT conducted by Svartberg et al. (2004), psychodynamic psychotherapy (40 sessions) was compared with CBT (Table 15–1). Both psychodynamic psychotherapy and CBT yielded significant improvements in patients with DSM-IV (American Psychiatric Association 1994) Cluster C personality disorders (i.e., avoidant, obsessive-compulsive, or dependent personality disorder). Symptoms, interpersonal problems, and core personality pathology improved. The results were stable at 24-month follow-up. No significant differences were found between psychodynamic psychotherapy and CBT with regard to efficacy.

Muran et al. (2005) compared the efficacy of psychodynamic therapy, brief relational therapy, and CBT in the treatment of Cluster C personality disorders and personality disorders not otherwise specified. Treatments lasted for 30 sessions. With regard to mean changes in outcome measures, no significant differences were found between the treatment conditions at termination or at follow-up. Furthermore, no significant differences were seen between the treatments with regard to the patients achieving clinically significant change in symptoms, interpersonal problems, features of personality disorders, or therapist ratings of target complaints. At termination, CBT and brief relational therapy were superior to psychodynamic psychotherapy in one outcome measure (patient ratings of target complaints). However, this difference did not persist at follow-up. With regard to the percentage of patients showing change, no significant differences were found, either at termination or at follow-up, except in one comparison. At termination, CBT was superior to STPP with regard to improvements in interpersonal problems. Again, this difference did not persist at follow-up. The conclusion is that only a few significant differences were found between the treatments that did not persist at follow-up.

HETEROGENEOUS SAMPLES OF PATIENTS WITH PERSONALITY DISORDERS

Winston et al. (1994) compared STPP with brief adaptive psychotherapy or a waiting-list condition in a heterogeneous group of patients with personality disorders. Most of the patients had a Cluster C personality disorder. Patients with paranoid, schizoid, schizotypal, borderline, or narcissistic personality disorders were excluded. Mean treatment duration was 40 weeks. In both treatment groups, patients showed significantly more improvements than did the patients on the waiting list. No differences in outcome were found between the two forms of psychotherapy. Hellerstein et al. (1998) compared STPP with brief supportive therapy in a heterogeneous sample of patients with personality disorders. Again, most of the patients had a Cluster C personality disorder. The authors reported similar degrees of improvement both at termination and at 6-month follow-up.

Vinnars et al. (2005) reported that manualized psychodynamic psychotherapy (supportive-expressive therapy; Luborsky 1984, 1999a) of a 1-year duration was as efficacious as community-delivered psychodynamic psychotherapy in a mixed group of patients with personality disorders.

Abbass et al. (2008) compared psychodynamic psychotherapy (intensive short-term dynamic psychotherapy) with a minimal-contact group in a heterogeneous group of patients with personality disorders. The most common Axis II diagnoses were borderline (44%), obsessive-compulsive (37%), and avoidant (33%) personality disorder. Average treatment duration was 27.7 sessions. Psychodynamic psychotherapy was significantly superior to the control condition in all primary outcome measures. When control patients were treated, they experienced benefits similar to those of the initial treatment group. In the long-term follow-up 2 years after end of treatment, the whole group maintained their gains and had an 83% reduction in personality disorder diagnoses. In addition, treatment costs were thrice offset by reductions in medication and disability payments. This preliminary study of intensive short-term dynamic psychotherapy suggests that it is efficacious and cost-effective in the treatment of personality disorders.

Discussion

Evidence from RCTs, quasi-experimental studies, and meta-analyses indicates that psychodynamic psychotherapy is an effective treatment of personality disorders. Efficacy studies are available for BPD and for Cluster C personality disorders. For other specific forms of personality disorders (such as narcissistic or obsessive-compulsive personality disorders), no RCTs of psychodynamic psychotherapy are currently available. Furthermore, in the available studies, different forms of psychodynamic psychotherapy were applied. The criteria of empirically supported therapy proposed by Chambless and Hollon (1998) require at least two RCTs of different work groups in which the same method of treatment was applied. At present, a specific method of psychodynamic psychotherapy has been applied in only one study each, except for TFP and MBT. Thus, further studies of psychodynamic psychotherapy in personality disorders are required.

Evidence suggests that short-term psychotherapy is sufficiently effective for most subjects with acute distress (Kopta et al. 1994). Evidence, however, also indicates that short-term treatments are insufficient for a considerable proportion of patients with chronic mental disorders or personality disorders. According to the data reported by Kopta et al. (1994, p. 1014, Figure 2), about 70% of the patients with acute distress were rated as clinically significantly improved after 25 sessions. For patients with chronic distress, this was true for about 60% (Kopta et al. 1994). However, for patients with characterological distress (i.e., personality disorders), the data of Kopta et al. (1994) suggested that after 25 sessions, only slightly more than 40% of the patients were clinically significantly improved. These data suggest that more than 52 sessions are required for about 50% of these patients to have clinically significant improvement. However, the data of Kopta et al. (1994, p. 1014, Figure 2) do not allow for exact predictions of how many sessions are required for the response rates to surpass the 50% rate. Perry et al. (1999) estimated the length of treatment necessary for a patient to no longer meet the full criteria for a personality disorder (recovery). According to these estimates, 50% of patients with personality disorders would recover by 1.3 years or 92 sessions, and 75% would recover by 2.2 years or about 216 sessions (Perry et al. 1999, p. 1318). According to these data, most patients with acute distress benefit significantly from short-term psychotherapy, whereas for patients with chronic distress and personality disorders, short-term psychotherapy is not sufficient. For most patients with personality disorders, long-term treatments seem to be required. This is true not only of psychodynamic therapy but also of psychotherapeutic approaches that are usually short-term, such as CBT (Giesen-Bloo et al. 2006; Linehan et al. 1994, 2006).

Conclusion

A large meta-analysis of treatment outcome research for patients with complex mental disorders, including personality disorders, found that long-term psychodynamic psychotherapy showed significantly better results in regard to overall effectiveness, target problems, and personality functioning when compared with shorter forms of treatment (Leichsenring and Rabung 2008). Antisocial personality disorder in the mild to moderate psychopathic range is a reasonable targeted problem for both psychodynamic researchers and clinicians. Through careful diagnostic assessment, the consideration of psychodynamic principles, the application of psychodynamic techniques, and continuous observation of countertransference, there is room for therapeutic hope.

Key Clinical Concepts

- ◆ Evidence indicates that most patients with acute distress benefit significantly from short-term psychotherapy, whereas for many patients with chronic distress and personality disorders, short-term psychotherapy is not sufficient. For most patients with personality disorders, long-term treatments seem to be required.

- ◆ The need for long-term treatments of personality disorders pertains not only to psychodynamic therapy but also to psychotherapeutic approaches that are usually short-term, such as cognitive-behavioral therapy.

- ◆ Evidence suggests that psychodynamic psychotherapy is an effective treatment of personality disorders. Different forms of psychodynamic psychotherapy have proved to be efficacious (e.g., transference-focused therapy or mentalization-based therapy) for the treatment of borderline personality disorder.

- ◆ Further studies addressing the efficacy of specific forms of psychodynamic psychotherapy in specific types of personality disorders are required.

Suggested Readings

Allen JG, Fonagy PF, Bateman AW: Mentalizing in Clinical Practice. Washington, DC, American Psychiatric Publishing, 2008

Bateman A, Fonagy P: Effectiveness of psychotherapeutic treatment of personality disorder. Br J Psychiatry 177:138–143, 2000

Benson K, Hartz AJ: A comparison of observational studies and randomized, controlled trials. N Engl J Med 342:1878–1886, 2000

Clarkin J, Kernberg OF, Yeomans F: Transference-Focused Psychotherapy for Borderline Personality Disorder Patients. New York, Guilford, 1999

Concato J, Shah N, Horwitz RI: Randomized, controlled trials, observational studies, and the hierarchy of research designs. N Engl J Med 342:1887–1892, 2000

Gabbard GO: Psychodynamic Psychiatry in Clinical Practice, 3rd Edition. Washington, DC, American Psychiatric Press, 2000

Gabbard GO: Long-Term Psychodynamic Psychotherapy: A Basic Text. Washington, DC, American Psychiatric Publishing, 2004

Gabbard GO, Gunderson JG, Fonagy P: The place of psychoanalytic treatments within psychiatry. Arch Gen Psychiatry 59:505–510, 2002

Gunderson JG, Gabbard GO: Making the case for psychoanalytic therapies in the current psychiatric environment. J Am Psychoanal Assoc 47:679–704, 1999

Leichsenring F: Randomized controlled vs. naturalistic studies: a new research agenda. Bull Menninger Clin 68:137–151, 2004

Leichsenring F, Rabung S: The effectiveness of long-term psychodynamic psychotherapy: a meta-analysis. JAMA 300:1551–1564, 2008

Leichsenring F, Rabung S, Leibing E: The efficacy of short-term psychodynamic therapy in specific psychiatric disorders: a meta-analysis. Arch Gen Psychiatry 61:1208–1216, 2004

PDM Task Force: Psychodynamic Diagnostic Manual. Silver Spring, MD, Alliance of Psychodynamic Organizations, 2006

Roth A, Fonagy P: What Works for Whom? A Critical Review of Psychotherapy Research, 2nd Edition. New York, Guilford, 2005

Westen D, Novotny CM, Thompson-Brenner H: The empirical status of empirically supported psychotherapies: assumptions, findings, and reporting in controlled clinical trials. Psychol Bull 130:631–663, 2004

References

Abbass A, Sheldon A, Gyra J, et al: Intensive short-term dynamic psychotherapy for DSM-IV personality disorders: a randomized controlled trial. J Nerv Ment Dis 196:211–216, 2008

Abraham K: The influence of oral erotism on character-formation (1924), in Handbook of Character Studies: Psychoanalytic Explorations. Edited by Perzow SM, Kets de Vries MFR. Madison, CT, International Universities Press, 1991

American Psychiatric Association: Diagnostic and Statistical Manual of Mental Disorders, 4th Edition. Washington, DC, American Psychiatric Association, 1994

Barber J, Morse JO, Krakauer ID, et al: Change in obsessive-compulsive and avoidant personality disorders following time-limited supportive expressive therapy. Psychotherapy 34:133–143, 1997

Bateman A, Fonagy P: The effectiveness of partial hospitalization in the treatment of borderline personality disorder: a randomized controlled trial. Am J Psychiatry 156:1563–1569, 1999

Bateman A, Fonagy P: Effectiveness of psychotherapeutic treatment of personality disorder. Br J Psychiatry 177:138–143, 2000

Bateman A, Fonagy P: Treatment of borderline personality disorder with psychoanalytically oriented partial hospitalization: an 18-month follow-up. Am J Psychiatry 158:36–42, 2001

Bateman A, Fonagy P: Health service utilization costs for borderline personality disorder patients treated with psychoanalytically oriented partial hospitalization versus general psychiatric care. Am J Psychiatry 160:169–171, 2003

Bateman A, Fonagy P: 8-year follow-up of patients treated for borderline personality disorder: mentalization-based treatment versus treatment as usual. Am J Psychiatry 165:631–638, 2008

Bateman A, Fonagy P: Randomized controlled trial of outpatient mentalization-based treatment versus structured clinical management for borderline personality disorder. Am J Psychiatry 166:1355–1364, 2009

Benson K, Hartz AJ: A comparison of observational studies and randomized, controlled trials. N Engl J Med 342:1878–1886, 2000

Chambless DL, Hollon SD: Defining empirically supported treatments. J Consult Clin Psychol 66:7–18, 1998

Chambless DL, Ollendick TH: Empirically supported psychological interventions: controversies and evidence. Annu Rev Psychol 52:685–716, 2001

Clarkin J, Kernberg OF, Yeomans F: Transference-Focused Psychotherapy for Borderline Personality Disorder Patients. New York, Guilford, 1999

Clarkin JF, Levy KN, Lenzenweger MF, et al: The Personality Disorders Institute/Borderline Personality Disorder Research Foundation randomized control trial for borderline personality disorder. Am J Psychiatry 164:52–72, 2007

Cohen J: Statistical Power Analysis for the Behavioral Sciences. Hillsdale, NJ, Erlbaum, 1988

Concato J, Shah N, Horwitz RI: Randomized, controlled trials, observational studies, and the hierarchy of research designs. N Engl J Med 342:1887–1892, 2000

Crits-Christoph P, Barber JP: Long-term psychotherapy, in Handbook of Psychological Change: Psychotherapy Processes and Practices for the 21st Century. Edited by Ingram RE, Snyder CR. Hoboken, NJ, Wiley, 2000, pp 455–473

Doering S, Hörz S, Rentrop M, et al: A randomized-controlled trial of Transference-Focused Psychotherapy vs. treatment by experienced community psychotherapists for borderline personality disorder. Br J Psychiatry (in press)

Emmelkamp PM, Benner A, Kuipers A, et al: Comparison of brief dynamic and cognitive-behavioural therapies in avoidant personality disorder. Br J Psychiatry 189:60–64, 2006

Fenichel O: The Psychoanalytic Theory of Neurosis. New York, WW Norton, 1945

Fonagy P, Roth A, Higgitt A: Psychodynamic psychotherapies: evidence-based practice and clinical wisdom. Bull Menninger Clin 69:1–58, 2005

Gabbard GO: Long-Term Psychodynamic Psychotherapy: A Basic Text. Washington, DC, American Psychiatric Publishing, 2004

Giesen-Bloo J, van Dyck R, Spinhoven P, et al: Outpatient psychotherapy for borderline personality disorder: randomized trial of schema-focused therapy vs transference-focused psychotherapy. Arch Gen Psychiatry 63:649–658, 2006

Gregory R, Chlebowski S, Kang D, et al: A controlled trial of psychodynamic psychotherapy for co-occurring borderline personality disorder and alcohol use disorder. Psychotherapy 45:28–41, 2008

Hellerstein DJ, Rosenthal RN, Pinsker H, et al: A randomized prospective study comparing supportive and dynamic therapies, outcome and alliance. J Psychother Pract Res 7:261–271, 1998

Kernberg OF: Borderline personality organization. J Am Psychoanal Assoc 15:641–685, 1967

Kohut H: The Analysis of the Self: A Systematic Approach to the Psychoanalytic Treatment of Narcissistic Personality Disorders. New York, International Universities Press, 1971

Kopta S, Howard K, Lowry J, et al: Patterns of symptomatic recovery in psychotherapy. J Consult Clin Psychol 62:1009–1016, 1994

Korner A, Gerull F, Meares R, et al: Borderline personality disorder treated with the conversational model: a replication study. Compr Psychiatry 47:406–411, 2006

Lamb WK: A meta-analysis of outcome studies in long-term psychodynamic psychotherapy and psychoanalysis. Unpublished doctoral dissertation. University of California, Berkeley, 2005

Leichsenring F: Randomized controlled vs naturalistic studies: a new research agenda. Bull Menninger Clin 68:137–151, 2004

Leichsenring F: Are psychoanalytic and psychodynamic psychotherapies effective? A review. Int J Psychoanal 86:841–868, 2005

Leichsenring F: Applications of psychodynamic psychotherapy to specific disorders: efficacy and indications, in Textbook of Psychotherapeutic Treatments. Edited by Gabbard GO. Washington, DC, American Psychiatric Publishing, 2009, pp 97–132

Leichsenring F, Leibing E: The effectiveness of psychodynamic psychotherapy and cognitive-behavioral therapy in personality disorders: a meta-analysis. Am J Psychiatry 160:1223–1232, 2003

Leichsenring F, Leibing E: Fair play, please! (letter). Br J Psychiatry 190:80, 2006

Leichsenring F, Rabung S: Effectiveness of long-term psychodynamic psychotherapy: a meta-analysis. JAMA 300:1551–1565, 2008

Leichsenring F, Hiller W, Weissberg M, et al: Cognitive-behavioral therapy and psychodynamic psychotherapy: techniques, efficacy, and indications. Am J Psychother 60:233–259, 2006

Linehan MM, Tutek DA, Heard HL, et al: Interpersonal outcome of cognitive behavioral treatment for chronically suicidal borderline patients. Am J Psychiatry 151:1771–1776, 1994

Linehan MM, Comtois KA, Murray AM, et al: Two-year randomized trial and follow-up of dialectical behavior therapy vs therapy by experts for suicidal behaviors and borderline personality disorder. Arch Gen Psychiatry 63:757–766, 2006

Luborsky L: Principles of Psychoanalytic Psychotherapy: A Manual for Supportive Expressive Treatments. New York, Basic Books, 1984

Luborsky L, Diguer L, Kächele H, et al: A guide to the CCRT's methods, discoveries, and future. 1999a. Available at: http://sip.medizin.uni-ulm.de/abteilung/buecher/PDF/ccrt_guide.pdf Accessed March 17, 2010.

Luborsky L, Diguer L, Seligman DA, et al: The researcher's own therapy allegiances: a "wild card" in comparisons of treatment efficacy. Clinical Psychology: Science and Practice 6:95–106, 1999b

Messer SB, Warren CS: Models of Brief Psychodynamic Therapy: A Comparative Approach. New York, Guilford, 1995

Munroe-Blum H, Marziali E: A controlled trial of short-term group treatment for borderline personality disorder. J Pers Disord 9:190–198, 1995

Muran JC, Safran JD, Samstag LW, et al: Evaluating an alliance-focused treatment for personality disorders. J Psychother Pract Res 42:532–545, 2005

Nathan PE, Gorman JM (eds): A Guide to Treatments That Work, 2nd Edition. New York, Oxford University Press, 2002

Perry J, Banon E, Floriana I: Effectiveness of psychotherapy for personality disorders. Am J Psychiatry 156:1312–1321, 1999

Pocock SJ, Elbourne DR: Randomized trials or observational tribulations? N Engl J Med 342:1907–1909, 2000

Reich W: Character Analysis (1933). Translated by Carfagno VR. Köln, Germany, Kiepenheuer & Witsch, 1970

Rothwell PM: External validity of randomised controlled trials: "to whom do the results of this trial apply?" Lancet 365:82–92, 2005

Seligman M: The effectiveness of psychotherapy: the Consumer Reports study. Am Psychol 50:965–974, 1995

Shadish WR, Matt G, Navarro A, et al: The effects of psychological therapies under clinically representative conditions: a meta-analysis. J Consult Clin Psychol 126:512–529, 2000

Shadish WR, Cook TD, Campbell DT: Experimental and Quasi-Experimental Designs for Generalized Causal Inference. Boston, MA, Houghton Mifflin, 2002

Stevenson J, Meares R: An outcome study of psychotherapy for patients with borderline personality disorder. Am J Psychiatry 149:358–362, 1992

Svartberg M, Stiles T, Seltzer MH: Randomized, controlled trial of the effectiveness of short-term dynamic psychotherapy and cognitive therapy for Cluster C personality disorders. Am J Psychiatry 161:810–817, 2004

Task Force on Promotion and Dissemination of Psychological Procedures: Training and dissemination of empirically validated psychological treatments: report and recommendations. Clin Psychol 48:3–23, 1995

Vinnars B, Barber JP, Norén K, et al: Manualized supportive-expressive psychotherapy versus nonmanualized community-delivered psychodynamic therapy for patients with personality disorders: bridging efficacy and effectiveness. Am J Psychiatry 162:1933–1940, 2005

Wallerstein R: The psychotherapy research project of the Menninger Foundation: an overview. J Consult Clin Psychol 57:195–205, 1989

Westen D, Novotny CM, Thompson-Brenner H: The empirical status of empirically supported psychotherapies: assumptions, findings, and reporting in controlled clinical trials. Psychol Bull 130:631–663, 2004

Winston A, Laikin M, Pollack J, et al: Short-term psychotherapy of personality disorders. Am J Psychiatry 151:190–194, 1994

CHAPTER 16

Psychodynamic Treatment Planning and the Official Diagnostic System

Toward DSM-5

John M. Oldham, M.D., M.S.

A psychodynamic approach to treatment planning is a time-honored tradition in clinical psychiatry. During much of the last half of the twentieth century, clinical psychiatry was strongly linked to psychoanalytic theory and practice, and a psychodynamic formulation was considered an essential blueprint to explain disordered cognition, emotion, and behavior in any given patient. The formulation emphasized the formative nature of early development and attachment. Candidates for board certification in psychiatry frequently passed or failed their examinations as a result of the quality of their formulations of the patients they interviewed. In board examinations today, however, if a candidate is asked (usually by a senior examiner) to present a formulation of a patient, it is not unusual to see that "deer in the headlights" look, followed by a differential diagnosis linked to DSM-IV-TR (American Psychiatric Association 2000) criteria. Is this a transformation in the field? If so, what accounts for it, and is it good or bad?

Change is inevitable and necessary. The field of psychiatry, as all of medicine, appropriately evolves on the basis of new research findings and clinical experience. Evidence-based treatment has now, for the most part, replaced theory-based treatment, and progress in translational neuroscience is powerfully influencing our thinking. Table 16–1 portrays a simple schematic of how these developments might be considered. Although no exact demarcations between the different epochs are shown, the attempt here is to show selected overarching predominant influences in the field. From theory-based psychoanalytic emphasis on the importance of the dynamic unconscious to explain disordered behavior, the field shifted to focus on brain neurobiology and neurotransmitter imbalance. A consensus then developed recognizing the importance of a biopsychosocial approach, a framework that remains quite useful today (Gabbard 2005). New neuroscience research emphasizes the bidirectional nature of gene-environment interaction and greater recognition of the plasticity of the brain and the capacity of many treatment interventions, including psychotherapy, to change the brain.

Review of DSM Classification Systems for Personality Disorders

Contrary to assumptions commonly encountered, personality disorders have been included in every edition of the American Psychiatric Association's *Diagnostic and Statistical Manual of Mental Disorders*. Although not explicit in the narrative text, DSM-I reflected the general view of personality disorders at that time (American Psychiatric Association 1952), elements of which persist to the present. Generally, per-

TABLE **16–1.**   Changing stages in the field of psychiatry

Era	Predominant influence
1940s–1970s	Psychoanalytic (psychogenic)
1960s–present	Psychopharmacological (chemical imbalance)
1980s–present	Biopsychosocial
1990–2000	Decade of the brain (bidirectional gene-environment interaction)
2000–2010	Decade of discovery (genomics, proteomics, molecular neurobiology, "neuropsychotherapy")

sonality disorders were viewed as more or less permanent patterns of behavior and human interaction that were established by early adulthood and were unlikely to change throughout the life cycle. Thorny issues such as how to differentiate personality disorders from personality styles and traits, which remain actively debated today, were clearly identified at the time.

In DSM-II (American Psychiatric Association 1968), attempts were made to move away from theory-derived diagnoses and to reach consensus on the main constellations of personality that were observable, measurable, enduring, and consistent over time. The earlier view that patients with personality disorders did not experience emotional distress was discarded, as were the DSM-I subcategories of personality pattern, personality trait, and sociopathic personality disturbances. One new personality disorder was added—asthenic personality disorder—only to be deleted in the next edition of DSM.

DSM-III arrived in 1980 and introduced a multiaxial system (American Psychiatric Association 1980). Disorders classified on Axis I included those generally seen as episodic, characterized by exacerbations and remissions, such as psychoses, mood disorders, and anxiety disorders. Axis II was established to include the personality disorders and mental retardation; both groups were seen as composed of early-onset, persistent conditions, but mental retardation was understood to be "biological" in origin, in contrast to the personality disorders, which were generally regarded as "psychogenic." The stated reason for placing the personality disorders on Axis II was to ensure that "consideration is given to the possible presence of disorders that are frequently overlooked when attention is directed to the usually more florid Axis I disorders" (American Psychiatric Association 1980, p. 23). Three new personality disorder diagnoses were added in DSM-III: schizotypal personality disorder, borderline personality disorder, and narcissistic personality disorder. In contrast to initial notions that patients called "borderline" were on the border between the psychoses and the neuroses, the criteria defining borderline personality disorder in DSM-III emphasized emotional dysregulation, unstable interpersonal relationships, and loss of impulse control more than cognitive distortions and marginal reality testing, which were more characteristic of schizotypal personality disorder (Spitzer et al. 1979). Among many scholars whose work greatly influenced and shaped our understanding of borderline pathology were Kernberg (1975) and Gunderson (2008). Although concepts of narcissism had been described by Freud, Reich, and others, the essence of the current views of narcissistic personality disorder emerged from the work of Millon (1969), Kohut (1971), and Kernberg (1975).

DSM-III-R was published in 1987 (American Psychiatric Association 1987) after an intensive process to revise DSM-III involving widely solicited input from researchers and clinicians and following principles similar to those articulated in DSM-III, such as ensuring reliable diagnostic categories that were clinically useful and consistent with research findings, thus minimizing reliance on theory. Efforts were made for diagnoses to be "descriptive" and to require a minimum of inference, although the introductory text of DSM-III-R acknowledged that for some disorders, "particularly the Personality Disorders, the criteria require much more inference on the part of the observer" (American Psychiatric Association 1987, p. xxiii). No changes were made in DSM-III-R diagnostic categories of personality disorders.

DSM-IV was published in 1994 (American Psychiatric Association 1994) after an extensive process of literature review, data analysis, field trials, and feedback from the profession. DSM-IV introduced, for the first time, a set of general diagnostic criteria for any personality disorder, shown here in Table 16–2. DSM-IV-TR (American Psychiatric Association 2000) did not change the diagnostic terms or criteria for the personality disorders from those in DSM-IV.

Problems, Controversies, and New Directions for DSM-5

The general consensus is that the placement of the personality disorders on Axis II in DSM-III led to a significant increase in focused clinical and educational attention, as well as research, on these conditions. However, during the 30 years since the publication of DSM-III, new findings have enhanced our understanding of the personality disorders, appropriately providing guidance for change (Clark 2007). Three predominant lines of evidence have been most influential during this period: 1) carefully designed longitudinal studies of personality disorders, 2) examination of the construct validity of the DSM-defined personality disorders, and 3) evaluation of the relative utility of dimensional systems compared with the categorical diagnostic systems used in DSM-IV-TR. I consider each of these in turn, followed by a summary of current (mid-2009) discussions by the Work Group on Personality and Personality Disorders for DSM-5.

LONGITUDINAL STUDIES

As shown in Table 16–2, the general diagnostic criteria for a personality disorder in DSM-IV-TR emphasize that it is an "enduring pattern of in-

TABLE 16–2.   DSM-IV-TR general diagnostic criteria for personality disorder

A.   An enduring pattern of inner experience and behavior that deviates markedly from the expectations of the individual's culture. This pattern is manifested in two (or more) of the following areas:

  1.   Cognition (i.e., ways of perceiving and interpreting self, other people, and events)

  2.   Affectivity (i.e., the range, intensity, lability, and appropriateness of emotional response)

  3.   Interpersonal functioning

  4.   Impulse control

B.   The enduring pattern is inflexible and pervasive across a broad range of personal and social situations.

C.   The enduring pattern leads to clinically significant distress or impairment in social, occupational, or other important areas of functioning.

D.   The pattern is stable and of long duration, and its onset can be traced back at least to adolescence or early adulthood.

E.   The enduring pattern is not better accounted for as a manifestation or consequence of another mental disorder.

F.   The enduring pattern is not due to the direct physiological effects of a substance (e.g., a drug of abuse, a medication) or a general medical condition (e.g., head trauma).

ner experience and behavior" that is "inflexible and pervasive across a broad range of personal and social situations." Although *enduring* is not defined, the traditional view of the personality disorders assumes that they persist for decades, if not throughout the life cycle, and that this serves as one factor differentiating them from Axis I conditions, more often thought of as episodic. New research, however, does not support this view. In 2005, a special issue of the *Journal of Personality Disorders* was published dedicated to longitudinal studies. This special issue includes articles summarizing three seminal longitudinal studies: the Children in the Community (CIC) Study (Cohen et al. 2005), the McLean Study of Adult Development (MSAD; Zanarini et al. 2005), and the Collaborative Longitudinal Personality Disorders Study (CLPS; Skodol et al. 2005), along with commentaries about these studies by many experts in the field. As described by Clark (2005), the three studies support a strong consensus that personality disorders, as defined by DSM-IV-TR, are not as stable as underlying traits and that the criteria sets are "hybrids of more acute, 'Axis I–like' symptoms that resolve more quickly" and "longer-lasting affective, cognitive, and behavioral personality dysfunctions" (p. 524). The MSAD project focused on borderline personality disorder, finding that 74% of patients showed remission over the entire 6 years of the study, only 6% of whom experienced recurrences. The CLPS reported that surprising percentages of patients with schizotypal, borderline, avoidant, and obsessive-compulsive personality disorders showed remission after 2 years, with even more robust numbers after 4 years, even after defining *remission* as sustaining no more than two criteria for 12 consecutive months. Both research groups found that personality traits were more stable over time than categorical diagnoses and that impaired functioning persisted after categorical remission.

CONSTRUCT VALIDITY OF CURRENT CATEGORIES

Research studies examining the construct validity of DSM-IV-TR–defined personality disorders have focused mostly on schizotypal personality disorder, borderline personality disorder, and antisocial personality disorder. These personality disorders have been shown to have good internal consistency and diagnostic validity. Schizotypal personality disorder is generally agreed to be on the schizophrenia spectrum (Webb and Levinson 1993) but is not a precursor of schizophrenia. The decision made in DSM-III to "unpack" schizoid personality disorder into three diagnoses—schizotypal, schizoid, and avoidant—was based more on clinical consensus than on data. Good evidence showed that schizotypal personality disorder was genetically linked to schizophrenia and that these patients showed idiosyncratic eccentricities that led to patterns of isolation and deviation from social norms. Schizoid patients were seen as "loners," but it remains unclear how valid this diagnosis is and whether it is, as once thought, a prodromal condition to schizophrenia. Paranoid personality disorder is considered genetically linked to delusional disorder, paranoid type (Webb and Levinson 1993), but information about its "stand-alone" validity is limited and equivocal.

In Cluster B, evidence is sparse regarding both histrionic and narcissistic personality disorders, and it seems unlikely that the evidence base guiding DSM-5 will support retention of these conditions as diagnostic categories rather than as important traits or dimensions that could be present in many patients (the fate, already, of the former diagnosis passive-aggressive personality disorder). In Cluster C, some evidence indicates that obsessive-compulsive personality disorder has construct validity (Skodol and Gunderson 2008), although the literature is inconsistent on its differentiation from Axis I obsessive-compulsive disorder. Patients with avoidant personality disorder have been conceptualized as socially averse not because of choice but because of social anxiety.

Some evidence suggests that certain patients with this condition may be difficult to distinguish from those with the Axis I condition generalized social phobia, but primarily these two populations are distinct (Skodol and Gunderson 2008). Little evidence supports the validity or utility of dependent personality disorder, which, again, may be more useful as a trait dimension.

Some of the disorders currently on Axis II (paranoid, schizoid, and avoidant personality disorders) may have a scarce database because, by their very nature, patients with these conditions avoid interpersonal contact. They therefore do not readily seek treatment or participate in research studies.

DIMENSIONAL VERSUS CATEGORICAL APPROACHES

Dimensional structure implies continuity, whereas categorical structure implies discontinuity. For example, being pregnant is a categorical concept (either one is pregnant or one is not), whereas being tall or short might better be conceptualized dimensionally because there is no exact definition of either, notions of tallness or shortness may vary among different cultures, and all gradations of height exist along a continuum.

We know, of course, that the DSM system is referred to as categorical and is contrasted to any number of systems referred to as dimensional, such as the interpersonal circumplex (Wiggins 1982), the three-factor model (Eysenck and Eysenck 1975), the four-factor model (Livesley 2008), the "Big Five" (Costa and McCrae 1992), and the seven-factor model (Cloninger et al. 1993). Although the concept of discontinuity is implied by a categorical system, clinicians do not necessarily think in such dichotomous terms. Thresholds defining disease categories, such as hypertension, are in fact somewhat arbitrary, as is certainly the case with the personality disorders. In addition, the polythetic criteria sets for the DSM-IV-TR personality disorders contain an element of dimensionality because one can just meet the threshold or one can have all the criteria, presumably a more extreme version of the disorder. Widiger and Sanderson (1995) suggested that this inherent dimensionality in our existing system could be usefully operationalized by stratifying each personality disorder into subcategories of "absent, traits, subthreshold, threshold, moderate, and extreme," according to the number of criteria met. Certainly if an individual is one criterion short of being diagnosed with a personality disorder, clinicians do not necessarily assume that no element of the disorder is present; instead, prudent clinicians would understand that features of the disorder need to be recognized if present and may need attention (Oldham and Morris 1995; Oldham and Skodol 2000).

Prominent among the issues regarding the use of a categorical system for the personality disorders are that many of the categorical diagnoses are quite heterogeneous, that no clear differentiation is made between normal functioning and pathology, and that the overlap of many specific criteria across different diagnoses is extensive, so that a careful systematic evaluation for all personality disorders in a given patient quite frequently results in extensive diagnostic co-occurrence on Axis II.

An example of a "person-centered" dimensional system is the prototype matching approach described by Shedler and Westen in Chapter 4 of this volume. In this system, a patient is compared to a description of a prototypical patient with each disorder, and the "match" is rated on a 5-point scale from "very good match" to "little or no match."

New Directions for DSM-5

In 2007, the Personality and Personality Disorders Work Group for DSM-5 was appointed by the American Psychiatric Association. The members of the work group are listed in Table 16–3. Note the decision at the outset to label the work group as shown, encompassing personality traits and types, as well as personality disorders. There was strong support for this approach, not just within the work group but also by the entire DSM-5 Task Force. There was a shared recognition that the premorbid temperament or personality of individuals who eventually developed Axis I conditions such as major depressive disorder, bipolar disorder, an anxiety disorder, or other illnesses needed to be evaluated and described because it could well affect later treatment participation and treatment response.

Although the revisions to be proposed for the personality disorders for DSM-5 are still being discussed, it is clear that change is needed (Krueger et al. 2007; Skodol and Bender 2009; Widiger and Trull 2007). At the point of this writing (mid-2009), an emerging consensus has begun to develop that a dimensional approach would allow assessment of the full range of personality, from nonpathological traits or styles (yet important determinants of behavior) to substantial pathology involving significant impairment in functioning. The proposed changes described later in this section involve both a "variable-centered" dimensional approach (rating the degree to which multiple traits apply to a given individual) and a "person-centered" dimensional approach (rating the degree of "match" between a given patient and a limited set of personality disorder prototypes). The following questions about DSM-5 are being considered:

TABLE 16–3.   DSM-5 Personality and Personality Disorders Work Group

---

Andrew E. Skodol II, M.D., Chair

Renato D. Alarcón, M.D., M.P.H.

Carl C. Bell, M.D.

Donna S. Bender, Ph.D.

Lee Anna Clark, Ph.D.

Robert Krueger, Ph.D.

W. John Livesley, M.D., Ph.D.

Leslie Morey, Ph.D.

John N. Oldham, M.D., M.S.

Larry J. Siever, M.D.

Roel Verheul, Ph.D.

---

1. *Should a systematic way to assess an individual's level of functioning be introduced?* It has been recognized in the CLPS research (Skodol et al. 2005) and in other work that impairment in functioning can be substantial and persistent in patients with personality disorders. A systematic method to assess level of functioning could be organized to evaluate a patient's self-concept and interpersonal functioning.
2. *Should the overall definition of a personality disorder be revised?* In DSM-IV-TR, a personality disorder is defined in terms of deviations in thinking, feeling, and behavior that are stable and persistent over time and across situations. These defining features are, in fact, shared by many Axis I conditions, and the body of longitudinal research referred to earlier has determined that DSM-IV-TR–defined personality disorders show patterns of remission also characteristic of many Axis I disorders. A potential revision could emphasize that the core components of all personality disorders are adaptive failures leading to impaired functioning in the self and interpersonal domains. As in DSM-IV-TR, this definition requires that a personality disorder reflect an adaptive failure that differentiates it significantly from the expectations of the individual's culture. A patient with a personality disorder would be likely to have a poorly developed or poorly integrated identity or sense of self and/or low self-directedness, combined with chronic interpersonal dysfunction identified by poorly integrated images of others, impaired empathy, impaired capacity for close relationships, or failure to develop prosocial behavior. Other aspects of this general definition of a per-

sonality disorder likely will be similar to those in DSM-IV-TR, although it is as yet unclear if "stability over time" will be included.

3. *Should a set of prototypes or main categories of personality pathology be identified on the basis of available evidence?* A scaled measure of the degree of match, or fit, of a given patient could then be applied to each prototype. Current considerations for prototypes include the following:

   A. Schizotypal personality disorder
   B. Borderline personality disorder
   C. Psychopathic/antisocial personality disorder
   D. Avoidant personality disorder
   E. Obsessive-compulsive personality disorder

4. *Should a list of personality traits be introduced that could be assessed for all patients?* Individuals could then be assessed with respect to these traits, to clarify basic personality and temperament, relevant to treatment planning. Component traits (e.g., emotional dysregulation, insecurity, self-harm) could be organized under higher-order domains (e.g., emotionality) along the lines of several evidence-based rosters of key personality traits (Clark 1996). Each trait in each domain could then be elaborated with a brief description of the trait, and a clinician could then be asked to rate a given patient on each trait as follows:

   ◆ 0: Not applicable (the description does not fit the patient well or only a little)
   ◆ 1: Somewhat applicable (some aspects of the description are applicable, or the patient's behavior matches the description only in limited respects)
   ◆ 2: Clearly applicable (the description fits the typical behavior of the patient well)
   ◆ 3: Extremely applicable (the description is a hallmark characteristic of the patient)

5. *Should the placement of the personality disorders on Axis II be reconsidered?* It has not yet been decided whether a multiaxial system will be retained in DSM-5. There is, however, no persuasive conceptual argument to justify retaining the personality disorders in a different diagnostic section than the one for current Axis I disorders (Oldham and Skodol 2000), but for reasons of familiarity and continuity of research, some pragmatic elements should be considered.

A preliminary design for a field trial of these proposed changes has been developed, and tentative sites have been selected to conduct this field trial during 2009–2010. One overriding goal of the work group has been that any new model for personality disorders must have good clinical utility (First 2005; Rottman et al. 2009); evaluating this aspect of the proposed changes will be an important component of the field trial. In a recent survey (Spitzer et al. 2008), clinicians reported favorably on the use of a prototype matching system. Because the literature reviews by the work group did not support retention, as valid independent disorders, of several current personality disorders (paranoid, schizoid, narcissistic, histrionic, and dependent), another goal of the field trial will be to determine whether these areas will be adequately identified through the proposed trait assessment system.

Psychodynamic Treatment Planning and DSM-5

It has been well established that patients with personality disorders use multiple forms of psychosocial and psychopharmacological treatment extensively (Bender et al. 2001). Too often, the treatment histories of patients with personality disorders suggest erratic "polytherapy" (i.e., overloading highly symptomatic patients with multiple treatment efforts without an evidence-based road map). Increasingly, as the personality disorders are becoming better understood, thoughtful treatment strategies are emerging. In particular, an evidence-based practice guideline has been developed for borderline personality disorder (American Psychiatric Association 2001), which recommends psychotherapy as the primary or core treatment, combined with symptom-targeted, adjunctive pharmacotherapy. Randomized controlled trials have shown that different types of psychotherapy are effective for patients with borderline personality disorder, such as dialectical behavior therapy (Linehan 1993; Linehan et al. 2006) or mentalization-based therapy, a type of psychodynamic psychotherapy (Bateman and Fonagy 1999, 2001, 2008). In addition, new and promising treatments are being studied, such as transference-focused psychotherapy (Clarkin et al. 2007) and Systems Training for Emotional Predictability and Problem Solving (Blum et al. 2008). Among other psychotherapies of interest are cognitive-behavioral therapy (Beck et al. 2003), interpersonal psychotherapy (Markowitz 2005), and schema-based therapy (Young and Klosko 2005). Also, refinement of the most effective way to combine psychotherapy with pharmacotherapy continues to be quite important (Soloff 2009). It is increasingly clear that careful and systemic application of many types of psychotherapy can be effective (Leichsenring and Leibing 2003; Leichsenring and Rabung 2008), and the choice of type of therapy depends on variables such as therapist training and preference, patient preference, the degree of motivation of the patient, and the nature of the personality psychopathology in question.

As discussed earlier, DSM-5 is likely to emphasize the dimensional nature of psychopathology, particularly for the personality disorders, underscoring the continuity from nonpathological traits with adaptive utility to extreme expressions of these traits that can involve adaptive failures and impairment in functioning. One result of this shift could be to augment the growing interest in "personalized medicine." This term has emerged in the context of the "decade of discovery" involving exciting exponential progress in genomics and proteomics. The day may be just around the corner when any of us could afford to have a complete personal genome scan identifying individual heritable risk and protective factors.

However, not only individual differences in DNA account for interindividual variability. The usefulness of the stress-vulnerability model has become apparent in all of medicine, and this model applies equally to brain disorders and other medical disorders. We understand its bidirectional nature: that genes partially determine temperament and behavior, and environmental influences "turn on" latent genes. Some of these genes, dormant until expressed, contain heritable risk factors for disease, and sustained high levels of stress can be the "trigger" activating these genes and the cascade of events that culminates in disease.

Psychodynamic treatment planning involves informed recognition of the importance of heritable risk factors and of presumed neurobiological and neuroendocrinological imbalances. For example, patients with borderline personality disorder are thought to have heritable endophenotypes of affect dysregulation and impulsive aggression (Oldham 2009; Siever et al. 2002). Developmentally, these vulnerabilities may interfere with the crucial milestone of healthy attachment to a trustworthy caregiving figure. The stage is then set for an incomplete and nonintegrated sense of self, plus interpersonal difficulties that reinforce mistrust of others, leading to interpersonal hypersensitivity (Gunderson and Lyons-Ruth 2008) and impairment in social and occupational functioning. A psychodynamically oriented treatment plan is strengthened by recognition of these vulnerabilities, so that validation, empathic attunement, mentalization, reflective functioning, and cognitive-behavioral restructuring can all be considered individually in the context of the patient's specific needs.

How will the revisions forthcoming in DSM-5 in the section on personality and personality disorders play a role in psychodynamic treatment planning? If the final version of DSM-5 approximates the current thinking, then the new system could have a substantial effect:

♦ Clinicians will have to decide whether any given patient does or does not have a personality disorder. Although this requirement is not new, because the multiaxial nature of DSM-IV-TR requires a consideration of the personality disorders on Axis II, the new definition of a personality disorder will necessitate thinking about a patient's sense of identity and about the nature of a patient's relationships with others. A colleague of mine, Jon Allen, relies on the concept of "mentalizing" in developing treatment plans, and he typically initiates hospital-based treatment planning with patients (most of whom have personality disorders) as follows:

> I find that we can accomplish more in the relatively brief time frame for individual psychotherapy if we can agree on a central focus for therapy, that is, a written formulation of the main problems we are working on. I also find that coming up with a focus and formulation of the main problems is not necessarily easy. This is an example of a task that requires "mentalizing," by which we mean being aware of your own thoughts and feelings as well as the thoughts and feelings of others. Because the problems that typically bring people to treatment include not only difficulties within the individual but also conflicts in key relationships, we rely on mentalizing of both self and others to clarify these problems and to work on them. (Allen et al., in press)

As can be seen, a new general definition of a personality disorder focusing on impaired self-integrity and interpersonal functioning aligns naturally with an approach to treatment planning such as the previous one. Such a focus on self and others could be simplifying and clarifying to patients and clinicians and could be compatible with many existing forms of evidence-based treatment for personality disorders.

♦ Regardless of whether a personality disorder is determined to be present, clinicians will be encouraged to evaluate a patient on a list of traits within selected domains of behavior. This information will result in a profile of an individual's personality, which is relevant to treatment participation, treatment adherence, and treatment outcome.

♦ If a personality disorder *is* judged to be present, ratings against prototypes can help characterize the main descriptive patterns of the pathology, which could be dominated by a strong match with a single prototype, a mixture of several prototypes, or a combination of other traits from various domains that may not fit any of the prototypes. For example, the borderline prototype might be "strongly applicable" for a given patient, with some additional traits but no significant match with any other prototypes. A second patient might be characterized by a "clearly applicable" match for the avoidant prototype, with a "somewhat applicable" match for the obsessive-compulsive prototype, along with additional other traits. A third patient might be judged to have a personality disorder but not one that matches any of the prototypes, yet one particularly characterized by narcissistic and callous traits. Even if a patient is judged not to have a personality disorder, the trait information could be informative. For example, an individual with major depressive disorder who has narcissistic traits might benefit from strategic emphasis on the importance of completing the total course of recommended treatment for the depression, to counter the patient's usual response of "knowing better" and deciding to disregard or adjust the recommended plan. In contrast, a patient without a personality disorder but with major depressive disorder and dependent traits might adhere religiously to treatment recommendations but might need extra contact and reassurance.

Conclusion

I strongly believe that all psychiatric treatment planning, regardless of one's theoretical and clinical orientation, should be psychodynamically informed treatment planning. Such an approach derives from a biopsychosocial model and recognizes the combined importance of 1) heritable risk factors and irregularities in neurobiology, 2) the potential lasting effects of stressful environmental circumstances during development (such as sustained trauma) and during adulthood (such as loss of a loved one), and 3) the effect of one's social network (such as living in poverty in an urban culture characterized by violence and drug use). Will the proposed changes in the section on personality disorders in DSM-5 help remind our early-career colleagues, such as the candidates for board certification mentioned earlier, of the importance of a formulation for each patient as a blueprint for treatment planning? I hope so. At the very least, the emphasis on understanding each patient's sense of personal identity, and the nature of each patient's capacity (or lack of it) to trust others and form rewarding and stable relationships, could help "re-center" our focus to where it belongs.

Key Clinical Concepts

- ◆ A psychodynamically informed approach to treatment planning for the personality disorders (PDs) is recommended and consistent with anticipated recommendations for changes in the PD section of DSM-5.

- ◆ The overall definition of a personality disorder in DSM-5 will likely focus on adaptive failure to achieve an integrated sense of self and a capacity to form mature, mutually satisfying interpersonal relationships.

- ◆ Personality trait structure will likely be emphasized in DSM-5, along with descriptions of selected specific PD prototypes.

- ◆ PDs should be understood as the result of heritable risk factors and environmental stressors, as is the case for many diseases or disorders in medicine.

Suggested Readings

Allen JG, Fonagy P, Bateman A: Mentalizing in Clinical Practice. Washington, DC, American Psychiatric Publishing, 2008

Gabbard GO: Mind, brain, and personality disorders. Am J Psychiatry 162:648–655, 2005

Oldham JM: Personality disorders: recent history and the DSM system, in Essentials of Personality Disorders. Edited by Oldham JM, Skodol AE, Bender DS. Washington, DC, American Psychiatric Publishing, 2009, pp 3–11

Oldham JM, Skodol AE: Charting the future of Axis II. J Pers Disord 14:17–29, 2000

Skodol AE, Bender DS: The future of personality disorders in DSM-V? Am J Psychiatry 166:388–391, 2009

References

Allen JG, O'Malley F, Freeman C, et al: Promoting mentalization in brief treatment, in Handbook of Mentalizing in Mental Health Practice. Edited by Bateman AW, Fonagy P. Washington, DC, American Psychiatric Publishing (in press)

American Psychiatric Association: Diagnostic and Statistical Manual: Mental Disorders. Washington, DC, American Psychiatric Association, 1952

American Psychiatric Association: Diagnostic and Statistical Manual of Mental Disorders, 2nd Edition. Washington, DC, American Psychiatric Association, 1968

American Psychiatric Association: Diagnostic and Statistical Manual of Mental Disorders, 3rd Edition. Washington, DC, American Psychiatric Association, 1980

American Psychiatric Association: Diagnostic and Statistical Manual of Mental Disorders, 3rd Edition, Revised. Washington, DC, American Psychiatric Association, 1987

American Psychiatric Association: Diagnostic and Statistical Manual of Mental Disorders, 4th Edition. Washington, DC, American Psychiatric Association, 1994

American Psychiatric Association: Diagnostic and Statistical Manual of Mental Disorders, 4th Edition, Text Revision. Washington, DC, American Psychiatric Association, 2000

American Psychiatric Association: Practice guideline for the treatment of patients with borderline personality disorder. Am J Psychiatry 158 (Oct suppl), 2001

Bateman A, Fonagy P: Effectiveness of partial hospitalization in the treatment of borderline personality disorder: a randomized controlled trial. Am J Psychiatry 156:1563–1569, 1999

Bateman A, Fonagy P: Treatment of borderline personality disorder with psychoanalytically oriented partial hospitalization: an 18-month follow-up. Am J Psychiatry 158:36–42, 2001

Bateman A, Fonagy P: 8-Year follow-up of patients treated for borderline personality disorder: mentalization-based treatment versus treatment as usual. Am J Psychiatry 165:631–638, 2008

Beck A, Freeman A, Davis D: Cognitive Therapy of Personality Disorders, 2nd Edition. New York, Guilford, 2003

Bender DS, Dolan RT, Skodol AE, et al: Treatment utilization by patients with personality disorders. Am J Psychiatry 158:295–302, 2001

Blum N, St. John D, Pfohl B, et al: Systems Training for Emotional Predictability and Problem Solving (STEPPS) for outpatients with borderline personality disorder: a randomized controlled trial and 1-year follow-up. Am J Psychiatry 165:468–478, 2008

Clark LA: Convergence of two systems for assessing specific traits of personality disorders. Psychol Assess 8:294–303, 1996

Clark LA: Stability and change in personality pathology: revelations of three longitudinal studies. J Pers Disord 19:524–532, 2005

Clark LA: Assessment and diagnosis of personality disorder: perennial issues and an emerging reconceptualization. Annu Rev Psychol 58:227–257, 2007

Clarkin JF, Levy KN, Lenzenweger MF, et al: Evaluating three treatments of borderline personality disorder: a multiwave study. Am J Psychiatry 164:922–928, 2007

Cloninger CR, Svrakic DM, Przybeck TR: A psychobiological model of temperament and character. Arch Gen Psychiatry 50:975–990, 1993

Cohen P, Crawford TN, Johnson JG, et al: The Children in the Community Study of developmental course of personality disorder. J Pers Disord 19:466–486, 2005

Costa PT, McCrae RR: The five-factor model of personality and its relevance to personality disorders. J Pers Disord 6:343–359, 1992

Eysenck HJ, Eysenck SBG: Manual of the Eysenck Personality Questionnaire. San Diego, CA, Educational and Industrial Testing Service, 1975

First MB: Clinical utility: a prerequisite for the adoption of a dimensional approach in DSM. J Abnorm Psychol 114:560–564, 2005

Gabbard GO: Mind, brain, and personality disorders. Am J Psychiatry 162:648–655, 2005

Gunderson JG: Borderline Personality Disorder: A Clinical Guide, 2nd Edition. Washington, DC, American Psychiatric Publishing, 2008

Gunderson JG, Lyons-Ruth K: BPD's interpersonal hypersensitivity phenotype: a gene-environment developmental model. J Pers Disord 22:22–41, 2008

Kernberg O: Borderline Conditions and Pathological Narcissism. New York, Jason Aronson, 1975

Kohut H: The Analysis of the Self. New York, International Universities Press, 1971

Krueger RF, Skodol AE, Livesley WJ, et al: Synthesizing dimensional and categorical approaches to personality disorders: refining the research agenda for DSM-V Axis II. Int J Methods Psychiatr Res 16 (suppl 1):S65–S73, 2007

Leichsenring F, Leibing E: The effectiveness of psychodynamic therapy and cognitive behavior therapy in the treatment of personality disorders: a meta-analysis. Am J Psychiatry 160:1223–1232, 2003

Leichsenring F, Rabung S: Effectiveness of long-term psychodynamic psychotherapy: a meta-analysis. JAMA 300:1551–1565, 2008

Linehan MM: Cognitive-Behavioral Treatment of Borderline Personality Disorder. New York, Guilford, 1993

Linehan MM, Comtois KA, Murray AM, et al: Two year randomized controlled trial and follow-up of dialectical behavior therapy vs therapy by experts for suicidal behaviors and borderline personality disorder. Arch Gen Psychiatry 63:757–766, 2006

Livesley J: Toward a genetically informed model of borderline personality disorder. J Pers Disord 22:42–71, 2008

Markowitz JC: Interpersonal therapy, in The American Psychiatric Publishing Textbook of Personality Disorders. Edited by Oldham JM, Skodol AE, Bender DS. Washington, DC, American Psychiatric Publishing, 2005, pp 321–334

Millon T: Modern Psychopathology. Philadelphia, PA, WB Saunders, 1969

Oldham JM: Borderline personality disorder comes of age. Am J Psychiatry 166:1–3, 2009

Oldham JM, Morris LB: The New Personality Self-Portrait. New York, Bantam, 1995

Oldham JM, Skodol AE: Charting the future of Axis II. J Pers Disord 14:17–29, 2000

Rottman BM, Ahn WK, Sanislow CA, et al: Can clinicians recognize DSM-IV personality disorders from five-factor model descriptions of patient cases? Am J Psychiatry 166:427–433, 2009

Siever LJ, Torgersen S, Gunderson JG, et al: The borderline diagnosis, III: identifying endophenotypes for genetic studies. Biol Psychiatry 51:964–968, 2002

Skodol AE, Bender DS: The future of personality disorders in DSM-V? Am J Psychiatry 166:1–4, 2009

Skodol AE, Gunderson JG: Personality disorders, in The American Psychiatric Publishing Textbook of Clinical Psychiatry, 5th Edition. Edited by Hales RE, Yudofsky SC. Washington, DC, American Psychiatric Publishing, 2008, pp 821–860

Skodol AE, Gunderson JG, Shea MT, et al: The Collaborative Longitudinal Personality Disorders Study (CLPS): overview and implications. J Pers Disord 19:487–504, 2005

Soloff PH: Somatic treatments, in Essentials of Personality Disorders. Edited by Oldham JM, Skodol AE, Bender DS. Washington, DC, American Psychiatric Publishing, 2009, pp 267–288

Spitzer RL, Endicott J, Gibbon M: Crossing the border into borderline personality and borderline schizophrenia. Arch Gen Psychiatry 36:17–24, 1979

Spitzer RL, First MB, Schedler J, et al: Clinical utility of five dimensional systems for personality diagnosis: a "consumer preference" study. J Nerv Ment Dis 196:356–374, 2008

Webb CT, Levinson DF: Schizotypal and paranoid personality disorder in the relatives of patients with schizophrenia and affective disorders: a review. Schizophr Res 11:81–92, 1993

Widiger TA, Sanderson CJ: Toward a dimensional model of personality disorder, in The DSM-IV Personality Disorders. Edited by Livesley WJ. New York, Guilford, 1995, pp 433–458

Widiger TA, Trull TJ: Plate tectonics in the classification of personality disorder: shifting to a dimensional model. Am Psychol 62:71–83, 2007

Wiggins J: Circumplex models of interpersonal behavior in clinical psychology, in Handbook of Research Methods in Clinical Psychology. Edited by Kendall P, Butcher J. New York, Wiley, 1982, pp 183–221

Young J, Klosko J: Schema therapy, in The American Psychiatric Publishing Textbook of Personality Disorders. Edited by Oldham JM, Skodol AE, Bender DS. Washington, DC, American Psychiatric Publishing, 2005, pp 289–306

Zanarini MC, Frankenburg FR, Hennen J, et al: The McLean Study of Adult Development (MSAD): overview and implications of the first six years of prospective follow-up. J Pers Disord 19:505–523, 2005

Index

Page numbers printed in **boldface** type refer to tables or figures. Page numbers followed by *n* refer to footnotes.

CPSIA information can be obtained
at www.ICGtesting.com
Printed in the USA
LVHW080425070522
717770LV00003B/3